E. Alt H. Klein J. C. Griffin (Eds.)

The Implantable Cardioverter/ Defibrillator

With 69 Figures and 30 Tables

Springer-Verlag
Berlin Heidelberg New York
London Paris Tokyo
Hong Kong Barcelona
Budapest

Prof. Dr. med. Eckhard Alt
I. Medizinische Klinik, Klinikum Rechts der Isar
der Technischen Universität München
Ismaninger Strasse 22, D-8000 München 80, FRG

Prof. Dr. med. Helmut Klein
Medizinische Hochschule Hannover,
Abteilung Kardiologie
Konstanty-Gutschow-Strasse 8, D-3000 Hannover 61, FRG

Prof. Dr. med. Jerry C. Griffin
Cardiovascular Research Institute, Room 312,
Moffit Hospital, UCSF, Third and Parnassus
San Francisco, CA 94143, USA

ISBN-13:978-3-642-76577-3 e-ISBN-13:978-3-642-76575-9
DOI: 10.1007/978-3-642-76575-9

Library of Congress Cataloging-in-Publication Data. Implantable cardioverter/defibrillator / E. Alt, H. Klein, J.C. Griffin (eds.). Includes bibliographical references and index. ISBN-13:978-3-642-76577-3
1. Ventricular tachycardia – Treatment. 2. Defibrillators. 3. Cardiac pacing. I. Alt, E. (Eckhard) II. Klein, H. (Helmut) III. Griffin, Jerry C. [DNLM: 1. Death, Sudden – epidemiology. 2. Electric Countershock. 3. Heart Surgery. 4. Implants, Artificial. 5. Tachycardia – mortality. 6. Tachycardia – therapy. WG 330 I34] RC685.T33I58 1992 616.1'28 – dc20 DNLM/DLC

Typesetting: K+V Fotosatz, D-6124 Beerfelden, FRG

19/3130-5 4 3 2 1 0 – Printed on acid-free paper

Foreword

Use of the implantable cardioverter/defibrillator is the most significant advance in the management of patients with life-threatening cardiac arrhythmias. This device represents both an important practical as well as conceptual breakthrough in arrhythmia management. It places on firm footing use of non-pharmacologic tools for clinicians. The text, Implantable Cardioverter/Defibrillator, represents contributions by the leading clinicians in this field from both sides of the Atlantic and is a welcome addition to the library of clinical electrophysiologists as well as cardiac surgeons. The editors have well collated the critical issues related to current use of device therapy in a meaningful and practical fashion. The text amply reminds us that we are in the early growth phases of a technology that promises to completely change our approach to the cure of patients with actual or potentially life-threatening ventricular dysrhythmias. It also reminds us that Dr. Mirwoski's dream continues to live and remains as a perpetual challenge to clinicians and engineers alike to better perfect and utilize device therapy for our patients. I commend the authors and editors for a superb and timely effort.

San Francisco, CA, USA *Melvin M. Scheinman*, M.D.

Preface

Treatment of patients with ventricular tachycardia and prevention of sudden arrhythmic death is one of the most challenging tasks of modern cardiology. Ten years ago antiarrhythmic drug therapy was the medical tool used most frequently in the management of patients with life-threatening ventricular tachyarrhythmias. The long-term result of drug therapy alone, however, proved to be disappointing and most unreliable.

Since the implantable defibrillator was first introduced by Dr. Michel Mirowsky in 1980, electrical therapy of ventricular tachyarrhythmias has become increasingly important, as is shown by implantations in more than 20000 patients 10 years after the first implantation. As with pacemaker therapy there has been enormous technical progress in defibrillator therapy, with several manufacturers introducing increasingly more complex devices. However, there are not only obvious technical advances, but also clinical aspects of antitachycardia management requiring reconsideration.

It has been for this reason that technical and clinical issues of defibrillator therapy have been undergone extensive considerations by leading authors in this field. Results and issues of defibrillator therapy are discussed by distinguished scientists and cardiologists, and this book contains their contributions to this rapidly growing field of clinical electrophysiology.

The book has been divided into six sections comprising several chapters each that deal with various aspects of theoretical and clinical issues of the automatic implantable cardioverter/defibrillator. The first section is devoted to the history of the development of the implantable defibrillator. The second section deals with the identification of the patient at risk for sudden arrhythmic death and discusses the various non-invasive and invasive techniques used to determine possible candidates for defibrillator treatment. An attempt has been made to set up a treatment algorithm including all non-pharmacological approaches that are currently available.

The third section describes the technical aspects of defibrillator therapy. Renowned scientists here explain the basic physical principles of defibrillation and discuss methods and problems of tachycardia detection. Long-term results and clinical issues of the implantable defibrillator are reviewed in the fourth section, including the subject of antitachycardia pacing that will play an important part in future defibrillator devices. A further section provides practical information on various surgical aspects of defibrillator implantation; it also deals with lead systems and discusses optimum energy delivery. The last section is a guide to correct follow-up, describing trouble-shooting and management of the defibrillator patient and also including social and psychological aspects of treatment.

We would like to express our gratitude to the many authors who sent us their excellent contributions and reviews that are now presented in this volume. This book is dedicated to Dr. Michel Mirowski, whose pioneering work in this field became a milestone in modern cardiology. Despite his early death, his ideas and philosophy will continue to guide defibrillator therapy even in the future.

The Editors

Contents

Part III: Technical and Electrophysiological Aspects of the Automatic Implantable Cardioverter Defibrillator

Part IV: The Role of the Automatic Implantable Cardioverter Defibrillator in the Treatment of Ventricular Tachyarrhythmia

List of Contributors

Eckhard Alt, M.D.
I. Medizinische Klinik
Technical University of Munich
Ismaningerstr. 22
D-8000 München 80, FRG

Stanley M. Bach, Jr., M.D.
Cardiac Pacemakers, Inc.
4100 Hamline Avenue North
St. Paul, MN 55112-5798, USA

Serge Barold, M.D.
Genesee Hospital
University of Rochester
School of Medicine and Dentistry
224 Alexander Street
Rochester, NY 14607, USA

Yaver Bashir
Department of
Cardiological Sciences
St. George's Hospital
Medical School
London SW17 0RE, UK

Martin Borggrefe, M.D.
Medizinische Klinik und
Poliklinik, Innere Medizin C
(Kardiologie, Angiologie)
Westfälische Wilhelms-Universität
Albert-Schweitzer-Straße 33
D-4400 Münster, FRG

Günter Breithardt, M.D., F.E.S.C.
Medizinische Klinik und
Poliklinik, Innere Medizin C
(Kardiologie, Angiologie)
Westfälische Wilhelms-Universität
Albert-Schweitzer-Straße 33
D-4400 Münster, FRG

Richard F. Brodman, M.D.
Montefiore Hospital
111 E. 210th Street
Bronx, NY 10467, USA

A. John Camm
Department of
Cardiological Sciences
St. George's Hospital
Medical School
London SW17 0RE, UK

Randolph A. S. Cooper, M.D.
Basic Arrhythmia Laboratory
P.O. Box 3140
Duke University Medical Center
Durham, NC 27710, USA

James P. Daubert, M.D.
Basic Arrhythmia Laboratory
P.O. Box 3140
Duke University Medical Center
Durham, NC 27710, USA

Debra S. Echt, M.D.
Vanderbilt University
School of Medicine
Cardiology Division Room
CC2218 MCN
Nashville, TN 37232-2170, USA

Scott A. Feeser, M.S.
Basic Arrhythmia Laboratory
P.O. Box 3140
Duke University Medical Center
Durham, NC 27710, USA

Kevin J. Ferrick, M.D.
Montefiore Hospital
111 E. 210th Street
Bronx, NY 10467, USA

John D. Fisher, M.D.
Cardiology Division
Arrhythmia Offices
Montefiore Hospital
111 E. 210th Street
Bronx, NY 10467, USA

Richard N. Fogoros, M.D.
Alleghany General Hospital
320 E North Avenue
Pittsburgh, PA 15212, USA

Seymour Furman, M.D.
Montefiore Hospital
111 E. 210th Street
Bronx, NY 10467, USA

Jerry C. Griffin, M.D.
University of California
Room 312, Moffitt Hospital
San Francisco, CA 94143, USA

Lawrence S.C. Griffith
Division of Cardiology
Sinai Hospital of Baltimore
Belvedere at Greenspring Avenue
Baltimore, MD 21215, USA

Jay Gross, M.D.
Montefiore Hospital
111 E. 210th Street
Bronx, NY 10467, USA

Thomas Guarnieri, M.D.
Division of Cardiology
Sinai Hospital of Baltimore
Belvedere at Greenspring Avenue
Baltimore, MD 21215, USA

Wilhelm Haverkamp, M.D.
Medizinische Klinik und
Poliklinik, Innere Medizin C
(Kardiologie, Angiologie)
Westfälische Wilhelms-Universität
Albert-Schweitzer-Straße 33
D-4400 Münster, FRG

Gerhard Hindricks, M.D.
Medizinische Klinik und
Poliklinik, Innere Medizin C
(Kardiologie, Angiologie)
Westfälische Wilhelms-Universität
Albert-Schweitzer-Straße 33
D-4400 Münster, FRG

J.C. Hsung, Ph.D.
Cardiac Pacemakers, Inc.
4100 Hamline Avenue North
St. Paul, MN 55112-5798, USA

Raymond E. Ideker, M.D., Ph.D.
Duke University Medical Center
P.O. Box 3140
Durham, NC 27710, USA

Werner Irnich, Ph.D.
Department of Medical
Engineering
Aulweg 123
D-6300 Giessen, FRG

Juan Juanteguy, M.D.
Division of Cardiology
Sinai Hospital of Baltimore
Belvedere at Greenspring Avenue
Baltimore, MD 21215, USA

Soo G. Kim, M.D.
Montefiore Hospital
111 E. 210th Street
Bronx, NY 10467, USA

Helmut Klein, M.D.
Medizinische Hochschule
Hannover
Abteilung Kardiologie
Konstanty-Gutschow-Str. 8
D-3000 Hannover 61, FRG

Douglas J. Lang, Ph.D.
Cardiac Pacemakers, Inc.
4100 Hamline Avenue North
St. Paul, MN 55112-5798, USA

Richard Lewis, M.D.
Division of Cardiology
Sinai Hospital of Baltimore
Belvedere at Greenspring Avenue
Baltimore, MD 21215, USA

Anthony W. Nathan, M.D.
St. Bartholomew's Hospital
West Smithfield
London EC1A 7BE, UK

Seah Nisam, BSEE
Cardiac Pacemakers, Inc.
4100 Hamline Avenue North
St. Paul, MN 55112-5798, USA

James A. Roth, M.D.
Montefiore Hospital
111 E. 210th Street
Bronx, NY 10467, USA

Sanjeev Saksena, M.D.
Newark Beth Israel
Medical Center
201 Lyons Avenue
Newark NJ 08060, USA

J. Edward Shapland, Ph.D.
Cardiac Pacemakers, Inc.
4100 Hamline Avenue North
St. Paul, MN 55112-5798, USA

Francesco Siclari, M.D.
Thorax-, Herz-, Gefäßchirurgie
Medizinische Hochschule
Hannover
Konstanty-Gutschow-Straße 8
D-3000 Hannover 61, FRG

Gerhard Steinbeck, M.D.
Klinikum Großhadern
Medizinische Klinik I
Marchioninistr. 15
D-8000 München 70, FRG

David K. Swanson, Ph.D.
Cardiac Pacemakers, Inc.
4100 Hamline Avenue North
St. Paul, MN 55112-5798, USA

Gordon Tomaselli, M.D.
Division of Cardiology
Sinai Hospital of Baltimore
Belvedere at Greenspring Avenue
Baltimore, MD 21215, USA

Joachim Trappe, M.D.
Medizinische Hochschule
Hannover
Abteilung Kardiologie
Konstanty-Gutschow-Str. 8
D-3000 Hannover 61, FRG

Paul J. Troup, M.D.
Sinai-Samaritan Medical Center
950 North Twelfth Street
G309, Milwaukee, WI 53233, USA

Enrico P. Veltri, M.D.
Division of Cardiology
Sinai Hospital of Baltimore
Belvedere at Greenspring Avenue
Baltimore, MD 21215, USA

Levi Watkins, Jr., M.D.
Division of Cardiology
Sinai Hospital of Baltimore
Belvedere at Greenspring Avenue
Baltimore, MD 21215, USA

J. Marcus Wharton, M.D.
Basic Arrhythmia Laboratory
P.O. Box 3140
Duke University Medical Center
Durham, NC 27710, USA

PART I

Historical Evolution of the Automatic Implantable Cardioverter Defibrillator

Historical Evolution of the Automatic Implantable Cardioverter Defibrillator in the Treatment of Malignant Ventricular Tachyarrhythmias

S. Nisam, S. Barold

"The advantages and disadvantages of the [automatic implantable defibrillator] approach ... to the prevention of sudden coronary death merit careful study. One would hope that the time necessary for establishing its feasibility and practicality will be brief, as we have little else to offer today to patients with high risk of dying suddenly ..." [1].

Although many workers contributed to the development of the automatic implantable cardioverter defibrillator (AICD), Dr. Michel Mirowski (see Fig. 1) is widely acknowledged as the father of the device now implanted in man; his single-minded perseverance, in the face of

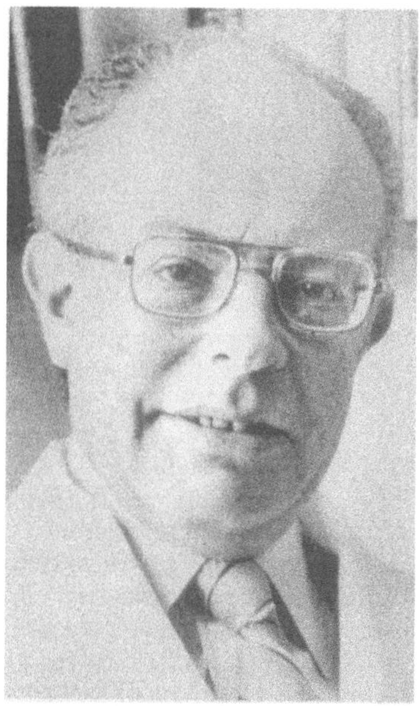

Fig. 1. M. Mirowski, M.D. (1924–1990)

great technological and other obstacles, continued long after the AICD's clinical introduction in 1980, and is largely responsible for the present degree of worldwide acceptance of this therapy, now being used to protect thousands of patients from sudden death. So his passing from among us, just a few months ago, adds particular significance to this review of the historical evolution of the AICD.

Historical Milestones

Two centuries ago, in 1788, Charles Kite's adaptation of a "Ramsden"-type plate electrostatic generator returned life to the body of a 3 year old child [2]. It took yet another century before John MacWilliams' British Heart Journal article *"Cardiac Failure and Sudden Death"* first linked sudden death to ventricular fibrillation (VF) [3].

In 1899 Prevost and Batteli induced VF in dogs and were the first to employ electrical currents (4800 volts for 1–2 s) directly applied to the canine heart to terminate VF [4]. Little more was done until 1933, when Hooker's experimental work demonstrated the feasibility of using alternating current (AC) to terminate VF [5]. Their initial studies suggested AC shocks were more effective, a concept prevalent for the next 30 years. In 1947 the first defibrillation in humans was achieved by Beck et al., who used 110 V AC directly applied to the heart, to convert VF during a thoracic surgery [6]. The era of transthoracic defibrillation was initiated when Zoll et al. applied AC current via copper electrodes on the chest wall of a patient to terminate four cardiac arrests [7]. Several years later, Lown et al. used a capacitor to store direct current and demonstrated that its discharge was as effective as AC for terminating tachyarrhythmias, and significantly less arrhythmogenic [8].

Table 1. Selected historical milestones

1788	First human defibrillation (Kite's electrostatic generator)
1889	MacWilliams' publication links sudden death to VF
1947	Beck uses AC current to convert VF intraoperatively
1954	Transthoracic defibrillation (Zoll)
1967	Pantridge et al. (Belfast) show value and feasibility of out-of-hospital resuscitation
1969	Mirowski, Mower et al. prototype implantable defibrillator
1973/74	Identification of VF, not acute myocardial infarction (AMI), as predominant cause of sudden cardiac death (SCD); recognition of high SCD recurrence rate
1980	First human implanted with automatic implantable defibrillator
1988	First chronic human implant of transvenous AICD system

In the next 20 years, with the advent of coronary care units (CCU) in the early 1960s, external cardioversion/defibrillation became more and more commonplace in the hospital [9]. During the mid-1970s, Cobb and others were instrumental in demonstrating that VF, not acute myocardial infarction, was the predominant cause of out of hospital cardiac arrest, and that prompt defibrillation could achieve high "salvage" rates [10–13]. This finding led naturally to the extensive use of ambulance and even bystander involvement in cardiopulmonary resuscitation (CPR), in attempts to reach more and more patients within the critical few minutes of their arrest [14, 15] (Table 1).

The Mirowski Era

Dr. Mirowski's conception of an implantable defibrillator began with the death in 1967 of his long-time Chief of Medicine, Professor Harry Heller, who had been having bouts of ventricular tachycardia (VT). John Kastor's *Historical Study* [16] quotes Mirowski:

> "How could we have prevented Heller's death at that time; keep him forever in the CCU, or follow him around with a defibrillator? Both solutions were obviously impossible. So, I reasoned, let's create a similar kind of implantable device to monitor for VF and automatically shock the patient back to sinus rhythm. Should be simple enough".

> "I talked to some cardiologists who know more about such devices. They all told me that defibrillators couldn't be miniaturized. In those days, a defibrillator weighed 30 to 40 pounds; it was preposterous to reduce it to the size of a cigarette box. But I had been challenged by the problem, because of the death of a man I admired very much, but also because people told me it couldn't be done".

Original Laboratory Prototype

Mirowski's own intuition overcame the greatest initial obstacle, energy requirements: he reasoned that the 400 watt-seconds required for transthoracic defibrillation could be reduced many fold simply by applying the shock directly to the heart, thereby minimizing the energy dissipated to chest wall muscles and tissues. As no literature existed in support of this hypothesis, Mirowski's group built and tested several electrode systems, some of which were partially and some completely intravascular, and with which they demonstrated in 1969–1970 the feasibility of terminating VF in animals with as little as 5–20 J [17, 18]! Dr. Mirowski, Dr. Morton Mower – close friend and major contributor to

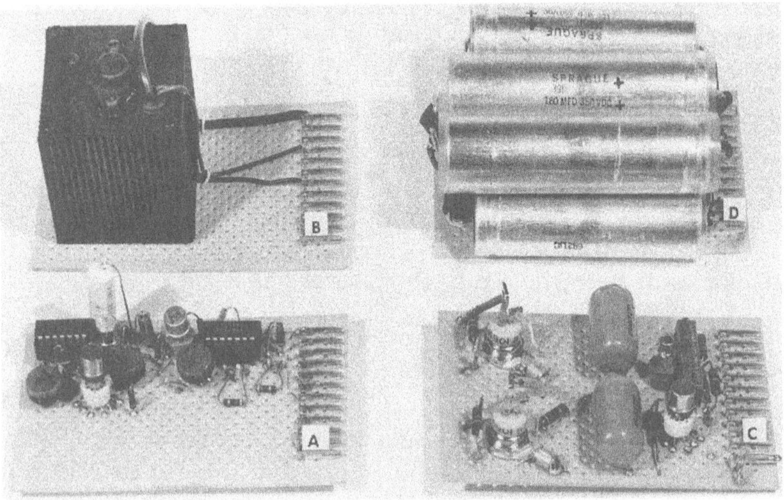

Fig. 2A–D. The first experimental prototype of the automatic defibrillator displayed on 3×4 inch circuit boards. **A** sensing circuit; **B** high-voltage converter; **C** switching circuit; **D** capacitor bank. The batteries, as large as this entire array, are not shown. Reproduced with permission. (From Mirowski et al. 1970 [1])

the project from the onset – and co-workers built their first experimental automatic defibrillator model (Fig. 2), in the basement of Sinai Hospital in Baltimore and successfully tested it in a dog in 1969 [1, 19]. This initial model's electrode configuration consisted of an anode located on a catheter within the heart, paired with a dispersive, sub-cutaneous, left chest wall plate as the cathode. Later prototypes utilized Schuder's truncated exponential waveform [20] to deliver outputs ranging from 30–50 J. For sensing, the original measured the right ventricular pressure via a transducer attached to the distal portion of the transvenous right ventricular catheter. VF persisting ≥*6 s* initiated charging of the capacitor, resulting in a countershock delivered through the defibrillating electrodes. The 20 s diagnostic-therapeutic sequence in an experimental animal is illustrated in Fig. 3. Mirowski's group continued to develop a completely intravascular lead, and from 1971–1973 actually utilized a variation of the lead to achieve defibrillation during cardiac surgery in 11 patients; doing so, in fact, with ≤*15 J* in 9 of the 11 [21]. In order to simulate the geometry of a single intravascular catheter system, one electrode was made a part of the superior vena cava canula used for the cardiopulmonary bypass, and the other electrode was a stiff hand-held probe placed by the surgeon through an atriotomy into the

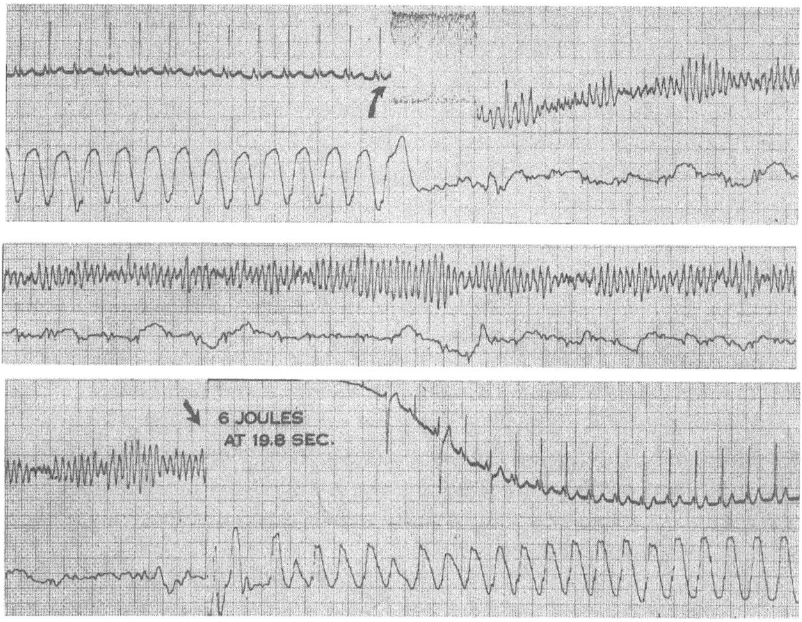

Fig. 3. Simultaneous electrocardiographic and right ventricular pressure curves recorded during operating cycle of the prototype. Ventricular fibrillation is induced in a dog with low-level alternating current (*upper arrow*); 19.8 s later, an intracardiac catheter discharge of 6 J is automatically delivered (*lower arrow*), resulting in resumption of sinus rhythm. The strips are continuous. Reproduced with permission. (From Mirowski et al. 1972 [19])

right ventricular apex. At the time when defibrillation of the patient would ordinarily have been needed, it was accomplished by delivering the shocks through this system rather than through paddles as was ordinarily done during such surgery.

Mirowski later recalled that, from the beginning, "...the very idea of an automatic implantable defibrillator was poorly received by both the engineering and the cardiological communities [22]. The need for such a device was not recognized and the validity of the assumptions underlying this concept was vigorously questioned... (Ironically,) many years ago, Rushmer [23] had already observed that '...at times scientific progress depends less upon the acqisition of new knowledge than upon the removal of conceptual obstacles' ".

Thus, while Mirowski, Mower, and their co-workers were solving their technological problems, one by one, they encountered two major setbacks in 1972: a highly critical editorial in *Circulation* by the eminently influential Dr. Bernard Lown [24]; and the decision, by the pacemaker company who had been working on the project, to drop it, essentially deeming the "market" too small and the technical problems too great.

So Mirowski and co-workers found themselves not only without outside funding, but also opposed conceptually by many in their own field. Fortuitously, that same year, Dr. Mirowski met Dr. Stephen Heilman, a physician and engineer, whose angiography company (Medrad, Pittsburgh) took an interest in funding the study and providing technical support*. His interaction subsequently played a decisive role in transforming the early experimental models into a reliable, sophisticated clinical device. A major contribution towards miniaturization came from Mower et al. who established the "critical mass" hypothesis, demonstrating that successful defibrillation did not require stopping all the VF activation fronts [25]. Garrey's classical work had established the basis for Mower's conclusions [26]. Subsequently, Zipes and associates confirmed this important hypothesis via a series of experiments in which electrical shocks and injections of potassium to limited portions of the myocardial cells in the dog terminated VF [27].

By 1976, the Mirowski group had a model ready for long-term implantation and testing in dogs [28]. The lead system was very similar to the early model except that the intravascular catheter introduced through the right external jugular vein was placed in the superior vena cava, and the second electrode was in the form of a flexible conformed patch which was placed via thoracotomy directly on the left ventricular surface. An implantable *fibrillator*, a magnetically triggered alternating current generator was also placed. VF could then be repeatedly induced in these active, conscious dogs. Without interfering with the dog's activity, a magnet placed over the implanted fibrillator would transmit current to the animal's heart through a right ventricular catheter, to initiate ventricular fibrillation. This constituted a convenient and reliable experimental model of sudden arrhythmic death in active animals. The chronically implanted automatic *defibrillator* then promptly diagnosed and terminated the VF within seconds.

With a picture being worth a thousand words, a movie, rather than another paper, demonstrated vividly the experimental sequence. Several fibrillation-defibrillation sequences were filmed in alert, nonanesthesized dogs with implanted fibrillators and defibrillators (Fig. 4). In some, the dog's ECG was added along the bottom of the film synchronized to the action. The arrhythmia and its conversion could be clearly

---

* In 1981, Heilman eventually created a new company, Intec, devoted solely to the implantable defibrillator project.

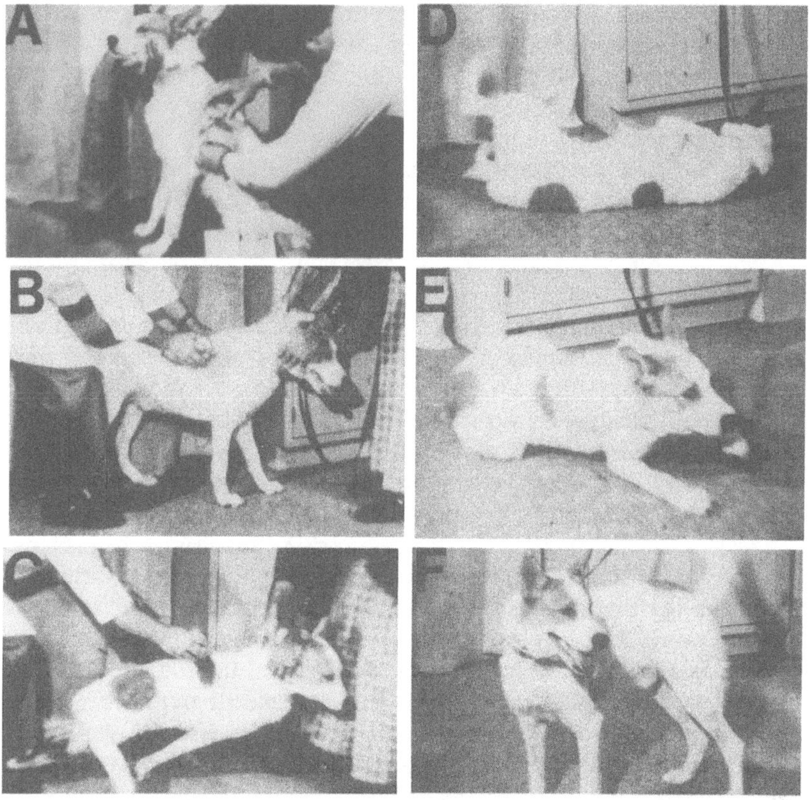

Fig. 4. Demonstration of a dog being fibrillated (**A**, **B**), losing consciousness in ventricular fibrillation **C**), shocked by the automatic implantable defibrillator (**D**), and recovering (**E**, **F**). In similar later episodes, a continuously running electrocardiogram was superimposed on the film during processing. Reproduced with permission. (From Excerpta Medica International Congress Series 458:660, 1978)

correlated with the dog's collapse and recovery. Those who saw the movie will recall it as an unforgettable experience.

Mirowski felt that this movie, seen by many at medical meetings in the late 1970s, played a major role in overcoming the reigning skepticism: "For the first time one could actually witness experimental sudden cardiac death due to ventricular fibrillation, with the arrhythmia being automatically diagnosed and terminated not just once but over and over again, and with the dog cheerfully playing with us only moments after each resuscitation" [22].

For those who saw the film, very few could predict that in only a few years, similar fibrillation-defibrillation sequences would become a routine event during clinical electrophysiological (EP) studies, and indeed written into the American College of Cardiology (ACC) and American Heart Association guidelines for testing AICDs [29]. This practice, as carried out by Mirowski et al. in their project and now routinely in EP laboratories everywhere, indicates just how far electrophysiology has evolved in just a few years. For Dr. Lown's 1972 editorial was in fact reflecting generally accepted contemporary attitudes: "Even in this age of derring and do and erosion of ethical constraints, it is unlikely that VF will be induced deliberately to ascertain performance [of the implanted device]" [24].

The group was then ready to convert the canine unit into a device more suitable for human implantation. Over the next 4 years, bench and environmental stress testing as well as long-term implantation in animals were carried out to qualify the device for human use. During this time, experimental observations were also made in the operating room to determine optimal energy levels and electrode positioning for internal defibrillation in humans.

The first sensing mechanism was based on the analysis of the probability density function (PDF) and was specific for ventricular fibrillation [30]. The system identified the arrhythmia electrically and therefore directly, rather than by monitoring indirect parameters of cardiac activity such as arterial pressure, R waves, or electrical impedance. The logic circuitry measured the time spent by the input electrogram between two amplitude limits located near zero potential. In essence, ventricular fibrillation was characterized by a striking absence of isoelectric potential segments.

Following extensive laboratory testing of both the sensing and automatic defibrillation functions and long-term effectiveness of the internal electrode system, the U.S. Federal Food and Drug Administration (FDA) granted the right to begin human trials, which began at the Johns Hopkins Medical Center in Baltimore, with the first implant on February 4, 1980 [31].

In a sense, the greatest task had been accomplished by 1980. The 1st generation Automatic Implantable Defibrillator (AID) can possibly be compared to the early VOO pacemaker. Both were lifesaving and further technological refinements, while improving the quality of life, ease of use, etc., might be expected to have little *further* impact upon survival.

In the next decade, unfortunately Dr. Mirowski's last, numerous expected refinements were added (see Fig. 5) [32]; more importantly, from a standpoint of impact on therapy, while "only" 800 patients were treated with the AICD for the 5 years prior to the FDA approval for market release in 1985, over 10000 received AICDs in the next 5 years!

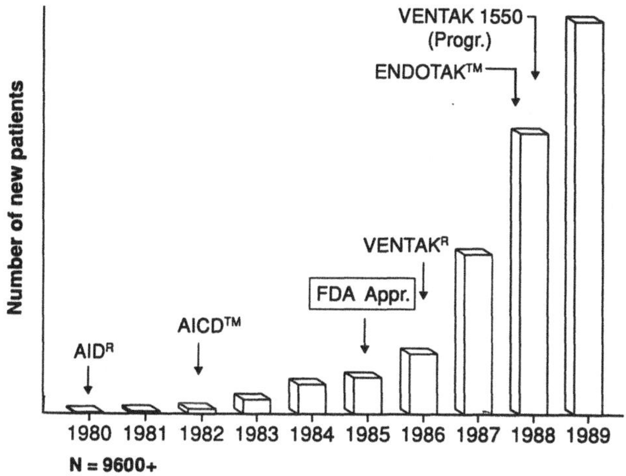

Fig. 5. Growth in number of AICD patients, starting with the first implant in 1980, and major technological developments during the first decade of AICD therapy

Clinical and Technological Developments of the 1980s

The Models AID-B and BR, introduced in 1982, added synchronous cardioversion and a rate-counting channel to the original "AID". It had become evident that in many of the patients, ventricular tachycardia rather than ventricular fibrillation was the initiating event, with the latter rhythm noted only later if at all. It was thought that these patients could be helped by earlier application of the countershock, thus preventing the further degeneration of the rhythm. Physicians were offered a range of "cut-off rates" preset at the factory, as well as the option between "rate only" or "rate plus PDF" for VT/VF detection. The pulse generator and lead system, external accessories, as well as the sensing algorithms, shock delivery sequence and surgical techniques have been amply described [33–38].

Winkle et al. [39] were among the first to emphasize the importance of *Defibrillation Threshold* (DFT) testing, in a remarkable study which demonstrated:

(a) Shocks below 10 J rarely convert VF and polymorphic VT, whose percentage of successful conversions increases linearly, as shock energies increase, from 10 to 25 J;
(b) for monomorphic VT, the success rate is essentially the same at all energies in the 1–25 J range;

(c) the risk of acceleration of VT is about the same at all energies from 1 to 25 J. The most important clinical implication of Winkle's work, confirmed subsequently by others, is that conversion for VF is essential, even if the patient's primary arrhythmia were to be VT only.

The importance of "adequate DFT" to ensure sufficient safety margins, the stability of DFT over time, and the impact of drugs and other factors on DFT have been extensively documented [40–45]. The use of biphasic waveforms has been reported to reduce DFT, although it is not yet clear whether this improvement holds for the particularly problematic "high DFT" cases [46–48]. For patients on chronic amiodarone, reported problems due to either increase in DFT and/or postoperative recovery have led many institutions to stop amiodarone well before AICD implantation [49–51].

The most recent technological improvements, in devices beginning clinical evaluation at the end of the first decade, aim primarily at

(a) improving the specificity of VT detection, via various sensing algorithms [52–55];
(b) the use of programmable lower energy shocks and/or antitachycardia pacing to minimize the patient discomfort associated with high energy shocks [56–58];
(c) back-up bradycardia pacing;
(d) extensive memory/telemetry, primarily to ascertain the arrhythmia(s) triggering the device; and
(e) capability of non-invasive EP testing.

From the time of his initial concept in 1967 through the next several years, Dr. Mirowski's talks often alluded to the need for an "implantable CCU". As preposterous as the idea may have seemed two decades ago, it is now evident that systems such as described above will in fact closely approach that concept.

Lastly, and probably most importantly, there is great optimism that lead systems obviating a thoracotomy, already envisioned by Mirowski and Mower in the early 1970s, may soon be clinically available [21, 59–60]; this important breakthrough, a transvenous AICD system, would make therapy accessible to a substantial number of patients, many of whom are now in a very high risk category even for a thoracotomy. It would also significantly reduce hospital stay and associated costs [6]. In late 1986, Troup implanted the first transvenous unit (Endotak, CPI St. Paul, MN), and the clinical investigation of this system began in earnest in 1988 [62]. The preliminary results were encouraging in that acceptable DFTs ($\leq 15\ J$) were achieved in 38 patients out of the 55 in whom it was tried. In all of these 38 chronically-implanted patients, predischarge EP testing was repeated again at approximately 3 months postimplant and demonstrated efficacious defibrillation. Several patients also had one or more spontaneous arrhythmias converted. Due to a number of lead fractures, it has had to be redesigned and clinical trials resumed September 1990.

Role of the AICD Today and in the Future

Patient Selection

The initial criteria for entry into the study were most stringent, specifically candidates for implantation had to have survived at least two episodes of cardiac arrest, not associated with acute myocardial infarction, with life-threatening arrhythmia documented at least once [30]. Later, as technical improvements were made in the device and its clinical efficacy vis-a-vis drugs and other alternatives came to be well known (see Impact on Survival, below), the criteria for implantation were liberalized somewhat.

Both the ACC (American College of Cardiology) and NASPE (North American Society of Pacing and Electrophysiology) have recommended Guidelines (see Tables 2 and 3) for patient selection for AICD therapy [63–64]. Historically, most patients have had one or more documented cardiac arrests and been found refractory to medical management under electrophysiological tests. While cardiac arrest continues to constitute an almost absolute indication, the category of patients presenting with symptomatic VT, nonresponsive to drug management and not considered amenable to surgical ablation, represents a growing proportion of AICD candidates. Implantation of an AICD is therefore no longer regarded as therapy of last resort.

Implications of Cardiac Arrhythmia Suppression Trial (CAST)

> "The Cardiac Arrhythmia Suppression Trial (CAST)... has shaken the confidence of the cardiologic community in the ability of antiarrhythmic therapy to prevent sudden cardiac death..." [65]

The tone of numerous discussions at medical meetings following the CAST results indicates that the view expressed above has already become a part of therapeutical decision-making. The significant increase in new AICD implants, post-CAST, may in fact be one of the manifestations of

Table 2. Guidelines for AICD patient selection

Indicated by general agreement

(A) Following one or more episodes of spontaneously occurring and inducible VF or syncopal or hypotensive VT which is:
- not associated with AMI
- not due to a remediable cause (e.g., drug toxicity, electrolyte disturbance, ischemia)
- neither controlled by acceptable drug therapy after multiple trials nor amenable to definitive therapy (e.g., surgical ablation)

(B) Following recurrent, spontaneously occurring but noninducible, documented syncopal or hypotensive VF which was not due to 1 – 3 above

(C) Following VT/VF cardiac arrest which was not due to 1 – 3 above

(D) Following surgery for VT or VT if the ventricular tachyarrhythmia remains inducible

(E) Following implantation of an antitachycardia pacemaker for recurrent inducible VT

Possibly indicated (patient characteristics determine appropriateness)

(A) Following one or more episodes of spontaneously occurring and inducible VF or syncopal or hypotensive VT which are:
- associated with an AMI (within 1 month but more than 2 days after the infarct)
- not due to a remediable cause
- neither controlled by acceptable drug therapy after multiple trials nor amenable to definitive treatment

(B) Following unexplained syncope, which by history and clinical circumstances is likely to be of cardiac origin, and in the presence of reproducible, inducible, syncopal or hypotensive VT or VF which is not due to 1 – 3 above

(C) Following recurrent VF or syncopal or hypotensive VT which is apparently controlled by drug, surgical, or ablative therapy, but in which the results of treatment are considered too unpredictable to justify withholding AICD therapy

AICD not indicated

(A) Other disease processes which clearly and severely limit life expectancy

(B) Incessant or very frequent VT which is not suppressed by medical, surgical, or ablative therapy such that the frequency of the arrhythmia would result in an excessive number of AICD discharges

(C) Asymptomatic VT or VT/VF which is:
- associated with AMI (within 2 weeks)
- due to remediable cause, controlled by acceptable drug therapy
- amenable to definitive treatment

VF, ventricular fibrillation; VT, ventricular tachycardia; AMI, acute myocardial infarction

Table 3. Indications for AICD implantation[a,b]

Class I (little or no controversy)
- One or more documented episodes of hemodynamically significant ventricular tachycardia (HSVT) or ventricular fibrillation in a patient in whom electrophysiologic testing and Holter monitoring cannot be used to accurately predict efficacy of therapy
- One or more documented episodes of HSVT or ventricular fibrillation in a patient in whom no drug was found to be effective or no drug currently available and appropriate was tolerated
- Continued inducibility at electrophysiologic study of HSVT or ventricular fibrillation despite the best available drug therapy, or despite surgery/catheter ablation if drug therapy has failed

Class II (no uniform agreement among experts)
- One or more documented episodes of HSVT or ventricular fibrillation in a patient in whom drug efficacy testing is possible
- Recurrent syncope of undetermined etiology in a patient with HSVT or ventricular fibrillation induced at electrophysiologic study in whom no effective or no tolerated drug is available or appropriate

Class III (generally not regarded as sufficient)
- Recurrent syncope of undetermined cause in a patient without inducible tachyarrhythmias
- Arrhythmias not due to HSVT or ventricular fibrillation

[a] ACC position paper.
[b] It should be noted that improvements in AICD design and results of well-designed clinical trials may alter indications for the AICD in the near future.

this evolving perception in the treatment of ventricular tachyarrhythmias. While CAST has not yet disproven the premise that PVC suppression reduces arrhythmic mortality, it has already undermined cardiologist's confidence that that is the case. The fact that two of the most potent PVC-suppressive drugs significantly increased arrhythmic (and total) mortality, vis-a-vis placebo, lays the burden of proof squarely on any drug to show the contrary. Perhaps just as significant is the clear evidence from CAST that PVC-suppression *per se* is not a reliable indicator, thus obligating physicians to consider further diagnostic tests for their high risk patients [66].

Patient Characteristics

The characteristics of the implantees and the therapy concomitant with their AICD implantation are summarized in Table 4. With regard to drug

Table 4. AICD patient characteristics[a]

Patients (*n*)	9807
Male/female (%)	80.7/19.3
Mean age	60.9
Mean EF (%)	33
Coronary artery disease (%)	75.3
Concomitant antiarrhythmic drugs (%)	55.1
Concomitant surgery (mostly CABG) (%)	20.3

[a] CPI medical records as of Feb. 15, 1990.

therapy, many centers prefer to discharge their AICD implantees off antiarrhythmic drugs, only resorting to them when and if the number or gravity of the VT episodes requires it [67–69]. A good example of this tendency is the Kelly et al. series of 94 patients, of whom only 14% were on amiodarone after AICD implantation, compared to 63% before [68]. Conceivably in the future the management of patients with VT considered to be the high risk group might even begin with the implantation of an AICD, followed by trials of drug therapy if necessary.

Impact on Survival

While the degree of benefit – in terms of arrhythmic and total survival – may vary as a function of patient selection and other factors, essentially all investigators acknowledge that the AICD has dramatically improved survival in high arrhythmic risk patients. This very fact has made prospective, randomized trials of the AICD versus other alternatives ethically impossible for most physicians. In lieu of such trials, there are many powerful indices of the AICD's contribution to improved survival. It is widely accepted that the 1 and 4 year actuarial sudden death rates are under 2% and 5%, respectively, compared to over 20% for similar drug-refractory patients obtained from historical controls, such as those projected (see Fig. 6) [70–71]. Overall, several published series, including the largest one by Winkle et al. (see Table 5), show about 80% total survival (considering all causes of death) at 4 years [67–69].

Ruskin et al. (see Table 6) reported on 285 aborted cardiac arrest patients over a 10 year period (1978–1988), treated medically or with the AICD during successive 5 year periods in the two reporting institutions [72]. The AICD group had a lower mean ejection fraction (EF 31% vs 43%) and only 15% responded to drugs vs 77% in the medically treated group. Despite the apparent risk bias in favor of the medically managed

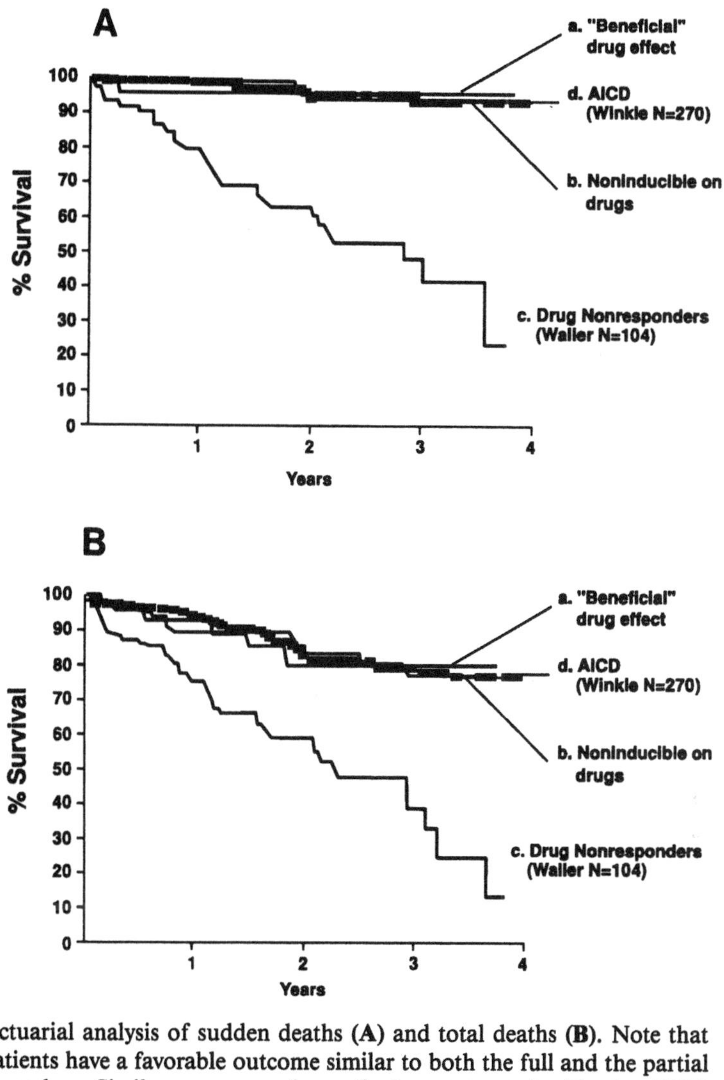

Fig. 6. Actuarial analysis of sudden deaths (**A**) and total deaths (**B**). Note that AICD patients have a favorable outcome similar to both the full and the partial drug responders. Similar nonresponder patients not treated with the AICD (*lower curves*) have a much poorer prognosis. *Curve a*, "Beneficial" ($N = 51$): patients who remained inducible on drugs, but whose VT rates were slowed down and who remained hemodynamically stable. *Curve b*, "Noninducible" ($N = 103$): drugs successfully supressed VT inducibility. *Curve c*, "Nonresponders" ($N = 104$): drugs were unable to slow VT rate or prevent hemodynamic compromise. *Curve d*, AICD patients ($N = 270$). Curves a–c replotted from Waller et al. (1987) [71]; d from Winkle et al. (1989) [67]

Table 5. AICD patient survival (Kaplan-Meier)

	CPI database (n = 9807 patients)					Winkle et al. 1989 [67] (n = 270)				
Year	1	2	3	4	5	1	2	3	4	5
Sample size	5392	2646	1094	564	292	188	113	69	51	52
Sudden cardiac death (%)	98.4	97.5	96.9	95.8	95.5	99.1	96.9	95.6	95.6	95.6
Non-sudden cardiac death (%)	97.2	95.4	93.5	92.5	91.3	93.8	87.0	86.1	84.7	79.7
Total cardiac death (%)	95.6	93.0	90.5	88.6	87.1	93.0	84.4	82.2	80.9	76.2
Death from all causes (%)	92.6	88.5	84.6	81.4	78.6	92.3	83.7	81.6	80.3	74.8

Table 6. AICD vs EP-guided drug therapy (285 survivors of cardiac arrest). From Tordjman-Fuchs et al. [72]

	1978–1983	1983–1988
N	195	90
Therapy	AARx	AICD
Mean EF (%)	43	31
Drug responders (% non-inducible on AARx)	77	15
Total cardiac death (%)		
1 year	15	4
5 year	37	16

patients, the AICD group showed significantly lower total mortality at 1 year (4% vs 15%) and at 5 years (18% vs 37%) vis-a-vis the drug-treated patients.

Future Indications

Patient populations such as survivors of acute myocardial infarction and patients with cardiomyopathy may someday provide additional candidates for prophylactic implantation [73, 74]. A number of multicenter, prospective studies in patients who have not had previous clinical (arrhythmic) events are or will soon be under way with the goal of establishing which subgroups demonstrate benefit. An example of one such imminent study will look prospectively at patients with EF ≤ 0.35 already destined for CABG to determine whether the AICD significantly improves subsequent survival (Medical Sciences Department, Cardiac Pacemakers Inc., St. Paul, personal communication, 1990).

It would be rather prophetic, if – as many now believe – the AICD's ultimate role will someday be primarily prophylactic, since that was precisely Dr. Mirowski's vision. It was by no means evident in 1967 that he would soon have a "pool" of resuscitated cardiac arrest victims who would provide the primary test for his device. The degree to which the AICD has essentially eradicated the risk for subsequent sudden death in this group is in fact the strongest justification for considering this therapy *prophylactically* for the majority of patients whose first episode would otherwise likely be fatal.

Acknowledgement. We wish to thank Dr. Morton Mower for his valuable inputs on historical details; and Ms. Joanne Vollhaber for her secretarial help in preparing this manuscript.

References

1. Mirowski M, Mower M, Staewen W, Tabatznik B, Mendeloff A (1970) Standby automatic defibrillator. An approach to prevention of sudden coronary death. Arch Intern Med 126:158–161
2. Lyons A, Petrucelli R (1978) In: Medicine. An illustrated history. Abrams, New York
3. MacWilliams J (1889) Cardiac failure and sudden death. Br Med J 1:6–8
4. Prevost J, Battelli F (1899) La mort par les courants electriques. J Physiol Pathol Gen 1:427–422
5. Hooker D, Kouwenhoven W, Langworthy O (1933) The effect of alternating electrical currents on the heart. Am J Physiol 103:444–454
6. Beck C, Pritchard W, Veil H (1947) Ventricular fibrillation of long duration abolished by electric shock. JAMA 135:985–986
7. Zoll P, Linenthal A, Gibson W et al. (1956) Termination of ventricular fibrillation in man by externally applied electric countershock. N Engl J Med 254:727–732
8. Lown B, Neuman J, Amarasingham R et al. (1962) Comparison of alternating current with direct current electroshock across the chest. Am J Cardiol 10:223–233
9. Pantridge J, Geddes J (1967) A mobile intensive care unit in the management of myocardial infarction. Lancet ii:271–273
10. Liberthson R, Nagel E et al. (1974) Prehospital ventricular defibrillation – prognosis and follow-up course. N Engl J Med 291:317–321
11. Baum R, Alvarez H, Cobb L (1974) Survival after resuscitation from out-of-hospital ventricular fibrillation. Circulation 50:1231–1235

12. Cobb L et al. (1980) Sudden cardiac death: a decade's experience with out-of-hospital resuscitation. Mod Concepts Cardiovasc Med 49:31–36
13. Myerburg R, Conde C, Sung R et al. (1980) Clinical, electrophysiologic and hemodynamic profile of patients resuscitated from prehospital cardiac arrest. Am J Med 68:568–576
14. Macintosh A, Crabb M, Grainger R, Williams J, Chamberlain D (1978) The Brighton resuscitation ambulances: a review of 40 consecutive survivors of out-of-hospital cardiac arrest. Br M J i:115–118
15. Eisenberg M, Copass M, Hallstron A et al. (1980) Treatment of out-of-hospital cardiac arrests with rapid defibrillation by emergency medical technicians. N Engl J Med 302:1379–1383
16. Kastor J (1989) Historical study. Michel Mirowski and the automatic implantable defibrillator. Am J Cardiol 63:977–982
17. Mower M, Mirowski M, Denniston RH (1972) Intraventricular defibrillation in dogs with impaired coronary artery circulation. Clin Res 20:388 (abstr)
18. Mirowski M, Mower M, Staewen W et al. (1971) Ventricular defibrillation through a single intravascular catheter electrode system. Clin Res 19:328 (abstr)
19. Mirowski M, Mower MM, Staewen WS, Denniston RH, Mendeloff AI (1972) The development of the transvenous automatic defibrillator. Arch Intern Med 129:773–779
20. Schuder J, Stoeckle H, Gold J et al. (1970) Experimental ventricular defibrillation with an automatic and completely implanted system. Trans Am Soc Artif Int Organs 16:207–212
21. Mirowski M, Mower M et al. (1973) Feasibility and effectiveness of low-energy catheter defibrillation in man. Circulation 47:79–85
22. Mirowski M, Mower M (1987) The automatic implantable defibrillator: some historical notes. In: Brugada P, Wellens H (eds) Cardiac arrhythmias: where do we go from here? Futura, Mt Kisco, pp 665–672
23. Rushmer R, Van Citters R, Franklin D (1963) Some axioms, popular notions, and misconceptions regarding cardiovascular control. Circulation 27:118–141
24. Lown B, Axelrod P (1972) Implanted standby defibrillators. Circulation 46:637–639 (editorial)
25. Mower M, Mirowski M, Spear J, Moore N (1974) Patterns of ventricular activity during catheter defibrillation. Circulation 149:858–861
26. Garrey W (1914) The nature of fibrillary contraction of the heart. Its relation to tissue mass and form. Am J Physiol 33:397–414
27. Zipes D, Fischer J, King R et al. (1975) Termination of ventricular fibrillation in dogs by depolarizing a critical amount of myocardium. Am J Cardiol 36:37–44
28. Mirowski M, Mower M, Langer A, Heilman S, Schreibman J (1978) A chronically implanted system for automatic defibrillation in active conscious dogs. Experimental model for treatment of sudden death from ventricular fibrillation. Circulation 58:90–94
29. Zipes D, Akhtar M et al. (1989) Guidelines for clinical intracardiac electrophysiologic studies. J Am Coll Cardiol 14:1827–1842

30. Langer A, Heilman S, Mower M, Mirowski M (1976) Considerations in the developments in the development of the automatic implantable defibrillator. Med Instrum 10:163–167
31. Mirowski M, Reid P, Mower M et al. (1980) Termination of malignant ventricular arrhythmics with an implanted automatic defibrillator in human beings. N Engl J Med 303:322–324
32. Cardiac Pacemakers Jnc (CPI) (1990) Clinical data base and device registry. CPI, St Paul
33. Mower M, Reid P, Watkins L et al. (1984) Automatic implantable defibrillator structural characteristics. PACE 7:1331–1337
34. Winkle R, Bach S, Echt D et al. (1983) The automatic implantable defibrillator: local ventricular bipolar sensing to detect ventricular tachycardia and fibrillation. Am J Cardiol 52:265–270
35. Nisam S (1987) The automatic implantable cardioverter defibrillator (AICD) – a clinical and technical review. J Med Eng Technol 11:97–102
36. Watkins L, Guarnieri T, Griffith L et al. (1986) Implantation of the automatic defibrillator: current surgical techniques. Clin Prog Electrophysiol Pacing 4:286–291
37. Jacobs M, Vlahakes G, Buckley M, Kelly P (1988) Automatic defibrillator implantation: surgical considerations. Arrhyth Clin 5(3):33–36
38. Lawrie G, Griffin J, Wyndham C (1984) Epicardial implantation of the automatic defibrillator by left subcostal thoracotomy. PACE 7:1370–1374
39. Winkle R, Stinson E, Bach S et al. (1984) Cardioversion/defibrillation thresholds using a truncated expotential waveform and an apical patch & SVC spring electrode configuration. Circulation 69:766–771
40. Troup P, Chapman P, Olinger G, Kleinman L (1985) The implanted defibrillator: relation of defibrillating lead configuration and clinical variables to defibrillation threshold. J Am Coll Cardiol 6:1315–1321
41. Wetherbee J, Chapman P, Troup P et al. (1989) Long-term internal cardiac defibrillation threshold stability. PACE 12:443–450
42. Guarnieri T, Levine J, Veltri E et al. (1987) Success of chronic defibrillation and the role of antiarrhythmic drugs with the automatic implantable cardioverter defibrillator. Am J Cardiol 60:1061–1064
43. Marchlinski F, Flores B, Miller J et al. (1988) Relation of the intraoperative debrillation threshold to successful postoperative defibrillation with an automatic implantable cardioverter defibrillator. Am J Cardiol 62:393–398
44. Echt D, Black J, Barbey J et al. (1989) Evaluation of antiarrhythmic drugs on defibrillation energy requirements in dogs. Circulation 79:1106–1117
45. Blakeman B, Pifarre R, Scanlon P, Wilbur D (1989) Coronary revascularization and implantation of the automatic cardioverter defibrillator. Reliability of immediate interoperative testing. PACE 12:86–91
46. Winkle R, Mead H, Ruder M et al. (1989) Improved low-energy defibrillation effiacy in man with the use of biphasic truncated exponential waveform. Am Heart J 117:122–127
47. Flaker G, Schuder J, McDaniel J et al. (1989) Superiority of biphasic shocks in the defibrillation of dogs with epicardial patches and catheter electrodes. Am Heart J 118:288–291

48. Bardy G, Ivey T, Allen M (1989) A prospective randomized evaluation of biphasic versus monophasic waveform pulses on defibrillation efficacy in humans. J Am Coll Cardiol 14:728–733
49. Haberman R, Veltri E, Mower M et al. (1988) The effect of amiodaroe on defibrillation threshold. J Electrophysiol 2:415–423
50. Fogoros R (1984) Amiodarone-induced refractoriness to cardioversion. Ann Intern Med 100:699–700
51. Myerburg R, Luceri R, Thurer R et al. (1989) Time to first shock and clinical outcome in patients receiving an automatic implantable defibrillator. J Am Coll Cardiol 14:508–514
52. Camm J, Davies W, Ward D (1987) Tachycardia recognition by implantable electronic devices. PACE 10:1175–1190
53. Langberg J, Gibb W, Auslander D, Griffin J (1988) Identification of ventricular tachycardia with use of the morphology of the endocardial electrogram. Circulation 77:1363–1369
54. Tomaselli G, Scheinman M (1987) The utility of timing algorithms for distinguishing ventricular from supraventricular tachycardias. PACE 10:415 (abstr)
55. Schuger C, Jackson K, Steinman R, Lehmann M (1988) Atrial sensing to augment ventricular tachycardia detection by the automatic implantable cardioverter defibrillator: a utility study. PACE 11:1456–1464
56. Wever E, Bakker P, Hauer R et al. (1989) First experience with the multiprogrammable Ventak P automatic implantable cardioverter defibrillator. Eur Heart J 10:212 (abstr)
57. Theis R, Bach S, Barstad J et al. (1989) Initial clinical experience with the Ventak P AICD: the programmable implantable cardioverter defibrillator. PACE 12:117 (abstr)
58. Winkle R, Mead H, Fain E et al. (1990) Initial clinical experience with an implantable tiered therapy defibrillator. J Am Coll Cardiol 15:60A (abstr)
59. Winkle R, Bach S et al. (1988) Comparison of defibrillation efficacy in humans using a new catheter and superior vena cava spring left ventricular patch electrode. J Am Coll Cardiol 11:365–370
60. Saksena S, Parsonnet V (1988) Implantation of a cardioverter defibrillator without thoracotomy using a triple electrode system. JAMA 259:69–72
61. Kupperman M, Luce B, McGovern B, Podrid P, Bigger T, Ruskin J (1990) An analysis of the cost effectiveness of the implantable defibrillator. Circulation 81:91–100
62. Bach S, Barstadt J, Harper N et al. (1989) Initial clinical experience: Endotak™ implantable transvenous system. J Am Coll Cardiol 13:65A (abstr)
63. North American Society of Pacing and Electrophysiology (NASPE) (1989) Executive committee recommendations on guidelines for AICD implantation
64. ACC Statement/Position Paper (1990) Indications for implantation of the automatic implantable cardioverter defibrillator (AICD). Adopted by ACC Board of Trustees, 17 March 1990

65. Winkle R, Cannom D (1990) The automatic implantable cardioverter-defibrillator: current applications and future directions. In: Barold S, Mugica J (eds) New perspectives in cardiac pacing, 2nd edn. Futura, Mt Kisco
66. CAST Investigators (1989) Preliminary report: effect of encainide and elecainide on mortality in a randomized trial of arrhythmia suppression after myocardial infarction. N Engl J Med 321:406–412
67. Winkle R, Mead H, Ruder M et al. (1989) Long-term outcome with the automatic implantable cardioverter-defibrillator. J Am Coll Cardiol 13:1353–1361
68. Kelly P, Cannom D, Garan H et al. (1988) The automatic implantable cardioverter defibrillator. Efficacy, complications, and survival in patients with malignant ventricular arrhythmias. J Am Coll Cardiol 11:1278–1286
69. Tchou P et al. (1988) Automatic implantable cardioverter defibrillators and survival of patients with left ventricular dysfunction and malignant ventricular arrhythmias. Ann Intern Med 109:529–534
70. Swerdlow C, Winkle R, Mason J (1983) Determinants of survival in patients with ventricular tachyarrhythmias. N Engl J Med 36:1436–1442
71. Waller T, Kay H et al. (1987) Reduction in sudden death and total mortality by antiarrhythmic therapy evaluated by electrophysiologic drug testing: criteria of efficacy in patients with sustained ventricular tachyarrhythmia. J Am Coll Cardiol 10:83–89
72. Tordjman-Fuchs T, Garan H et al. (1989) Out of hospital cardiac arrest: improved long-term outcome in patients with automatic implantable cardioverter defibrillator (AICD). Circulation 80(4):II–121
73. Mower M, Nisam S (1988) AICD indications (Patient selection): past, present and future. PACE 11:2064–2070
74. Brooks R, Garan H, McGovern B, Ruskin J (1990) The automatic implantable cardioverter defibrillator (AICD): early development, current utilization, and future directions. In: Braunwald E (ed) Heart disease, 3rd edn. Saunders, Philadelphia, pp 193–206

PART II

Identification of the Patient at High Risk for Sudden Cardiac Death

The Role of Ambulatory ECG Monitoring in the Prediction of Sudden Cardiac Death

Y. Bashir, A. J. Camm

Introduction

Sudden cardiac death represents arguably the greatest challenge in the field of cardiovascular medicine today, with some 400000 cases per annum in the USA alone. Advances in arrhythmia management, particularly the development of implantable defibrillators, provide only one component of an effective strategy to prevent sudden death. An equally important requirement is for an accurate but practical risk-stratification scheme to discriminate patients at high risk of treatable life-threatening arrhythmias. This was well illustrated by the recent Cardiac Arrhythmia Suppression Trial [1], in which failure of the risk-stratification scheme resulted in an annual sudden death rate of only 3% in placebo-treated patients: in such a low-risk population, it would have been extremely difficult to detect a positive beneficial effect of any form of antiarrhythmic therapy. Clearly, an expensive, high-technology approach such as prophylactic defibrillator-implantation would impose far more stringent requirements on the process of patient selection to have any prospect of overall success.

Ambulatory ECG monitoring has many advantages as a primary screening technique for target populations (e.g. post-infarction patients): it is non-invasive, widely available and relatively simple and inexpensive. It was one of the earliest risk-stratification methods to be evaluated because of the intuitive assumption that detecting asymptomatic ventricular arrhythmias would provide an accurate indication of a patient's propensity to life-threatening rhythm disturbances in the future. Although this viewpoint has been largely discredited, the repertoire and potential of Holter monitoring as a tool for risk-stratification has been much enhanced by recent technological advances.

Thus, future integrated Holter systems may incorporate additional capabilities including:

(1) algorithms for spectral/non-spectral analysis of heart rate variability, providing information about cardiac sympathovagal balance,

(2) detection of silent myocardial ischaemia by monitoring ST segment shifts,
(3) high-resolution signal-averaging techniques for recording ventricular late potentials,
(4) monitoring of diurnal QT interval variation, an index of the dynamic interaction between autonomic tone and ventricular repolarization.

In this review, we will examine the prognostic value of traditional Holter indices (ventricular ectopic frequency/complexity) and how this has been enhanced by the newer modalities, particularly analysis of heart rate variability and detection of late potentials. To date, most research has addressed stratification in survivors of acute myocardial infarction, but other high-risk populations include patients with congestive heart failure, hypertrophic cardiomyopathy and those who have sustained a cardiac arrest out of hospital.

Mechanism of Sudden Death

Risk-stratification schemes examine ventricular vulnerability to life-threatening arrhythmias, with the implicit assumption that the primary mechanism in most cases of sudden death is ventricular tachycardia or ventricular fibrillation rather than ischaemia/infarction, a bradyarrhythmia or electromechanical dissociation. This is supported by analysis of 157 cases of sudden death during ambulatory ECG recording [2], which showed that VT degenerating to VF was the commonest mechanism (62.4%), with primary VF and Torsades de Pointes accounting for about 20% of cases and bradyarrhythmias only 16.5%. Unfortunately, the findings on this unselected series of patients cannot be extrapolated to specific populations. For example, Luu et al. reported that among 21 cardiac arrests in patients with severe but stable congestive heart failure, VT/VF was the underlying arrhythmia in only 8 cases (38%) with bradycardia or electromechanical dissociation accounting for the other 13 (62%) [3].

Most sudden deaths occur without any electrocardiographic documentation and in this situation, the method of classification can significantly influence the sensitivity and specificity of any risk-stratification scheme. Among post-infarction patients, it has been suggested that use of traditional temporal criteria alone to define sudden death (usually death within 1 h of onset of symptoms) will result in misclassification in over 25% of cases. More sophisticated schemes such as the one employed by the CAPS Investigators [4] exclude patients with deteriorating ventricular function or re-infarction but it remains an act of faith that sudden deaths classified as 'arrhythmic' are truly due to reversible ventricular tachyarrhythmias. Confirmation of this may eventually come from future trials of prophylactic defibrillator implantation in 'high-risk' patients, provided that devices with adequate Holter capabilities are used.

Holter Monitoring for Post-Infarction Risk Stratification

The early post-infarction period is associated with an increased risk of malignant ventricular arrhythmias, with an arrhythmic event rate (sudden death, VF or sustained VT) of around 5%–10% in the first 6 months. Thus, survivors of acute myocardial infarction represent the biggest and most important target population for strategies to prevent sudden death. To date, beta-blockade is the only form of therapy that has been shown to reduce (albeit modestly) post-infarction arrhythmic mortality [5], and there is now conclusive evidence that Class I drugs can increase the risk of sudden death [1]. Multicentre trials are presently being undertaken to evaluate the possible benefits of amiodarone, but it seems increasingly likely that there will be a role for prophylactic implantation of automatic defibrillators in carefully selected high-risk patients. It is important to stress that, since a significant proportion of arrhythmic episodes develop within the first few weeks, no risk-stratification scheme can be truly effective unless the results are available by the time of discharge from hospital, allowing early intervention if appropriate.

Ventricular Ectopic Activity

Pre-discharge ambulatory ECG recording discloses frequent (>10/h) or complex ventricular ectopic activity in 15%–25% of patients, and it has long been recognized that this finding is associated with increased mortality during follow-up [6]. Although it used to be thought that the prognostic value of ventricular ectopic activity was due to its association with left ventricular dysfunction [7], two large prospective infarct surveys, the Multicentre Investigation of Limitation of Infarct Size (MILIS) [8] and the Multicentre Post-Infarction Research Group (MPRG) [9], have confirmed that ventricular arrhythmias and LV function are independently related to all-cause cardiac mortality. However, numerous studies [8–12] have shown that high grade ventricular ectopy alone is not a good predictor of sudden death and life-threatening arrhythmias (Table 1), with a sensitivity of 35%–70% and a positive predictive accuracy below 15% in most surveys. Two groups have examined the relative merits of dif-

Table 1. Relationship of ventricular ectopic activity to life-threatening arrhythmic events during follow-up

	N	Criterion	End point	Sensitivity	Specificity	PPA	Relative risk
MRPG 1984	766	VE>10/h	SD[a]	33	80	12	1.8
MILIS 1984	533	VE>10/h	SD	34	87	13	3.1
BHAT 1987	1640	Complex VE	SD	68	61	8	3.1
Kuchar et al. 1987 [11]	210	Complex VE	Arrhythmic episodes	71	68	13	4.3
Farrell et al. 1990 [12]	416	VE>10/h	Arrhythmic episodes[b]	54	82	16	5.1

VE, ventricular ectopics; SD, sudden death
[a] Hinkle Class I.
[b] Sudden death, VF, or sustained VT.

ferent categories of ventricular ectopic frequency or complexity. In MILIS, grouping by repetitive forms (couplets/non-sustained VT) or by VPC frequency (>10/h) made virtually no difference to sensitivity or predictive accuracy [8]. Kostis et al. analysed seven different categoric definitions of ventricular ectopic activity among 1640 patients in the placebo arm of the Beta-Blocker Heart Attack Trial (BHAT) and noted that, although there was a reciprocal relationship between sensitivity and specificity, the positive predictive accuracy for sudden death varied only slightly (5%–11%) [10].

Furthermore, there is little evidence that measurement of LV function (widely regarded as a 'gold standard' investigation in post-infarction risk stratification) in combination with ventricular ectopic activity significantly improves prediction of arrhythmic events. In MILIS [8], the addition of LV dysfunction (EF<40%) to ventricular ectopic activity (>10/h) only increased positive predictive accuracy from 13% to 18% (relative risk from 3.4 to 11), whereas sensitivity fell from 34% to 24%. Similar findings have emerged from the St. George's Hospital Infarct Survey [12]: positive predictive accuracy increased from 16% to 22% (relative risk from 5.1 to 8.9) and sensitivity was reduced to 33% from 54%.

In conclusion, it seems that no category of ventricular ectopic activity on the ambulatory ECG recording is adequate for assessing future arrhythmic propensity, even if combined with measurement of LV function.

Signal-averaged ECG

An important development has been the introduction of high-resolution surface electrocardiography for recording low amplitude potentials arising from areas of delayed myocardial conduction. These 'late potentials' are believed to indicate the presence of an anatomical substrate for re-entrant ventricular arrhythmias [13] and several post-infarction studies have confirmed that late potentials are associated with increased risk of life-threatening arrhythmic events during follow-up [14, 15]. The sensitivity of the technique is quite high (typically 70%–90%) but with a positive predictive accuracy below 20% in most series. Much of the work to date has been performed with dedicated bedside recording systems, but advances in signal processing now permit detection of late potentials from ambulatory ECG recordings, and integrated Holter systems with this capability are becoming commercially available. Three recent studies [11, 12, 16] have examined the prognostic value of combinations of ventricular ectopic activity and late potentials and their relationship to LV function (Table 2); all of these have used arrhythmic episodes (sudden death, VF or sustained VT) as the primary endpoint. There was general agreement that the late potential/ventricular ectopy combination improves positive predictive accuracy to over 30% at the expense of some

Table 2. Prognostic value of combinations of Holter monitoring, signal averaged ECG and LV function in three series

	N	Criteria	Sensitivity	Specificity	PPA	Relative risk
Kuchar et al.	210	VEA only	71	68	13	4.3
1987 [11]		LP only	93	65	17	23.6
		VEA + LP	65	89	31	NA
		LP + LVEF	80	89	34	NA
Gomes et al.	102	VEA only	80	68	23	4.3
1987 [16]		LP only	87	63	29	11
		VEA + LP	60	80	35	15.7
		LP + LVEF	67	79	36	30.1
Farrell et al.	416	VEA only	54	82	16	5.1
1990 [12]		LP only	63	81	17	6.6
		VEA + LP	38	94	29	15.2
		LP + LVEF	25	94	19	7.4

VEA, ventricular ectopic activity (>10/h); LP, ventricular late potentials; LVEF, reduced LV ejection fraction (<40%)

reduction in sensitivity (40%–60%). However, both Kuchar [11] and Gomes [16] reported excellent results with the late potential/LV dysfunction combination (sensitivity 80% and 67%, PPA 34% and 36%) whereas in the larger series of Farrell [12] this combination was much less successful (sensitivity 25%, PPA 19%). The series of Gomes contained an unusually high proportion (>50%) of patients with an ejection fraction below 40%, which may be one reason for the discrepant results.

Heart Rate Variability

In recent years, there has been increasing recognition of the important role played by disturbances of cardiac sympathovagal balance in the genesis of malignant ventricular arrhythmias in the post-infarction period. Formal measurement of baroreflex sensitivity has been proposed as one approach to risk stratification [17, 18] and this is being evaluated in a multicentre study (ATRAMI). However, the methodology is complex and highly operator-dependent and would be unlikely to gain widespread acceptance for routine clinical work. An alternative approach for assessment of cardiac autonomic function is analysis of heart rate variability. Physiologists have long recognized that periodic oscillations in heart rate reflect the dynamic interaction of sympathetic and vagal drives to the sinus node [19] and a variety of spectral and nonspectral techniques have been used to study this phenomenon. The prognostic significance of reduced heart rate variability was first reported by Wolf in 1978, using variance of RR intervals over 30 consecutive sinus beats [20]. With increased application of computer analysis techniques for ambulatory ECG recordings, indices of heart rate variability can be easily derived and several Holter systems with this capability are already commercially available. Interest in the use of heart rate variability for risk stratification stems largely from an influential report by Kleiger on behalf of the MPRG in 1987 [21]: calculation of mean and standard deviation for all normal RR intervals among 808 patients with tapes suitable for analysis showed that reduced heart rate variability is associated with increased allcause cardiac mortality (relative risk 7.0 for SD < 50 ms) during follow-up. This association was independent of mean heart rate and LV function. Magid et al. reported reduced heart rate variability in 21 patients resuscitated from sudden death due to VF or VT compared to 18 patients with coronary artery disease and high-grade ventricular ectopy but no inducible arrhythmias at programmed stimulation [22]. The same group has subsequently reported lower heart rate variability among 10 patients succumbing to sudden cardiac death compared to 15 patients with recurrent VT [23].

Table 3. Prognostic value of combinations based on heart rate variability and LV function in the St. George's Hospital Infarct Survey

	Sensitivity	Specificity	PPA	NPA	Relative risk
HRV only	92	86	19	77	34.1
HRV + LVEF	42	90	22	91	54.0
HRV + VEA	50	94	34	96	110.8
HRV + LP	59	93	33	93	90.9
LVEF only	46	75	10	75	2.8
LVEF + VEA	33	93	22	93	9.0
LVEF + LP	25	94	19	94	7.4

HRV, reduced heart rate variability (<20 ms); LVEF, LP, VEA, as for Table 2.

The value of heart rate variability in risk stratification for arrhythmic events has now been prospectively evaluated among 416 consecutive patients in the St. George's Hospital Infarct Survey [12]. Heart rate variability was measured by the method of minimum square difference interpolation [24], with 20 ms used as the dichotomy point. Reduced heart rate variability emerged as the strongest univariate predictor of arrhythmic events during follow-up (sensitivity 92%, positive predictive accuracy 19%, relative risk 34.1). Furthermore, in multivariate analysis, only heart rate variability followed by late potentials were found to be independent predictors of arrhythmic risk, whereas all other variables (including LV function) were not. Combinations based on heart rate variability were consistently superior to those incorporating LV function (Table 3) and, in particular, the presence of reduced heart rate variability plus late potentials yielded a sensitivity of 59% with a positive predictive accuracy of 33% and a relative risk ratio of 90.9.

The heart rate variability/late potential combination has a sound rationale in that it examines two key factors in arrhythmogenesis, the presence of anatomical substrate and permissive autonomic tone. With integrated Holter technology incorporating automatic computer analysis, the information can be simply and quickly obtained from a single ambulatory ECG recording. By contrast, the expense and complexity of techniques such as radionuclide angiography would preclude the routine measurement of pre-discharge LV ejection fraction in many hospitals. The heart rate variability/late potential combination appears to select a small group of patients (approximately 10% of the post-infarction population) at high risk of future life-threatening arrhythmias, but if necessary, these patients could be further stratified by programmed ventricular stimulation, to meet the exacting requirements for a trial of prophylactic defibrillator-implantation.

Although several different methods for non-spectral quantification of heart rate variability have been proposed, little is known about their relative merits/drawbacks. However, the method of triangular interpolation of the RR frequency distribution is less affected by noise and misrecognition artefact [25] and therefore has the important advantage of requiring less editing/technician time. It also remains to be seen if spectral analysis into low frequency (sympathetically mediated) and high frequency (vagally mediated) components will confer any additional prognostic information over crude heart rate variability indices [26, 27].

Diurnal QT Variation

Heart rate variability reflects the influence of autonomic tone on the sinus node, whereas arrhythmogenesis results from the interaction of neural mechanisms and ventricular myocardium. Another parameter modulated by autonomic tone is QT interval [28]. QT prolongation in post-infarction patients probably reflects dispersion of ventricular recovery time, a substrate for re-entrant arrhythmias, but previous studies have reached differing conclusions about the prognostic significance of the QT interval in survivors of acute myocardial infarction [29–31]. These discrepancies might be resolved by examining the diurnal variation of QT interval in ambulatory ECG recordings, possibly a better guide to the dynamic interaction of autonomic tone and ventricular repolarization.

Bayes de Luna et al. have recently compared hourly corrected QT interval measurements in Holter tapes of post-infarction patients with and without a history of malignant ventricular arrhythmias (outside the acute infarct period) [32]. The groups were matched for age, sex, infarct site, degree of heart failure, etc. Although there was no difference in the mean global value of QT, the arrhythmia group exhibited a significantly higher proportion of corrected QT measurements over 500 ms. Presumably, this reflected periods of increased vulnerability to ventricular arrhythmias according to prevailing autonomic tone. This approach to risk-stratification looks promising, but further development of the requisite Holter technology and prospective studies are needed.

Silent Myocardial Ischaemia

The development of techniques for monitoring ST segments shifts on ambulatory ECG recordings has led to increased awareness of the

prevalence and prognostic significance of silent myocardial ischaemia in patients with coronary artery disease [33]. Many clinicians have long suspected a role for myocardial ischaemia in the genesis of malignant arrhythmias, but outside the acute phase of myocardial infarction there is little hard evidence to support this viewpoint. Among 157 cases of sudden death during ambulatory monitoring [2], myocardial ischaemia did not appear to be an important triggering mechanism for lethal ventricular tachyarrhythmias, even though most of the patients (84%) suffered from coronary artery disease. In keeping with this, data from the CASS registry suggests that coronary artery surgery has little influence on the incidence of arrhythmic death [34].

In a recent study, Gomes et al. found that among 14 patients with coronary artery disease and sustained ventricular arrhythmias during ambulatory ECG recording, silent ischaemia preceded the onset of tachycardia in only 2 patients, whereas among 15 patients with silent ischaemic episodes and inducible VT, only one episode of ST segment shift precipitated a ventricular arrhythmia [35]. Similarly, Hausmann et al. reported that among 97 patients with coronary artery disease and a positive exercise test, only 5% of episodes of silent ischaemia were associated with ventricular arrhythmias, all non-sustained [36]. In conclusion, it seems unlikely that ambulatory ST segment monitoring will greatly contribute to post-infarction stratification of arrhythmic risk although as yet there are no satisfactory prospective studies examining this issue.

Holter Monitoring in Congestive Heart Failure

Despite advances in therapy, advanced congestive heart failure is associated with an annual mortality of 40%–50%. Approximately half of these deaths occur suddenly, and because asymptomatic ventricular arrhythmias are commonplace in patients with heart failure, it has been suggested that the terminal event is often a sustained ventricular tachyarrhythmia [37, 38]. However, as discussed above, the validity of this assumption has been challenged by the report of Luu et al. [3] which suggested that the mechanism of death is more often a bradyarrhythmia. Nevertheless, there may be a role for implantable defibrillators with antibradycardia pacing capability, particularly if the implantation mortality of 6%–8% in patients with poor LV function could be reduced by the development of transvenous systems. By contrast, conventional antiarrhythmic drugs would be expected to exacerbate bradyarrhythmias, quite apart from negative inotropic and proarrhythmic effects, and this may account for the disappointing results reported even for amiodarone [39].

Several studies have now established that high-grade ventricular ectopic activity, particularly the presence of nonsustained VT, is an independent risk factor for sudden death and total cardiac mortality in heart failure, even after allowing for traditional prognostic variables such as LV function, exercise capacity and neurohormonal indices [36, 37, 40]. This association has been noted both for ischaemic heart disease and heart failure due to other causes, mainly idiopathic dilated cardiomyopathy. However, these asymptomatic arrhythmias may only be markers of overall disease severity, since patients with nonsustained VT on Holter monitoring are just as likely to die from progressive haemodynamic deterioration [41]. Thus, even if sudden arrhythmic death could be prevented these patients would probably still succumb from heart failure. It is not known if susceptibility to malignant arrhythmias and progressive haemodynamic deterioration are inextricably linked in advanced heart failure, or if newer methods of risk stratification such as heart rate variability analysis and signal-averaged ECG can identify patients specifically at risk of sudden death. In the future, there will probably be greater emphasis on targeting patients with mild heart failure or asymptomatic LV dysfunction.

Holter Monitoring in Hypertrophic Cardiomyopathy

The annual sudden death rate associated with hypertrophic cardiomyopathy is 2%–4% in adults and 4%–6% in children/adolescents [42]. Although ultimately these sudden deaths are related to the susceptibility of disordered myocardium to sustain ventricular fibrillation, diverse triggering mechanisms may be involved, with interactions between exercise, abnormal autonomic reflexes, supraventricular arrhythmias, myocardial ischaemia and haemodynamic instability. Nevertheless, among adults with hypertrophic cardiomyopathy, the finding of nonsustained VT during ambulatory ECG monitoring is the most useful marker of increased vulnerability to sudden death. In two major series, the sensitivity was 69% with a specificity of 80% and positive predictive accuracy of 22% [43, 44]. The sensitivity would probably have been increased by routine use of more prolonged (>48 h) ambulatory recording.

Signal-averaged ECG recording in 64 patients with hypertrophic cardiomyopathy detected ventricular late potentials in 13 (20%) [45], and there appeared to be an association with markers of electrical instability (history of cardiac arrest or nonsustained VT on Holter). Prospective studies are needed to establish whether or not this method will improve prediction of sudden death. Analysis of heart rate variability and QT fluctuations may also be of value, since abnormal autonomic function appears to play an important role in this condition.

Conclusions

The advent of new, computer-based methods of electrocardiographic analysis for detection of late potentials, quantification of heart rate variability, etc., has greatly enhanced the potential of Holter monitoring as a tool for assessing vulnerability to life-threatening arrhythmias in various patient populations, particularly survivors of acute myocardial infarction. Integrated Holter systems incorporating these newer capabilities are becoming commercially available. Holter monitoring offers a simple, noninvasive but accurate approach to risk stratification, without the requirement for measurement of left ventricular function. It is likely to be increasingly used to select high-risk patients for interventions such as defibrillator implantation.

References

1. CAST Investigators (1989) Preliminary report: effect of encainide and flecainide on mortality in a randomized trial of arrhythmia suppression after myocardial infarction. N Engl Med 321:406–412
2. Bayes de Luna A, Coumel P, Leclerq JF (1989) Ambulatory sudden cardiac death: mechanisms of production of fatal arrhythmia on the basis of data from 157 cases. Am Heart J 117:151–159
3. Luu M, Stevenson WG, Stevenson LW et al. (1989) Diverse mechanisms of unexpected cardiac arrest in advanced heart failure. Circulation 80:1675–1680
4. Greene HL, Richardson DW, Barker AH et al. (1989) Classification of deaths after myocardial infarction as arrhythmic or nonarrhythmic (the Cardiac Arrhythmia Pilot Study). Am J Cardiol 63:1–6
5. Yusuf S, Peto R, Lewis J, Collins R, Sleight P (1985) Beta-blockade during and after myocardial infarction. An overviews of the randomized trials. Prog Cardiovasc Dis 27:335–351
6. Bigger JT, Coromilas J, Rolnitzky LM, Weld FM (1986) Ventricular arrhythmias after myocardial infarction: significance of findings in 24-hour ECG recordings. In: Kulbertus HE (ed) Medical management of cardiac arrhythmias. Churchill Livingstone, Edinburgh, pp 218–227
7. Schulze RA, Strauss HW, Pitt B (1977) Sudden death in the year following myocardial infarction. Relation to ventricular premature contractions in the late hospital phase and left ventricular ejection fraction. Am J Med 62:192–199
8. Mukharji J, Rude RE, Poole K et al. (1984) Risk factors for sudden death after acute myocardial infarction: two-year follow-up. Am J Cardiol 54:31–36
9. Bigger JT, Fleiss JL, Kleiger R et al. (1984) The relationships among ventricular arrhythmias, left ventricular dysfunction and mortality in the 2 years after myocardial infarction. Circulation 69:250–258

10. Kostis JB, Byington R, Friedman LM et al. (1987) Prognostic significance of ventricular ectopic activity in survivors of acute myocardial infarction. J Am Coll Cardiol 10:231–242
11. Kuchard DL, Thorburn CW, Sammel NL (1987) Prediction of serious arrhythmic events after myocardial infarction: signal-averaged electrocardiogram, Holter monitoring and radionuclide ventriculography. J Am Coll Cardiol 9:531–538
12. Farrell TG, Bashir Y, Cripps TR et al. (1991) A simple method of risk-stratification for arrhythmic events in post-infarction patients based on heart rate variability and the signal-averaged ECG. J Am Coll Cardiol (vol 18, in press)
13. Borbola J, Erzi MD, Denes P (1988) Correlation between the signal-averaged electrocardiogram and electrophysiological study findings in patients with coronary artery disease and sustained ventricular tachycardia. Am Heart J 115:816–824
14. Breithardt G, Borggrefe M, Haarten K (1984) Role of programmed stimulation and non-invasive recording of ventricular late potentials for the identification of patients at risk of ventricular arrhythmias after acute myocardial infarction. In: Zipes DP, Jalife J (eds) Cardiac electrophysiology and arrhythmias. Grune and Stratton, Orlando, pp 553–561
15. Denniss AR, Richard DA, Cody DV et al. (1986) Prognostic significance of ventricular tachycardia and fibrillation induced at programmed stimulation and delayed potentials detected on the signal-averaged electrocardiograms of survivors of acute myocardial infarction. Circulation 74:731–745
16. Gomes JA, Winters SL, Stewart D et al. (1987) New noninvasive index to predict sustained ventricular tachycardia and sudden death in the first year after myocardial infarction: based on signal-averaged electrocardiogram, radionuclide ejection fraction and Holter monitoring. J Am Coll Cardiol 10:349–357
17. LaRovere MT, Specchia G, Mortara A, Schwartz PJ (1986) Baroreflex sensitivity, clinical correlates and cardiovascular mortality among patients with first myocardial infarction. Circulation 78:816–824
18. Farrell TG, Paul VE, Cripps TR et al. (1991) Baroreflex sensitivity after myocardial infarction: clinical and electrophysiologic correlates. Circulation 83:945–952
19. Akselrod S, Gordon D, Ubel FA et al. (1981) Power spectrum analysis of heart rate fluctuations: a quantitative probe of beat-to-beat cardiovascular control. Science 213:220–230
20. Wolf MW, Varigos GA, Hunt D, Sloman JG (1978) Sinus arrhythmia in acute myocardial infarction. Med J Aust 2:52–53
21. Kleiger RE, Millar P, Bigger JT et al. (1987) Decreased heart rate variability and its association with increased mortality after acute myocardial infarction. Am J Cardiol 59:256–262
22. Magid NM, Martin GJ, Kehoe RF et al. (1985) Diminished heart rate variability in patients with sudden cardiac death. Circulation 72 [Suppl III]:241, A964
23. Van Hoogenhuyze D, Martin GJ, Weiss JS et al. (1989) Heart rate variability 1989: an update. J Electrocardiol 22 [Suppl]:256–262

24. Malik M, Farrell TG, Cripps TR, Camm AJ (1989) Heart rate variability in relation to prognosis after myocardial infarction. Eur Heart J 10:1060–1074
25. Malik M, Cripps TR, Farrell TG, Camm AJ (1989) Prognostic value of heart rate variability after myocardial infarction. A comparison of different data-processing methods. Med Biol Eng Comput 27:603–611
26. Lombardi F, Sandrome G, Pernpruner S et al. (1987) Heart rate variability as an index of sympathovagal interaction after acute myocardial infarction. Am J Cardiol 60:1238–1245
27. Bigger JT, LaRovere MT, Steinman RC et al. (1989) Comparison of heart period variability and baroreflex sensitivity after myocardial infarction. J Am Coll Cardiol 15:1511–1518
28. Bexton RS, Vallin HO, Camm AJ (1986) Diurnal variation of the QT interval-influence of the autonomic nervous system. Br Heart J 55:253–258
29. Ahnve S, Gilpin E, Madsen EB et al. (1984) Prognostic importance of QT_c interval at discharge after acute myocardial infarction: a multicentre study of 865 patients. Am Heart J 108:395–400
30. Schwartz PJ, Wolf S (1978) QT interval prolongation as a predictor of sudden death in patients with myocardial infarction. Circulation 57:1074–1077
31. Wheelan K, Mukharji J, Rude RE et al. (1986) Sudden death and its relation to QT prolongation after acute myocardial infarction: two-year follow-up. Am J Cardiol 57:745–750
32. Bayes de Luna A, Marti V, Songa V et al. (1989) Value of dynamic QT_c measurement to stratify prognosis in cardiac patients. In: Schwartz PJ, Butrous GS (eds) Aspects of ventricular repolarization. 389–394
33. Tzivoni D, Stern S (1989) Prognostic significance of silent ischaemia. J Ambul Monit 2:115–121
34. Holmes RD, Davis K, Gersh BJ, Mock MB, Pettinger MB (1989) Risk factor profiles of patients with sudden cardiac death and death from other cardiac causes: a report from the Coronary Artery Surgery Study (CASS). J Am Coll Cardiol 13:524–530
35. Gomes JA, Alexopoulos D, Winters SL et al. (1989) The role of silent ischaemia, the arrhythmic substrate and the short long sequence in the genesis of sudden cardiac death. J Am Coll Cardiol 14:1618–1625
36. Hausmann D, Nikutta P, Trappe HJ et al. (1990) Incidence of ventricular arrhythmias during transient myocardial ischaemia in patients with stable coronary artery disease. J Am Coll Cardiol 16:49–54
37. Bigger JT (1987) Why patients with congestive heart failure die: arrhythmias and sudden cardiac death. Circulation 75 [Suppl IV]:28–35
38. Francis GS (1988) Should asymptomatic ventricular arrhythmias in patients with congestive heart failure be treated with antiarrhythmic drugs? J Am Coll Cardiol 12:274–283
39. Stewart RA, McKenna WJ, Polonieckie JD et al. (1989) Prospective randomized double-blind placebo-controlled trial of low dose amiodarone in patients with severe heart failure and frequent ventricular ectopy. Eur Heart J 10 [Suppl]:1158

40. Gradman A, Deedwania P, Cody R et al. (1989) Predictors of total mortality and sudden death in mild-to-moderate heart failure. J Am Coll Cardiol 14:564–570
41. Wilson JR, Schwartz JS, Sutton MSJ et al. (1983) Prognosis in severe heart failure: relation to haemodynamic measurements and ventricular ectopic activity. J Am Coll Cardiol 2:403–410
42. McKenna WJ, Camm AJ (1989) Sudden death in hypertrophic cardiomyopathy. Circulation 80:1489–1492
43. Maron BJ, Savage DD, Wolfson JK, Epstein SE (1981) Prognostic significance of 24 hour ambulatory electrocardiographic monitoring in patients with hypertrophic cardiomyopathy. Am J Cardiol 48:252–257
44. McKenna WJ, England D, Doi YL et al. (1981) Arrhythmia in hypertrophic cardiomyopathy: 1. Influence on prognosis. Br Heart J 46:168–172
45. Cripps TR, Counihan PJ, Frenneaux MP et al. (1990) Signal-averaged electrocardiography in hypertrophic cardiomyopathy. J Am Coll Cardiol 15:956–961

Identification of the Patient at High Risk for Sudden Cardiac Death: The Value of Ventricular Late Potentials

G. Breithardt, M. Borggrefe, W. Haverkamp, G. Hindricks

Introduction

Sudden cardiac death is still one of the major causes of cardiac death, mostly occurring in patients after myocardial infarction. Early identification of such patients is therefore of great clinical significance. The major parameters that identify patients at increased risk of sudden cardiac death are:

1) A previous myocardial infarction
2) The degree of left ventricular impairment
3) The frequency and type of spontaneously occurring ventricular arrhythmias
4) The modulation by the autonomous nervous system
5) The persistence or new appearance of ischemia.

In addition, patients who have already survived an episode of sustained ventricular tachycardia or of out-of-hospital cardiac arrest are at increased risk for subsequent recurrences. This also applies to patients who do not respond to electropharmacologic testing [1–3].

With the advent of new non-pharmacologic approaches to the management of ventricular tachyarrhythmias such as map-guided antitachycardia surgery, catheter ablation of ventricular tachycardia, and the implantable cardioverter-defibrillator, an improvement of our strategies for identification of high risk patients after myocardial infarction is even more mandatory. This is the more important since the results of the Cardiac Arrhythmia Suppression Trial (CAST) using flecainide and encainide have disappointingly shown the failure of these two drugs to improve prognosis; instead, there was a worsening of prognosis [4]. Recently, approaches that directly assess the presence of an "arrhythmogenic substrate" such as recording of ventricular late potentials or programmed ventricular stimulation have gained increasing recognition as tools to prospectively assess prognosis in post-myocardial infarction patients [5–10]. The purpose of this chapter will be to present some information, mostly based on our own experience, on the usefulness of signal-averaging for detection of late potentials and their prognostic implications.

High-gain amplification and subsequent signal-averaging for reduction of randomly occurring noise has attracted a great deal of interest for the detection of low-amplitude signals from the body surface since the initial reports by Fontaine et al. [11, 12] and Berbari et al. [13] and subsequent reports by Simson et al. [14, 15], Rozanski et al. [16], Breithardt et al. [17–20], Uther et al. [21] and Hombach et al. [22]. The latter authors presented their initial experience in patients with ventricular tachyarrhythmias. Since then, experimental and clinical studies have improved our understanding of the pathophysiologic mechanisms as well as of the clinical significance of ventricular late potentials [5].

Pathophysiological Background

The anatomic substrate for ventricular late potentials after myocardial infarction is interstitial fibrosis that forms insulating bounderies between muscle bundles [23, 24]. The fragmented electrograms recorded from these areas most probably represent asynchronous electrical activity in each of the separate bundles of surviving muscle. The slow activation might result from conduction over circuitous pathways caused by the separation and distortion of the myocardial fiber bundles. The low amplitude of the electrograms from the border zone of myocardial infarction probably results from the paucity of surviving muscle fibers [23]. The anatomic substrate for reentry seems to be present in regions where fragmented electrograms can be recorded. However, fragmented electrograms are probably found wherever myocardial fibers are separated by connective tissue, even if reentry does not occur in the region. This has been recently shown by Kienzle et al. [25] who concluded that these electrograms may be associated with, but are not specific for sites of origin of ventricular tachycardia.

Late Potentials in Patients Without Ventricular Tachyarrhythmias

Ventricular late potentials can be detected in a high percentage of patients with previously documented ventricular tachycardia. However, they can also be recorded in about one-third of patients without a history of ventricular tachycardia or fibrillation outside acute myocardial infarction [19, 20, 26–30]. This indicates that in these patients, there is a substrate for reentrant arrhythmias which, however, has not yet manifested

itself. Obviously, some additional trigger factor is needed to initiate ventricular tachycardia or fibrillation [7].

Prognostic Significance of Late Potentials

The major impact for the use of signal-averaging is not so much in the field of retrospective analysis of patients with documented sustained ventricular tachycardia [14–19, 21, 22, 26, 28–33] but in the prediction of the clinical course of patients after recent myocardial infarction who have been hitherto free of ventricular tachyarrhythmias. In recent years, several studies have addressed this issue [8, 10, 34–38; S. Kacet, C. Libersa, J. Caron, B. Bondoux d'Haute-Fenille, X. Marchand, J. Lekieffre, personal communication].

Our own experience is based on two prospective studies. The first prospective trial was initiated at Düsseldorf University in 1980. It used the methodology for recording of signal-averaged ECGs that had been developed in our department between 1978 and 1979. This system was primarily based on a hard-wired signal-averager [10, 18–20, 34]. The second study was started in January 1983. This study included only male patients after recent Q-wave myocardial infarction. Signal-averaging was performed using the software program by Simson [15] which includes bidirectional filtering and automated analysis of signal-averaged ECGs. This multicenter non-interventional study has been called the PILP-Study (Post-Infarction Late Potential-study). It has recently been completed after inclusion of almost 800 patients (manuscript in preparation).

The long-term results of our first study group has recently been reported in a preliminary fashion [6, 39, 40]. 628 patients without a history of sustained ventricular tachycardia or fibrillation outside the acute phase of myocardial infarction, without a history of syncope, and without complete bundle branch block were included. The patients were selected if they either had survived recent myocardial infarction or if they were referred to our department because of a clinical indication for coronary angiography to establish or exclude the presence of coronary artery disease. In the first subgroup, only patients with acute myocardial infarction were included that were admitted to the hospital on a primary referral basis. Thus, patients referred from other hospitals because of major complications of myocardial infarction were not included. Signal-averaging was done as previously described [18, 20]. Mean age of these patients was 54±7.6 years; 469 patients had a history of previous myocardial infarction; 258 patients were included within the first 4 weeks after myocardial infarction, another 52 patients within the second

month. The remaining 259 patients were studied after more than 2 months after their myocardial infarction. There were 379 patients (60%) who had no late potentials, 191 patients (30%) who had late potentials of less than 40 ms in duration and 58 patients (9%) who had late potentials of 40 ms duration or more.

Mean follow-up duration was 39±15.0 months. At the end of follow-up, 21 patients (3.3%) had died suddenly within 1 h, mostly occurring either instantaneously or during sleep whereas another 3 patients (0.5%) died within 1–24 h. There were another 14 cardiac deaths mostly due to reinfarction and myocardial failure. In addition, there were 14 patients (2.2%) who had survived an episode of symptomatic spontaneous sustained ventricular tachycardia that required some type of emergency intervention. Thus, in a total of 35 patients, a major arrhythmic event occurred during follow-up. The risk of major arrhythmic complications was 2.8 times greater in patients with late potentials of less than 40 ms duration than in those without and 9.3 times greater in those with a duration of 40 ms or more. The chance of sudden cardiac death within 1 h was 3.3 and 5.4 times greater, respectively, whereas the chance for symptomatic sustained ventricular tachycardia was 2.0 and 17.4 times greater, respectively, depending on the duration of late potentials (less than 40 ms or greater). The chance of major arrhythmic complications such as sudden cardiac death or sustained symptomatic ventricular tachycardia was greatest in those patients who were studied within the first 4–8 weeks after their qualifying myocardial infarction. The results of follow-up were significantly correlated with the presence and duration of late potentials, the site of (anterior wall) and the interval after myocardial infarction (1–2 months), and the degree of left ventricular dysfunction. The 4 year arrhythmic event-free rate in patients with late potentials was 72% (ejection fraction below 40%) and 93% (ejection fraction greater 40%) vs 98% in patients without late potentials. Thus, the presence of late potentials predicted the subsequent occurrence of arrhythmic events during long-term follow-up in post-myocardial infarction patients with impaired left ventricular function.

These results have been confirmed by other groups though different recording technologies were used [8, 9, 35, 36–38] in the subacute and late post-myocardial infarction period and in the early phase [41, 42].

Role of Thrombolytic Therapy

With an increasing use of thrombolytic therapy in the acute phase of myocardial infarction, there might be a change in the anatomical and functional substrate of infarction. This might have implications for the

evaluation of these patients and may also be the reason for the improved prognosis in many patients after acute thrombolysis in myocardial infarction. To address these questions, several studies were recently performed. Eldar and coworkers reported the effect of thrombolysis on the evolution of late potentials in the early post-infarction period [43]. During the first 10 days after acute myocardial infarction, 158 patients were prospectively studied. The study population consisted of two nonrandomized groups: 93 patients had been treated conservatively, whereas 65 patients had been treated by intravenous thrombolysis. The incidence of late potentials in the first 2 days after infarction was not significantly different between patients treated conservatively (14%) and patients treated by thrombolysis (11.8%). On days 7–10, the incidence of late potentials among patients who had undergone thrombolysis, had remained unchanged; however, it had increased significantly in the conservatively treated group from 11.8% to 22.5% ($p<0.01$). Another study also evaluated the time-course of late potentials after myocardial infarction [44]. They observed that in reperfused infarctions, development of late potentials was related to the presence of Q-waves and was independent of peak CPK and infarct location. Late potentials sometimes were present only in the early infarction period; they may represent areas of transiently delayed myocardial activation which resolve with infarct healing [44].

A similar study has recently been published by Gang et al. [45]. These authors studied 106 consecutive patients less than 75 years of age who were admitted to hospital with a first acute myocardial infarction. The 44 patients who had chest pain for less than 4 h received recombinant tissue plasminogen activator (t-PA), whereas another 62 patients who either did not qualify for or refused treatment with t-PA received conventional therapy. Thus, these patients were not a randomized sample of acute myocardial infarction patients. The two groups did not differ with respect to age, sex, site and size of myocardial infarction, extent of coronary artery disease or left ventricular ejection fraction. Signal-averaging was performed in all patients within 48 h of admission to the hospital and again in the surviving patients before discharge. In only 2 of the 44 patients (5%) treated with t-PA, late potentials were present as compared to 14 of 62 patients (23%) who did not receive t-PA ($p = 0.01$). Patency of the infarct-related coronary artery and administration of t-PA were found to be the only independent predictors of the presence of late potentials. Preliminary data by Riccio et al. [46] on 172 patients studied in the context of the GISSI-2 study point into a similar direction. Of 103 patients 20 (16.5%) treated with streptokinase or t-PA had late potentials as compared to 17 of 69 patients (28.9%) who did not receive thrombolytic therapy because of contraindications or late admission to the hospital.

Another very recent study by Turitto et al. [47] assessed the presence of an abnormal signal-average ECG in 118 patients 13±2 days after acute myocardial infarction [47]. Group 1 (46 patients) underwent intravenous thrombolysis within 6 h on the onset of symptoms, whereas group 2 (72 patients) did not. An abnormal signal-averaged ECG was seen in 15% of patients in group I and 21% of those in group 2 (n. s.). Comparing patients with ($n = 26$) or without ($n = 20$) angiographic patency of the infarct-related coronary artery after thrombolysis showed no significant difference in the prevalence of an abnormal signal-averaged ECG (8% vs 25%, respectively) and complex ventricular arrhythmias (19% vs 20% respectively). From these data, the authors concluded that thrombolysis did not seem to effect the prevalence of complex ventricular arrhythmias and of an abnormal signal-averaged ECG. However, the subset of patients in whom angiography was performed was probably too small to yield meaningful results.

The results of these still preliminary studies indicate that successful early reperfusion may prevent the formation of an arrhythmogenic substrate as evidenced by the presence of late potentials on high-resolution electrocardiography. However, the prognostic significance of these findings needs still to be elucidated.

Comparison with Other Parameters

Denniss et al. [48] recently assessed the relative values of signal-averaging and exercise testing in predicting death and arrhythmias after myocardial infarction in 250 clinically well patients age less than 66 years. Signal-averaging and exercise testing had been done within 2 months of myocardial infarction. An abnormal finding was defined as late potentials on the signal-averaged ECG being present, ST-segment changes of 2 mm or more or impaired hemodynamics or angina on exercise testing. Patients were followed for 3 years. They reported that the signal-averaged electrocardiogram was superior to exercise testing. The odds ratio for death or sustained ventricular tachycardia or fibrillation was 7.4 in patients with compared to those without late potentials; in contrast, it was only 1.5 in patients with compared to those without ST-segment depression or in those in whom any of these parameters (ST-segment depression or impaired hemodynamics or angina) were present.

Similar results were recently reported by Cripps et al. [49]. These authors prospectively investigated the relative value of exercise testing, late potentials recorded using the algorithm by Simson [15] and simple clinical assessment in predicting ischemic and arrhythmic events during follow-up after acute myocardial infarction. A series of 176 consecutive

patients surviving at least 7 days after acute myocardial infarction were studied. The presence of late potentials was defined as the presence of one or more of the following criteria: (1) filtered QRS-duration of 120 ms or more; (2) duration of the filtered QRS-complex after the voltage had decreased below 40 µV, of 40 ms or more and (3) a root mean square voltage during the last 40 ms of the filtered QRS-complex of 20 µV or less. A prolonged filtered QRS alone was not considered a positive result if QRS duration in the standard ECG was more than 120 ms in duration. Patients with bundle branch block were excluded. No investigations or therapy were instituted on the basis of the results of signal averaging, and no patient received prophylactic antiarrhythmic therapy before the occurrence of arrhythmic events. Treadmill exercise testing was carried out within 6 weeks of infarction. In 108 of 172 patients (63%), this was a symptom-limited test using the Bruce protocol and the test was carried out after discharge at about 1 month after infarction. In the remaining patients, exercise testing was carried out before discharge using a 9 min three stage protocol. The latter protocol was introduced after the death of a number of patients after discharge but before the time of the planned post-discharge exercise test. The age of the patients was 56±9 years (range 28–70), 20% of the patients were female. The site of infarction was anterior in 90 (52%), inferior or posterior or both in 76 (44%) and indeterminate in 8 patients (4%). Signal-averaging was performed 12±19 days after infarction in all 176 patients. Late potentials were present in 41 patients (24%). All but two of the patients with arrhythmic events (sudden death defined as witnessed instantaneous sudden death not preceded by chest pain or sustained ventricular tachycardia associated with symptomatic hypotension or requiring emergency intervention or both) had late potentials, whereas 32 of 165 patients without arrhythmic events had late potentials. However, only 5 of 23 patients with ischemic events (including coronary artery bypass grafting) had late potentials. Exercise testing was performed 21±14 days after infarction. There were two patients who where unable to perform the test due to cardiovascular instability at the time of the test. Test results were positive in 18 of 23 patients with ischemic events, but only in 6 of 11 patients with arrhythmic events. There were four positive exercise test results in 63 of 153 patients. The duration of follow-up was 15±7 months (range 3–24 months). Using multivariate analysis, the only independent variable predicting ischemic events was the exercise test result. Arrhythmic events were independent of the exercise test result but the Killip class on admission, presence of late potentials, previous infarction, occurrence of in-hospital complications and non-Q-wave infarction were independently associated with arrhythmic events. The independent variables predicting any event (reinfarction, coronary artery bypass grafting, symptomatic ventricular tachycardia, and sudden death) included, in the order of importance, Killip class, exercise test result, presence of late potentials and non-Q-wave infarction.

Based on these results, the authors [49] concluded that exercise testing is sensitive although of low positive predictive accuracy in predicting *ischemic* events and that, similarly, the presence of late potentials is sensitive yet inaccurate in predicting *arrhythmic* events. Only about one out of five patients with late potentials will suffer an arrhythmic event. Therefore, they suggested that more specific tests are required in the group identified by non-invasive screening. They suggested that the addition of clinical observations and the occurrence of a positive result in the exercise test also enhanced the predictive accuracy of this test. In contrast, patients at low risk were those free of complications during the acute phase of myocardial infarction, with a negative result in the exercise test and no late potentials. In the presence of this combination of parameters, a course free of subsequent arrhythmic or ischemic events could be predicted with a certainty of 99% [49].

In our prospective study, several parameters were evaluated in 552 patients with coronary artery disease but without a history of ventricular tachycardia or ventricular fibrillation outside the acute phase of myocardial infarction. Using a combination of signal-averaging and programmed ventricular stimulation, we were able to show that the predictive value for subsequent arrhythmic events could be markedly increased [10, 50]. During a mean follow-up period of 30 ± 19 months, 53 patients (10%) died. There were 21 sudden deaths and 16 patients had documented symptomatic sustained ventricular tachycardia (total arrhythmic event rate 7%). The prevalence of a subsequent arrhythmic event was 2.8% in patients without late potentials and without inducible ventricular tachycardia, whereas in patients with late potentials and inducible ventricular tachycardia the prevalence was 25%. Compared to patients without late potentials, the relative risk (odds ratio) of patients with late potentials was 2.6, of those with late potentials and inducible sustained ventricular tachycardia 4.5. The predictive value of these tests and the odds ratios were markedly higher if only the subgroup of patients with subsequent symptomatic sustained ventricular tachycardia was evaluated. In this subgroup, the relative risk of late potentials and inducible ventricular tachycardia was 19.4 compared to those without late potentials. This means that these patients had a 19.4 times greater chance of developing sustained symptomatic ventricular tachycardia than those without a positive finding. Thus, this combined approach helped to identify subgroups at very high risk of subsequent arrhythmic events. Using ejection fraction as an additional parameter, the predictive value of these parameters could even be increased (unpublished data).

Conclusions and Clinical Implications

Based on these presently available prospective studies, the presence of ventricular late potentials obviously heralds an increased risk for subsequent occurrence of sudden cardiac death or symptomatic sustained ventricular tachycardia. This mainly applies to patients who have been studied after recent myocardial infarction [34, 35; S. Kacet, C. Libersa, J. Caron, B. Bodoux d'Haute-Fenille, X. Marchand, J. Dagano, J. Lekieffre, personal communication; 37, 38], whereas patients who are included later and/or who are considered eligible for a cardiac rehabilitation program [36], obviously have a much lower incidence of arrhythmic events. Thus, the predictive value of the presence of ventricular late potentials largely depends on the clinical circumstances under which they can be detected. Patients who have survived for a long period after their myocardial infarction have a much lower risk of subsequent development of sudden cardiac death or symptomatic sustained ventricular tachycardia. This is obviously based on a selection process as patients at greater risk might have died in the meanwhile.

Since sudden cardiac death is a multifactorial problem, it seems unjustified to expect any single method to be able to identify the individual patient at risk of sustained ventricular tachycardia and/or sudden death. Instead, a combination of various parameters including late potentials, spontaneous ventricular arrhythmias during long-term ECG-recording, extent of myocardial contractile disturbance (ejection fraction), exercise test, electrophysiological study and estimates of central nervous activity [51, 52] might aid in further risk stratification in patients after recent myocardial infarction.

References

1. Breithardt G, Borggrefe M, Seipel L (1984) Selection of optimal drug treatment of ventricular tachycardia by programmed electrical stimulation of the heart. Ann NY Acad Sci 427:49–65
2. Borggrefe M, Breithardt G (1986) Predictive value of electrophysiologic testing in the treatment of drug-refractory ventricular arrhythmias with amiodarone. Eur Heart J 7:735–742
3. Borggrefe M, Trampisch HJ, Breithardt G (1988) Reappraisal of criteria for assessing drug efficacy in patients with ventricular tachyarrhythmias: complete versus partial suppression of inducible arrhythmias. J Am Coll Cardiol 12:140–149
4. Cardiac Arrhythmias Suppression Trial (CAST) (1989) Preliminary report: effect of encainide and flecainide on mortality in a randomized trial of arrhythmia suppression after myocardial infarction. N Engl J Med 321: 406–412

5. Breithardt G, Borggrefe M (1986) Pathophysiological mechanisms and clinical significance of ventricular late potentials. Eur Heart J 7:364–385
6. Breithardt G, Borggrefe M (1987) Recent advances in the identification of patients at risk of ventricular tachyarrhythmias: role of ventricular late potentials. Circulation 75:1091–1096
7. Breithardt G, Borggrefe M, Martinez-Rubio A, Budde T (1989) Pathophysiological mechanisms of ventricular tachyarrhythmias. Eur Heart J 10 [Suppl]:9–18
8. Denniss AR, Cody DV, Russell PA, Young AA, Ross DL, Uther JB (1984) Prognostic significance of inducible ventricular tachycardia after myocardial infarction. J Am Coll Cardiol 3:610
9. Denniss AR, Richards DA, Cody DV, Russell PA, Young AA, Cooper MJ, Ross DL, Uther JB (1986) Prognostic significance of ventricular tachycardia and fibrillation induced at programmed ventricular stimulation and delayed potentials detected on the signal-averaged electrocardiogram of survivors of acute myocardial infarction. Circulation 74:731–745
10. Breithardt G, Borggrefe M, Haerten K (1985) Role of programmed ventricular stimulation and noninvasive recording of ventricular late potentials for the identification of patients at risk of ventricular tachyarrhythmias after acute myocardial infarction. In: Zipes DP, Jaliffe J (eds) Cardiac electrophysiology and arrhythmias. Grune and Stratton, New York, pp 553–561
11. Fontaine G, Guiraudon G, Frank R (1978) Intramyocardial conduction defects in patients prone to ventricular tachycardia. III. In: Sandoe E, Julian DG, Bell JW (eds) Management of ventricular tachycardia – role of mexiletine. Excerpta Medica, Amsterdam, pp 67–69
12. Fontaine G, Frank R, Gallais-Hamonno F, Allali I, Phan-Thuc H, Grosgogeat Y (1978) Electrocardiographie des potentials tardifs du syndrome de postexcitation. Arch Mal Coeur 71:854–886
13. Berbari EJ, Scherlag BJ, Hope RR, Lazzara R (1978) Recording from the body surface of arrhythmogenic ventricular activity during the ST-segment. Am J Cardiol 41:697–702
14. Simson M, Horowitz L, Josephson M, Moore NE, Kastor J (1980) A marker for ventricular tachycardia after myocardial infarction. Circulation 62:III–262 (abstr)
15. Simson M (1981) Use of signals in the terminal QRS-complex to identify patients with ventricular tachycardia after myocardial infarction. Circulation 64:235–242
16. Rozanski JJ, Mortara D, Myerburg RJ, Castellanos A (1981) Body surface detection of delayed depolarizations in patients with recurrent ventricular tachycardia and left ventricular aneurysm. Circulation 63:1172–1178
17. Breithardt G, Becker R, Seipel L (1980) Non-invasive recording of late ventricular activation in man. Circulation 62:III–320 (abstr)
18. Breithardt G, Becker R, Seipel L, Abendroth RR, Ostermeyer J (1981) Non-invasive detection of late potentials in man – a new marker for ventricular tachycardia. Eur Heart J 2:1–11
19. Breithardt G, Borggrefe M, Karbenn U, Abendroth RR, Yeh HL, Seipel L (1982) Prevalence of late potentials in patients with and without ventricular

tachycardia: correlation to angiographic findings. Am J Cardiol 49: 1932–1937
20. Breithardt G, Borggrefe M, Quantius B, Karbenn U, Seipel L (1983) Ventricular vulnerability assessed by programmed ventricular stimulation in patients with and without late potentials. Circulation 68:275–281
21. Uther JB, Dennett CJ, Tan A (1978) The detection of delayed activation signals of low amplitude in the vectorcardiogram of patients with recurrent ventricular tachycardia by signal averaging. In: Sandöe E et al. (eds) Management of ventricular tachycardia – role of mexiletine. Excerpta Medica, Amsterdam, pp 80–82
22. Hombach V, Höpp HW, Braun V, Behrenbeck DW, Tauchert M, Hilger HH (1980) Die Bedeutung von Nachpotentialen innerhalb des ST-Segmentes im Oberflächen-EKG bei Patienten mit koronarer Herzkrankheit. Dtsch Med Wochenschr 105:1457–1462
23. Gardner PHJ, Ursell PHC, Pham TD, Fenoglio JJ, Wit AL (1984) Experimental chronic ventricular tachycardia: anatomic and electrophysiologic substrates. In: Josephson ME, Wellens HJJ (eds) Tachycardias: mechanisms, diagnosis, treatment. Lea and Febiger, Philadelphia, pp 29–60
24. Richards DA, Blake GJ, Spear JF, Moore EN (1984) Electrophysiologic substrate for ventricular tachycardia: correlation of properties in vivo and in vitro. Circulation 69:369–381
25. Kienzle MG, Miller J, Falcone R, Harken A, Josephson ME (1984) Intraoperative endocardial mapping during sinus rhythm: relationship to site of origin of ventricular tachycardia. Circulation 70:957–965
26. Kertes PJ, Glaubus M, Murray A, Julian DG, Campbell RWF (1984) Delayed ventricular depolarization-correlation with ventricular activation and relevance to ventricular fibrillation in acute myocardial infarction. Eur Heart J 5:974–983
27. Abboud S, Belhassen B, Laniado S, Sadeh D (1983) Non-invasive recording of late ventricular activity using an advanced method in patients with a damaged mass of ventricular tissue. J Electrocardiol 16:245
28. Höpp HW, Hombach V, Deutsch HJ, Osterspey A, Winter U, Hilger HH (1983) Assessment of ventricular vulnerability by Holter ECG, programmed ventricular stimulation and recording of ventricular late potentials. In: Steinbach K et al. (eds) Cardiac pacing. Steinkopff, Darmstadt, pp 625–632
29. Freedman RA, Gillis AM, Keren A, Soderholm-Difatte V, Mason JW (1984) Signal-averaged ECG late potentials correlate with clinical arrhythmia and electrophysiological study in patients with ventricular tachycardia or fibrillation. Circulation 70:II–252
30. Kanovsky MS, Falcone RA, Dresden CA, Josephson ME, Simson ME (1984) Identification of patients with ventricular tachycardia after myocardial infarction: signal-averaged electrocardiogram, Holter monitoring, and cardiac catheterization. Circulation 70:264–270
31. Cain ME, Ambos D, Witkowski FX, Sobel BE (1984) Fast-Fourier transform analysis of signal-averaged electrocardiograms for identification of patients prone to sustained ventricular tachycardia. Circulation 69:711–720

32. Poll DS, Marchlinski FE, Falcone RA, Simson MB (1984) Abnormal signal averaged ECG in nonischemic congestive cardiomyopathy: relationship to sustained ventricular tachyarrhythmias. Circulation 70:II–253
33. Cain ME, Ambos HD, Markham J, Fischer AE, Sobel BE (1985) Quantification of differences in frequency content of signal-averaged electrocardiograms in patients with compared to those without sustained ventricular tachycardia. Am J Cardiol 55:1500–1505
34. Breithardt G, Schwarzmaier J, Borggrefe M, Haerten K, Seipel L (1983) Prognostic significance of ventricular late potentials after acute myocardial infarction. Eur Heart J 4:487–495
35. Denniss AR, Cody DV, Fenton SM, Richards DA, Ross DL, Russell PA, Young AA, Uther JB (1983) Significance of delayed activation potentials in survivors of myocardial infarction. J Am Coll Cardiol 1:582 (abstr)
36. v Leitner ER, Oeff M, Loock D, Jahns B, Schröder R (1983) Value of non invasively detected delayed ventricular depolarizations to predict prognosis in post myocardial infarction patients. Circulation 68:III–83
37. Höpp HW, Hombach V, Osterspey A, Deutsch H, Winter U, Behrenbeck DW, Tauchert M, Hilger HH (1985) Clinical and prognostic significance of ventricular arrhythmias and ventricular late potentials in patients with coronary heart disease. In: Hombach V, Hilger HH (eds) Holter monitoring technique. Technical aspects and clinical applications. Liss, New York, pp 297–307
38. Kuchar D, Thorburn C, Sammel N (1985) Natural history and clinical significance of late potentials after myocardial infarction. Circulation 72:III–477
39. Breithardt G, Borggrefe M, Haerten K, Seipel L (1986) Value of electrophysiologic testing, recording of late potentials by averaging techniques and Holter monitoring for the identification of high risk patients after acute myocardial infarction. In: Kulbertus HE (ed) Medical management of cardiac arrhythmias. Churchill Livingstone, Edinburgh, pp 228–246
40. Breithardt G, Borggrefe M, Podczeck A, Schwarzmaier J, Karbenn U (1987) Prognostic significance of late potentials in patients with coronary heart disease. Circulation 76:IV–344 (abstr)
41. Eldar M, Leor J, Rotstein Z, Hod H, Truman S, Abboud S (1988) Signal averaging identifies increased mortality risk at early post-infarction period. Circulation 78 [Suppl II]:51
42. Hong M, Gang ES, Wang FZ, Siebert C, Xu YX, Simonson J, Peter T (1988) Ventricular late potentials are associated with ventricular tachyarrhythmias in the early phase of myocardial infarction. Circulation 78 [Suppl II]:302
43. Eldar M, Leor J, Hod H, Rotstein Z, Truman S, Kaplinsky E, Abboud S (1992) Effect of thrombolysis on the evolution of late potentials in the early post infarction period. Br Heart J (in press)
44. Volosin KJ, Beauregard LA, Kurnik BK, Fabiszewski R, Waxman HL (1989) Time course of ventricular late potential development after coronary reperfusion with tissue plasminogen activator. PACE 12 [Suppl I]:636

45. Gang ES, Lew AS, Hong M, Wang FZ, Siebert CA, Peter T (1989) Decreased incidence of ventricular late potentials after successful thrombolytic therapy for acute myocardial infarction. N Engl J Med 321:712–716
46. Riccio C, Cesaro F, Perrotta R, Romano S, Correale E, Corsini G (1990) Early thrombolysis, reperfusion arrhythmias and late potentials in acute myocardial infarction. New Frontiers Arrhythmias 6:157–161
47. Turitto G, Risa AL, Sanchi E, Prati TL (1990) The signal-averaged electrocardiogram and ventricular arrhythmias after thrombolysis for acute myocardial infarction. J Am Coll Cardiol 15:1270–1276
48. Denniss AR, Cody DV, Richards DA, Ross DL, Russell PA, Young AA, Uther JB (1988) Signal-averaged electrocardiogram is superior to exercise testing in predicting death and arrhythmias after myocardial infarction. Circulation 78 [Suppl II]:301
49. Cripps T, Bennett D, Camm J, Ward D (1988) Prospective evaluation of clinical assessment, exercise testing and signal-averaged electrocardiogram in predicting outcome after acute myocardial infarction. Am J Cardiol 62:995–999
50. Breithardt G, Borggrefe M, Haerten K, Martínez-Rubio A (1988) Value of late potentials and programmed ventricular stimulation in predicting long-term arrhythmic complications in patients with coronary artery disease. Circulation 78 [Suppl II]:301
51. Malliani A, Schwartz PJ, Zanchetti A (1980) Neural mechanisms in life-threatening arrhythmias. Am Heart J 100:705–715
52. Tavazzi L, Zotti AM, Rondanelli R (1986) The role of psychologic stress in the genesis of lethal arrhythmias in patients with coronary artery disease. Eur Heart J 7 [Suppl A]:99–106

Identification of the Patient at High Risk for Sudden Cardiac Death: The Value of Electrophysiological Studies

G. Steinbeck

Introduction

Pioneering electrophysiological studies in the 1970s by Wellens et al. [1] and Josephson et al. [2] showed that in the majority of patients who have survived an episode of sustained ventricular tachycardia (defined as tachycardia either lasting ≥30 s or needing prior termination by overdrive stimulation, drug administration or DC-cardioversion), the arrhythmia could be reproducibly initiated and terminated by programmed electrical stimulation under safe conditions in the catheterization laboratory. Later work demonstrated that this method could also be applied to patients who had survived an episode of cardiac arrest due to ventricular fibrillation, not associated with acute myocardial infarction [3]. As a consequence, programmed ventricular stimulation was recommended to assess the diagnosis of sustained ventricular tachyarrhythmia as well as the efficacy of antiarrhythmic agents. This report focuses on some aspects of this rapidly evolving, invasive method of clinical electrophysiology and also briefly reviews its present role for risk stratification of asymptomatic patients after acute myocardial infarction.

Methods

After withdrawal of antiarrhythmic drug therapy, an invasive electrophysiologic study is performed; several electrode catheters are passed via the right femoral or cubital vein to the right atrium, His bundle region and the apex of the right ventricle. These permit atrial stimulation, His bundle recording and ventricular stimulation. Rectangular stimuli of twice diastolic threshold are delivered by battery-powered programmable stimulators, and several intracardiac recordings from the right atrium, His bundle and right ventricle are simultaneously recorded with surface electrocardiographic leads (usually I, II, III, V1 and V6) on a multichannel recorder.

Programmed ventricular stimulation is performed by applying single premature stimuli during regular right ventricular basic drive starting in late diastole and moved earlier into diastole in steps of 10 ms until ventricular refractoriness is reached. Basic drive intervals are first usually slightly shorter than the sinus cycle length and then are continuously decreased down to 330 ms. If a sustained ventricular tachycardia cannot be induced, double premature impulses are applied.

If this sequence does not result in sustained tachycardia or fibrillation, the whole protocol of stimulation should first be repeated at another site (right ventricular septum of outflow tract). Thereafter, more aggressive modes of stimulation may be applied, such as application of three premature stimuli, stimulation in the left ventricle, administration of catecholamines, and, finally, burst stimulation.

If a sustained ventricular tachyarrhythmia is induced and electrocardiographically documented, overdrive stimulation with or without administration of antiarrhythmic drugs is usually able to terminate the tachyarrhythmia. However, in a substantial percentage of patients, application of DC-cardioversion is necessary. To evaluate the reproducibility of induction in a given patient, it may be appropriate to attempt induction of the arrhythmia at least twice.

In patients with sustained ventricular tachycardia or primary cardiac arrest based on coronary artery disease or dilated cardiomyopathy, the percentage of patients whose arrhythmia can be induced by the methods described above, ranges from 50% to 90% [4, 5]. If the arrhythmia is induced, the patient may be suitable for serial electrophysiologic testing. After intravenous or oral antiarrhythmic drug therapy, programmed electrical stimulation is repeated. For a repeat study on oral therapy, generally only one electrode catheter is reinserted after several days of drug administration. This procedure is repeated – if necessary – several times in order to find a drug under which tachycardia induction is suppressed. If this drug or combination of drugs is found, long-term antiarrhythmic therapy is started and the patient is discharged on that therapy. This protocol assumes that in cases of suppression of inducibility, the likelihood of a recurrence of the arrhythmia for the patient is very low, while this risk will be much higher in cases of continued inducibility. However, this may not be so for all patients and for all drugs tested. Recent studies indicate that although the arrhythmia might still be inducible under drug therapy, other parameters, such as the difficulty of inducing the arrhythmia and the cycle length of the tachycardia, might have prognostic implications [6, 7]. As an alternative to serial electrophysiologic testing, parallel drug testing has been proposed [8]. Using this approach, the patient is invasively studied during both control periods and antiarrhythmic drug therapy. However, long-term drug therapy is then instituted without taking into consideration the result of the second electrophysiological study on antiarrhythmic drugs. The results of this approach will form the basis of a scientific approach to future invasive electrophysiologic drug studies but this strategy has little to offer patients of today.

The invasive electrophysiologic study is associated with risks and emotional stress (both for the patient and for the doctor). However, in experienced hands, the method is associated with low morbidity and mortality [9].

For more detailed description of methodological details as well as indications of this method under various clinical conditions the reader is referred to the literature [10].

Patients with a History of Sustained Ventricular Tachycardia or Primary Cardiac Arrest

Serial electrophysiologic testing of a patient with sustained recurrent ventricular tachycardia on the basis of coronary artery disease is illustrated in Fig. 1. Under control conditions, double premature stimuli induced sustained ventricular tachycardia with a QRS morphology and rate very similar to the spontaneous episode of the arrhythmia. Oral drug therapy with disopyramide could not prevent induction whereas the combination of disopyramide and amiodarone could do so.

Using a protocol of stimulation with two extrastimuli, various drug studies have shown the following success rates (defined as suppression of inducibility of ventricular tachycardia): procainamide 10%–40% [11, 12], quinidine 10%–25% [11–13], disopyramide 8%–15% [12, 14], lidocaine 10% [12], phenytoin 21% [12], aprindine 21% [15], mexiletine 10%–26% [14, 16], amiodarone 8%–53% [17–20], and sotalol 44% [21]. The relationship between the result of the electrophysiologic study and follow-up should be carefully assessed for every drug. While it is generally held that electrophysiologic testing can predict long-term success or failure of that drug, this assertion is controversial in the case of amiodarone [17, 18, 22–24], and certain other drugs. While suppression of inducibility in most studies accurately predicts freedom from recurrence, future studies must focus on the central question of whether drug failure must be assumed in patients with continued inducibility.

In comparing the results of various groups of authors, differences between studies with respect to the definition of arrhythmia, inducibility and suppression of inducibility, as well as the protocol of stimulation have to be taken into account. The more aggressive the protocol of stimulation, the better the sensitivity for reproducing the clinical ar-

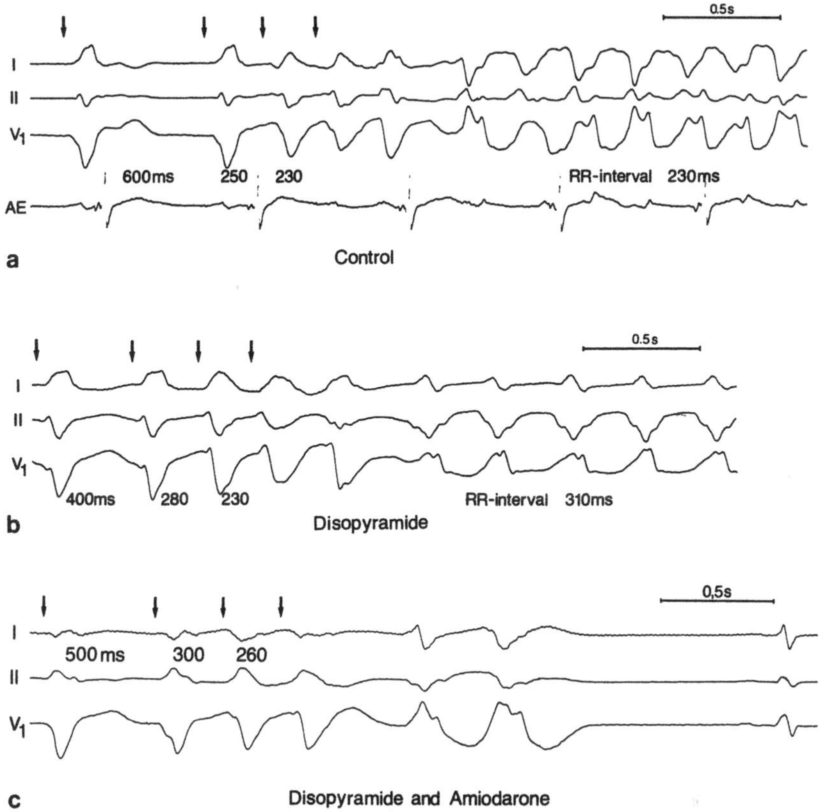

Fig. 1. a Programmed stimulation of antiarrhythmic drugs in a 52 year old patient with spontaneous, sustained ventricular tachycardia on the basis of coronary artery disease. *Leads I, II, V1* and a right atrial lead (*AE*) are recorded. Basic drive interval (S1-S1) is 600 ms; application of two premature stimuli (S1-S2 250 ms; S2-S3 230 ms) is followed by ventricular tachycardia with right bundle branch block morphology and a cycle length of 230 ms. Rate and QRS morphology are similar to the spontaneously occurring tachycardia. Tachycardia is terminated by bolus injection of lidocaine 60 mg intravenously. **b** Programmed stimulation under oral therapy with disopyramide 600 mg daily; same patient as in **a**. *Leads I, II and V1* are recorded. Basic drive interval (S1-S1) is 400 ms; two premature stimuli (S1-S2 280 ms; S2-S3 230 ms) are again followed by sustained ventricular tachycardia with right bundle branch block morphology; cycle length has increased (310 ms $\geq$ rate of 194 beats min^{-1}). Termination was performed by right ventricular overdrive stimulation. **c** Programmed stimulation under disopyramide (600 mg) and amiodarone (600 mg) orally per day for 14 days; same patient as in **a** and **b**. *Leads I, II and V1* are recorded. Basic drive interval (S1-S1) is 500 ms; two premature stimuli (S1-S2 300 ms; S2-S3 260 ms) are followed by, at most, two consecutive ventricular echo beats

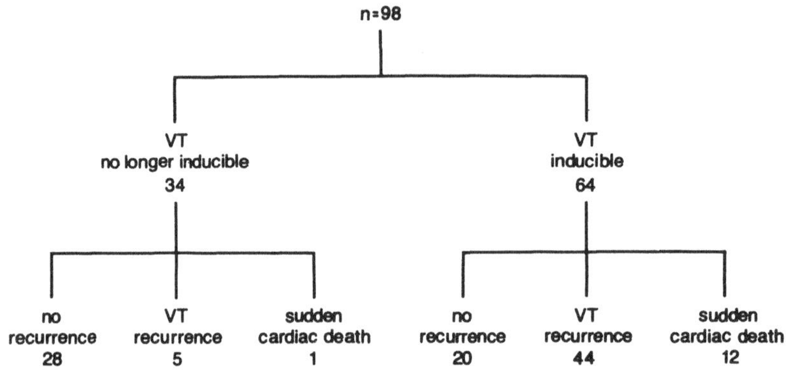

Fig. 2. Follow-up for a mean of 20 months of patients with recurrent sustained ventricular tachycardia, on the basis of 98 drug trials in 90 patients guided by serial electrophysiologic testing

rhythmia, but at the expense of specificity. While for patients with sustained ventricular tachycardia the sensitivity and specificity of a stimulation protocol might be assessed, it is much more difficult for patients with syncope, cardiac arrest, and even more difficult for all patients with unsustained arrhythmias.

Correlation between the final result of serial electrophysiologic testing under oral antiarrhythmic drug therapy and follow-up in a series of 98 patients with sustained ventricular tachyarrhythmias is illustrated in Fig. 2 [25]. Suppression of inducibility predicted freedom from recurrence in the vast majority, while two thirds of patients with continued inducibility had VT recurrence; in addition, 12 of 44 patients in the latter group died suddenly. However, 20 of the 64 patients remained asymptomatic despite continued inducibility; thus, prediction of drug failure is not established as well as prediction of drug success. Numerous other studies have reported the same or a similar relationship between inducibility of arrhythmia and outcome, based on arrhythmia recurrence and sudden death [3, 6, 11, 25–28]. In addition, left ventricular ejection fraction has a major impact on outcome of these patients [29]. It should be stressed that these results were obtained exclusively in patients with sustained ventricular tachyarrhythmias such as ventricular tachycardia or ventricular fibrillation complicating various heart diseases. In contrast to this relatively small number of patients referred to specialized centres for invasive electrophysiologic drug testing, it is generally thought at present that for the much larger group of patients with unsustained ventricular tachyarrhythmias, the invasive approach is unsuitable for reproducing arrhythmia and predicting antiarrhythmic drug efficacy.

For more detailed description of the results of electropharmacologic testing in patients with ventricular arrhythmias, the reader is referred to the survey article of Prystowsky [30].

Risk Stratification After Myocardial Infarction

Prompted by favorable results of programmed ventricular stimulation in patients with a history of sustained ventricular tachyarrhythmias, this method was also prospectively applied in asymptomatic patients who have survived acute myocardial infarction, in order to predict the future occurrence of sustained ventricular tachyarrhythmias or sudden cardiac death. In one such major study on 403 survivors of transmural myocardial infarction, programmed ventricular stimulation induced ventricular tachycardia in 20%, ventricular fibrillation in 14% and no sustained ventricular arrhythmias in 66% of patients. The probability of remaining incident-free (cardiac death, occurrence of nonfatal ventricular tachycardia or ventricular fibrillation) was 73% for patients with inducible ventricular tachycardia, compared to 93% of patients with inducible ventricular fibrillation and 92% of patients with noninducible arrhythmia [31].

Therefore, induction of ventricular fibrillation bears no adverse prognostic implication, as opposed to induction of sustained ventricular tachycardia, especially if the cycle length of the induced arrhythmias was ≥230 ms [31]; this result is depicted in Fig. 3.

Results of other studies have been quite variable, either confirming the results of Denniss and coworkers [32, 33] or finding no association between the results of programmed ventricular stimulation and outcome [34].

Explanations for the discrepancy of these results include the number of patients studied, differences in the protocol of stimulation, the reproducibility of the method, recruitment of patients and differences in the prevalence of sudden cardiac death or sustained ventricular tachyarrhythmias in the patient population studied.

Even in the study of Denniss et al. [31], inducible ventricular tachycardia for prediction of instantaneous death and/or nonfatal ventricular tachycardia or ventricular fibrillation had a sensitivity of 52% only and a specificity of 82%, a predictive accuracy of a positive test of 18% only, and of a negative test of 92%. Thus, in case antiarrhythmic therapy was based on the results of programmed ventricular stimulation, 82% of patients treated would remain asymptomatic without drugs, and in only 18% of patients the arrhythmia possibly prevented by drugs would occur. In fact, antiarrhythmic drug therapy instituted in a preliminary

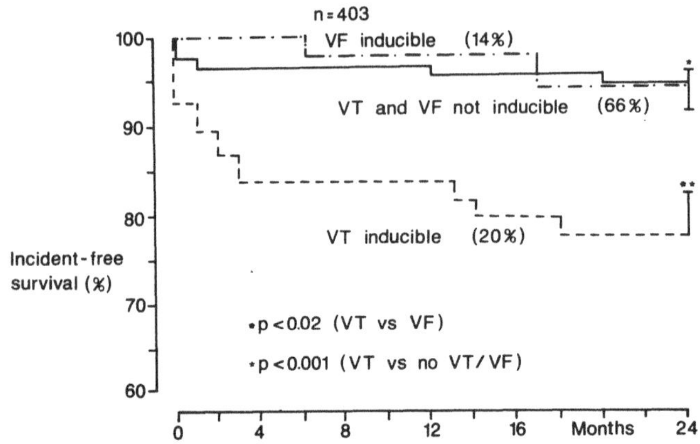

Fig. 3. Prediction of instantaneous death and/or nonfatal ventricular tachycardia or fibrillation (VT or VF) by programmed stimulation in 403 clinically well survivors of transmural infarction undergoing programmed stimulation (Denniss et al. 1986 [31])

study on the basis of programmed stimulation in patients after myocardial infarction has shown no benefit compared to those left untreated [35]. Future studies have to concentrate on answering the question whether programmed ventricular stimulation bears prognostic information dependent or independent of other factors such as left ventricular ejection fraction, signal averaging for detection of late potentials, exercise testing and Holter monitoring. Only if by combining several prognostic factors of importance it will be possible to definitely increase the predictive accuracy of the positive test, that is induction of sustained ventricular tachycardia, an antiarrhythmic intervention such as drugs or an automatic defibrillator (either implantable or external) will have a reasonable chance to prevent sudden cardiac death or life-threatening ventricular tachyarrhythmias in future prospective trials.

References

1. Wellens HJJ, Schuilenburg RM, Durrer D (1972) Electrical stimulation of the heart in patients with ventricular tachycardia. Circulation 46:216–226
2. Josephson ME, Horowitz LN, Farshidi A, Kastor JA (1978) Recurrent sustained ventricular tachycardia. I. Mechanisms. Circulation 57:431–440
3. Ruskin JN, DiMarco JP, Garan H (1980) Out-of-hospital cardiac arrest. Electrophysiologic observations and selection of long-term antiarrhythmic therapy. N Engl J Med 303:607–613

4. Naccarelli GV, Prystowsky EN, Jackman WM, Heger JJ, Rahilly GT, Zipes DP (1982) Role of electrophysiologic testing in managing patients who have ventricular tachycardia unrelated to coronary artery disease. Am J Cardiol 50:165–171
5. Bigger JT Jr, Reiffel JA, Livelli FD Jr, Wang PJ (1986) Sensitivity, specificity and reproducibility of programmed ventricular stimulation. Circulation [Suppl II] 73:73–78
6. Borggrefe M, Trampisch HJ, Breithardt G (1988) Reappraisal of criteria for assessing drug efficacy in patients with ventricular tachyarrhythmias: complete versus partial suppression of inducible arrhythmias. J Am Coll Cardiol 12:140–149
7. Waller TJ, Kay HR, Spielman SR, Kutalek SP, Greenspan AM, Horowitz LN (1987) Reduction in sudden death and total mortality by antiarrhythmic therapy evaluated by electrophysiologic drug testing: criteria of efficacy in patients with sustained ventricular tachyarrhythmias. J Am Coll Cardiol 10:83–89
8. Brugada P, Wellens HJJ (1986) Need and design of a prospective study to assess the value of different strategic approaches for management of ventricular tachycardia or fibrillation. Am J Cardiol 57:1180–1184
9. Horowitz LN, Kay HR, Kutalek SP et al. (1987) Risks and complications of clinical cardiac electrophysiologic studies: a prospective analysis of 1000 consecutive patients. J Am Coll Cardiol 9:1261–1268
10. Report of the American College of Cardiology/American Heart Association Task Force on Assessment of Diagnostic and Therapeutic Cardiovascular Procedures (Subcommittee to Assess Clinical Intracardiac Electrophysiologic Studies) (1989) Guidelines for clinical intracardiac electrophysiologic studies. Circulation 80:1925–1939
11. Horowitz LN, Josephson ME, Farshidi A, Spielman SR, Michelson EL, Greenspan AM, (1978) Recurrent sustained ventricular tachycardia. 3. Role of the electrophysiologic study in selection of antiarrhythmic regimens. Circulation 58:986–997
12. Horowitz LN, Josephson ME, Kastor JA (1980) Intracardiac electrophysiologic studies a s a method for the optimization of drug therapy in chronic ventricular arrhythmia. Prog Cardiovasc Dis 23:81–98
13. Ruskin JN, Garan H (1979) Chronic electrophysiologic testing in patients with recurrent sustained ventricular tachycardia. Am J Cardiol 43:400 (abstr)
14. Manz M, Steinbeck G, Nitsch J, Lüderitz B (1983) Treatment of recurrent sustained ventricular tachycardia with mexiletine and disopyramide: control by programmed ventricular stimulation. Br Heart J 49:222–228
15. Steinbeck G, Manz M, Lüderitz B (1982) Therapie chronisch rezidivierender ventrikulärer Tachykardien mit Aprindin. Verh Dtsch Ges Inn Med 88:182–185
16. DiMarco JP, Garan H, Ruskin JN (1981) Mexiletine for refractory ventricular arrhythmias: results using serial electrophysiologic testing. Am J Cardiol 47:131–138

17. Heger JJ, Prystowsky EN, Jackman WM et al. (1981) Amiodarone: clinical efficacy and electrophysiology during long-term therapy for recurrent ventricular tachycardia or ventricular fibrillation. N Engl J Med 305:539–545
18. McGovern B, Garan H, Malacoff RF et al. (1984) Long-term clinical outcome of ventricular tachycardia or fibrillation treaded with amiodarone. Am J Cardiol 53:1558–1563
19. Nademanee K, Singh BN, Henrickson J et al. (1983) Amiodarone in refractory life-threatening ventricular arrhythmias. Ann Intern Med 98:577–584
20. Steinbeck G, Manz M, Lüderitz B (1982) Amiodaron bei ventrikulären Tachykardien. Münch Med Wochenschr 124:723–727
21. Steinbeck G, Bach P, Haberl R (1986) Electrophysiologic and antiarrhythmic efficacy of oral sotalol for sustained ventricular tachyarrhythmias: evaluation by programmed stimulation and ambulatory electrocardiogram. J Am Coll Cardiol 8:949–958
22. Waxman HL, Groh WC, Marchlinski FE et al. (1982) Amiodarone for control of sustained ventricular tachyarrhythmia: clinical and electrophysiologic effects in 51 patients. Am J Cardiol 50:1066–1074
23. Mason JW, Swerdlow CD, Winkle RA et al. (1982) Programmed ventricular stimulation in predicting vulnerability to ventricular arrhythmias and their response to antiarrhythmic therapy. Am Heart J 103:633–637
24. Horowitz LN, Greenspan AM, Spielman SR et al. (1985) Usefulness of electrophysiologic testing in evaluation of amiodarone therapy for sustained ventricular tachyarrhythmias associated with coronary heart disease. Am J Cardiol 55:367–371
25. Steinbeck G, Manz M, Lüderitz B (1984) Neue Möglichkeiten in der Therapie bedrohlicher tachykarder Rhythmusstörungen: medikamentös – elektrisch – operativ. Internist 25:351–358
26. Mason JW, Winkle RA (1980) Accuracy of the ventricular tachycardia-induction study for predicting long-term efficacy and inefficacy of antiarrhythmic drugs. N Engl J Med 303:1073–1077
27. Swerdlow CD, Winkle RA, Mason JW (1983) Determinants of survival in patients with ventricular tachyarrhythmias. N Engl J Med 308:1436–1442
28. Breithardt G, Seipel L, Haerten K, Abendroth RR, Loogen F (1979) Effektivitätskontrolle der antiarrhythmischen Therapie bei Patienten mit chronisch-rezidivierenden ventrikulären Tachykardien mittels elektrophysiologischer Stimulationsverfahren. Z Kardiol 68:725–730
29. Wilber DJ, Garan H, Finkelstein D et al. (1988) Out-of-hospital cardiac arrest. Use of electrophysiologic testing in the prediction of long-term outcome. N Engl J Med 318:19–24
30. Prystowsky EN (1988) Electrophysiologic-electropharmacologic testing in patients with ventricular arrhythmias. PACE 11:225–251
31. Denniss AR, Richards DA, Cody DV et al. (1986) Prognostic significance of ventricular tachycardia and fibrillation induced at programmed stimulation and delayed potentials detected on the signal-averaged electrocardiograms of survivors of acute myocardial infarction. Circulation 74:731–745

32. Richards DA, Cody DV, Denniss AR, Russell PA, Young AA, Uther JB (1983) Ventricular electrical instability: A predictor of death after myocardial infarction. Am J Cardiol 51:75–80
33. Breithardt G, Borggrefe M, Haerten K, Trampisch HJ (1985) Prognostische Bedeutung der programmierten Ventrikelstimulation und der nichtinvasiven Registrierung ventrikulärer Spätpotentiale in der Postinfarktperiode. Z Kardiol 74:389–396
34. Roy D, Marchand E, Theroux P, Waters DD, Pelltier GB, Bourassa MG (1985) Programmed ventricular stimulation in survivors of an acute myocardial infarction. Circulation 72:487–494
35. Denniss AR, Ross DL, Cody DV, Russell PA, Young AA, Richards DA, Uther JB (1988) Randomized controlled trial of prophylactic antiarrhythmic therapy in patients with inducible ventricular tachyarrhythmias after recent myocardial infarction. Eur Heart J 9:746–757

PART III

Technical and Electrophysiological Aspects of the Automatic Implantable Cardioverter Defibrillator

Implantable Device Algorithms for Detection and Discrimination of Tachyarrhythmia

S. M. Bach, J. C. Hsung

Introduction

Automatic implantable treatment of ventricular tachyarrhythmias has been clinically utilized for more than 10 years. Devices for pacing and shock delivery have been recently combined into a single implantable unit. The biggest technical obstacle to proper clinical function of these units remains the accurate identification of normal and abnormal cardiac rhythms. Because the potentially severe consequences of not recognizing ventricular arrhythmias, devices have been designed to have a high sensitivity. The problem of good device specifity without sacrificing sensitivity is technically difficult and is only partially addressed in present day technology. The following discussion relates to tachyarrhythmia detection via interpretation of cardiac depolarization rate and morphology. Some of the techniques discussed are incorporated into present day devices while others are under active development.

The Cardiac Signal Source

Implantable device cardiac rate sensing begins at the electrode interface. The ideal rate signal for an analog amplifier would be one which unambiguously gave one discrete constant amplitude event per cardiac depolarization, irrespective of the underlying rhythm or depolarization wave direction. The transmembrane potential comes close to this ideal, but its measurement is impractical for an implanted electrode system. Somewhat less ideal is a 50 µm plunge bipolar electrode pair with electrode spacing on the order of 0.25 mm. This geometry gives a discrete narrow electrogram without much repolarization activity; it provides excellent far-field signal suppression while not degrading the near-field signal. However, this geometry is somewhat sensitive to the direction of wave front propagation. This signal's discrete nature is maintained during nearly all ventricular rhythms, even the early stages of ventricular fibrillation. An electrode placement close to the endocardium maintains the discrete nature of the electrogram at longer fibrillation durations than placement near the epicardium [1] (Fig. 1). This is advantageous for sensing amplifiers that must detect fibrillation rate after unsuccessful defibrillation shocks. The difficulty with a 0.25 mm bipolar electrogram is the signal amplitude, which tends to be in the order of 1 – 3 mV.

Increasing the electrode size to about 12 mm^2 and the electrode spacing to 1 cm results in a much larger signal amplitude (up to 30 mV). These advantages are offset by increased directional sensitivity, increased repolarization potentials, reduced frequency content, longer duration, and increased far-field sensing. Usually repolarization potentials that are present can be filtered by high-pass filters which cutoff at ≈ 30 Hz. Because they are directionally sensitive and contain some far-field signal, 1 cm bipolar signals contain morphologic features that can change with ventricular rhythm and thus offer the opportunity for additional signal analysis. However, 1 cm signals can become highly variable during ventricular fibrillation, necessitating the use of automatic gain or thresholding circuits [2].

True unipolar electrograms are theoretically the second derivative of the transmembrane potential [3]. Practically, they contain features (amplitude, slew rate, polarity, depolarization) that tend to change from rhythm to rhythm. Because of more repolarization activity, they tend not to be as good for rate counting as bipolar signals. Pseudo-unipolar signals, ones whose reference is a device shocking electrode, can have a discrete nature, but they may be significantly altered by a defibrillating shock because of high voltage gradients near the shocking electrode edge. Decrease in depolarization amplitude and slew rate, and appearance of injury potentials, coupled with repolarization changes, may cause difficulty for rate sensing amplifiers.

Great interest has been generated in floating electrode sensing, whereby two or more electrodes are in the blood pool, with no contact with the endocardium. Brownlee has recently described diagonal bipolar atrial electrodes that reside 1 cm apart and on opposite sides of a 3 mm diameter catheter [4]. The inherent assumption is that the primary direc-

Fig. 1A–C. Electrograms from a dog during and after cardiopulmonary bypass. In all panels the *first line* is lead II of the body surface electrocardiogram; *lines 2 through 5* are electrograms recorded 0.3, 2.7, 5.7 and 8.4 mm from the endocardial surface. Panels **A** and **B** were recorded 1 and 20 min after the induction of ventricular fibrillation (*VF*) on bypass. Both the endocardial and epicardial RR intervals remain constant. Panel **C** was recorded 5 min after termination of bypass. A marked gradient of activation rate has developed. Used by permission (Worley et al. 1985 [1])

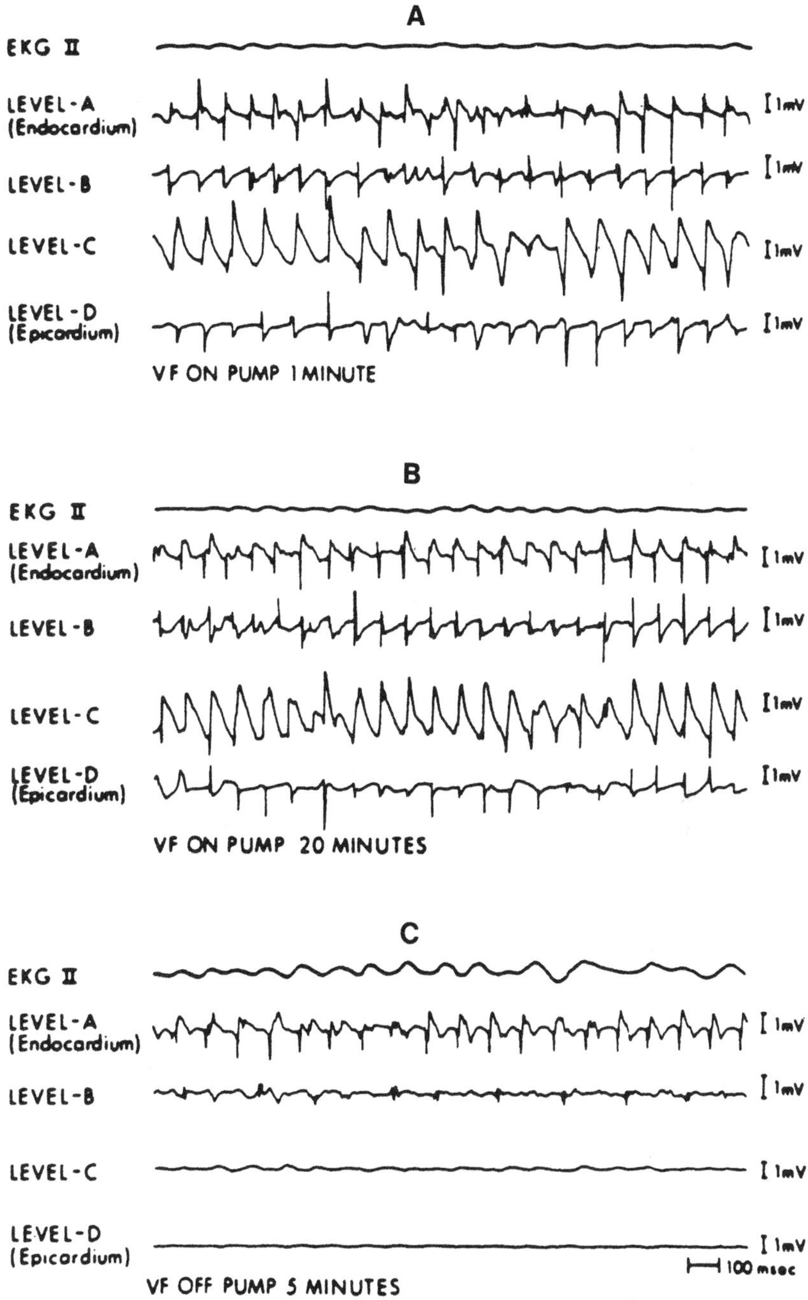
A
EKG II
LEVEL-A (Endocardium)
LEVEL-B
LEVEL-C
LEVEL-D (Epicardium)
1mV
VF ON PUMP 1 MINUTE
B
EKG II
LEVEL-A (Endocardium)
LEVEL-B
LEVEL-C
LEVEL-D (Epicardium)
1mV
VF ON PUMP 20 MINUTES
C
EKG II
LEVEL-A (Endocardium)
LEVEL-B
LEVEL-C
LEVEL-D (Epicardium)
1mV
100 msec
VF OFF PUMP 5 MINUTES

tion of atrial depolarization is along the natural path of the catheter. Chronic clinical electrograms using this geometry were double or singly deflected, short duration, high slew rate signals of 3 mV peak amplitude. In an attempt to make the sensed electrogram independent of the propagating wave front direction, Goldreyer et al. described an "orthogonal" sensing scheme in which 0.8 mm^2 electrodes were separated 90° or 120° around the circumference of a pacing catheter 2 cm from a contacting tip electrode [5]. Ventricular electrograms obtained from this lead were approximately 8 mV, of high slew rate, and contained little repolarization activity. Vector summation of electrograms was not actually done.

Finally, electrograms obtained from defibrillation shocking electrodes have been found to be unsatisfactory for cardiac rate determination [6]. They are often not discrete, and may contain significant features (P-wave, S-T segment, T-wave) which can be altered by the defibrillating shock.

Amplifier Control

Amplifier sensitivity or gain can be controlled by a menu of fixed settings selectable by a programmer or by a feedback-control loop known as an automatic gain control. When used in bradycardia pacemakers, a fixed sensitivity (gain) amplifier/detector generally deals with the same input signal. If ventricular ectopy is present, it may or may not be sensed depending upon sensing electrode orientation with respect to the depolarization wave front. Selecting a high sensitivity corrects this problem, but increases the chance than the repolarization signal will be detected. Extending the refractory period can avoid this problem. Amplifiers used in implantable antitachyarrhythmia devices must detect signals that have widely variable amplitude and slew rate. Accurate cardiac rate determination must take place over the range of 40–400 BPM (bradycardia to ventricular fibrillation), since devices are now designed to act both as a pacemaker and an implantable defibrillator. Amplitudes and slew rates frequently vary in excess of 5 : 1 during polymorphic rhythms. Sufficient depolarization counts must be generated during polymorphic rhythms in order to declare these rhythms as ones that need to be shocked.

This can be accomplished by a fixed high sensitivity; however, normal rhythm repolarization (T-wave) signals may also be sensed. Extension of the refractory period cannot be used to eliminate this T-wave sensing since upper rate limit of the device will be compromised. For instance, at a typical pacemaker refractory period of 330 ms, the maximum countable rate is $1/0.33 \times 60 = 182$ BPM. At rates faster than this, counting

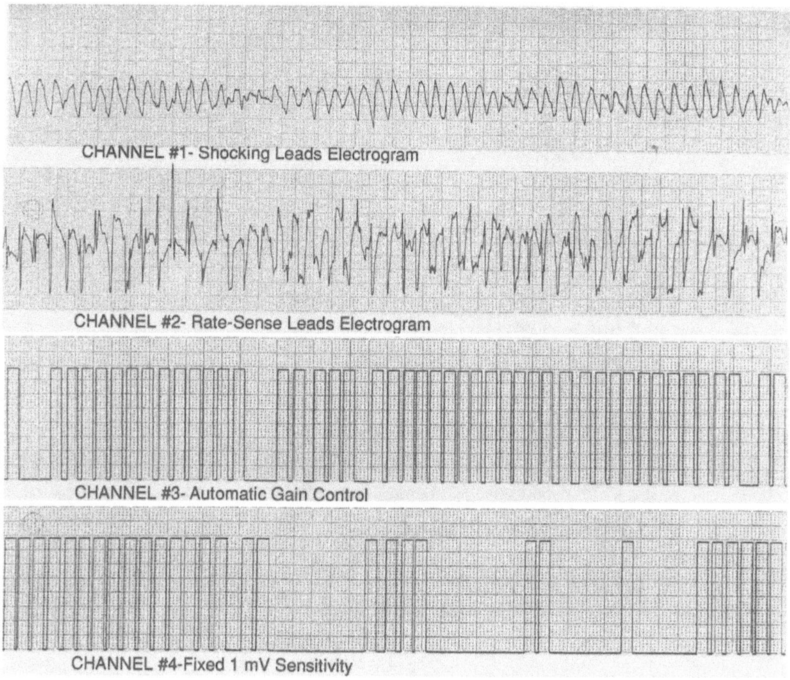

Fig. 2. Comparison of ventricular fibrillation rate counting using automatic gain control and 1 mV fixed sensitivity. The fixed sensitivity amplifier suddenly undersenses the signal. Each sensed event is an upright pulse of 120 ms duration

precipitously drops to one-half the actual rate ($\approx$95 BPM) since every other complex falls inside the refractory period. Thus, a tachyarrhythmia would not be sensed. Further, polymorphic rhythms are accompanied by severe ischemia, which electrically manifests itself as a progressive deterioration in electrogram amplitude and slew rate. Fixed sensitivity amplifiers cannot track this deterioration. Therefore, ineffective defibrillation shocks may compromise subsequent arrhythmia detection.

Figure 2 illustrates rate detection during fibrillation with 1 mV fixed and automatic gain sensing. Note that the fixed sensitivity amplifier initially detects properly, but then abruptly and severely undersenses the signal due to signal morphology changes. The automatic gain sensing amplifier circuit continues to sense a high number of counts. As noted in Fig. 3, these counts have a frequency distribution which may contain long cycle lengths. Device algorithms must make the distinction between these long cycle lengths and arrhythmia spontaneous termination.

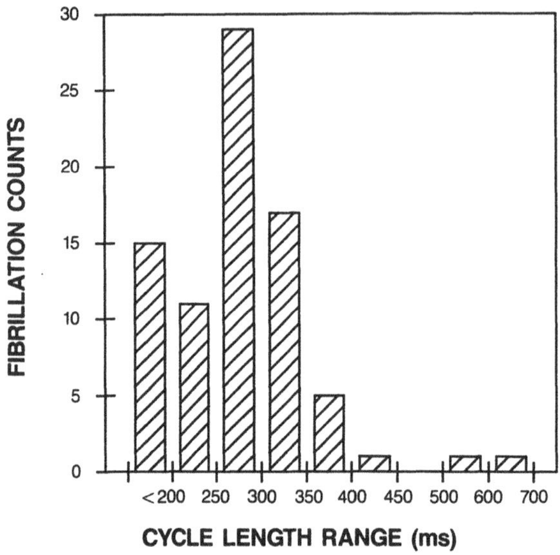

Fig. 3. Typical frequency distribution of interval counts resulting from automatic gain control sensing of ventricular fibrillation

Event Handling

The first clinical implantable defibrillators converted each detected cardiac event to a charge on an integrating capacitor with a fixed decay time constant. Therefore, each detected cardiac event was counted in proportion to its cycle length, since at low rates the integrating capacitor had more time to discharge than at high rates. Newer devices measure the time between events and classify the cycle length into one of several rate range bins. For instance, a cycle length may fall in a range to be classified as brady rhythm, normal rhythm, or one of several tachyarrhythmia rate ranges. If all cycle lengths within a given rate range are weighted equally by a device algorithm, the device arrhythmia recognition time can be radically different than with an averaging scheme. This is particularly true for a rhythm where rate is just below the lowest tachyarrhythmia recognition cutoff limit. In this case none of the accumulated cycle lengths contributes toward detection using the bin technique; however, with the averaging technique one additional slightly shorter cycle length may be enough to declare arrhythmia detection.

Digital techniques for handling sequences of cycle lengths fall into two categories: those which require a consecutive number of rapid of events for detection or those which allow some "forgiveness" by requiring a certain percentage of the most recent events to be shorter than a rate limit criterion. Practical algorithms combine the two techniques, and provide for a detection algorithm to progress through a sequence of states prior to actual arrhythmia declaration. For instance, the newest CPI device moves to a new state with three consecutive cycle lengths faster than the lowest rate limit. Once there, a certain number of fast, programmable cycle lengths are required before detection is declared. Isolated single cycle lengths below the lowest tachyarrhythmia rate limit are "forgiven" and counted as fast, whereas two consecutive cycle lengths below the lowest rate limit cause a detection reset. Therefore, if the automatic gain control momentarily fails to track the signal, a gain increase occurs that allows sensing of the next event. With the gain already at a higher level, a subsequent second consecutive long cycle length most likely represents a spontaneous rhythm termination. The Medtronic PCD requires a certain programmable number of consecutive cycle lengths for detection of slower, presumably monomorphic rhythms, but provides for only a certain percent of cycle lengths to be fast when they fall in the polymorphic rhythm rate range [7].

The Zone Concept

The newest combination antitachycardia pacemakers/defibrillators with bradycardia pacing stratify the entire range of rhythm rates into programmable discrete rate ranges known as zones in order to provide therapy appropriate for each rhythm. For instance, pacing treatment may be attempted more times for slow ventricular tachycardia than for fast ventricular tachycardia whose rate resides in a higher zone. A rhythm whose rate is even faster is treated with shock first. When zones are introduced into devices, the problem of rhythms whose rate falls on the boundary between two zones is increased by the number of additional zones programmed. In older defibrillators slow detection could sometimes be attributed to a tachycardia rate near the device rate limit. Without the introduction of certain rules of cycle length processing, the increase in the number of zone boundaries would cause indecision in the detection process. For instance, the newest CPI device requires four consecutive cycle lengths in the same zone for arrhythmia declaration. If this does not occur, then the arrhythmia continues to be monitored up to a maximum number of cycle lengths. If the maximum duration occurs, then the average of the last four cycle lengths is used to direct therapy.

Onset

The concept of onset discrimination is that pathologic rhythms begin abruptly, whereas physiologic rhythms begin more slowly. While generally true, there may be overlap in these rate changes as demonstrated by Fisher et al. in 1983 [8]. However, later work comparing onset for pathologic rhythms to that for bicycle exercise sprint in the same patient demonstrated no overlap [9]. One algorithm for onset discrimination is illustrated in Fig. 4. First, the algorithm retrospectively examines the maximum cycle length change between consecutive intervals beginning with the fifth cycle length that falls in the tachyarrhythmia rate zone(s). If this change (in % or ms) is large enough, then the algorithm identifies the shorter of the two intervals that caused the maximum change. This interval and the subsequent three intervals are each compared to the average of the four intervals that occurred two intervals prior to the maximum change interval. If at least three out of four tachyarrhythmia intervals differ from the average by more than the criterion, the onset of the rhythm is declared rapid.

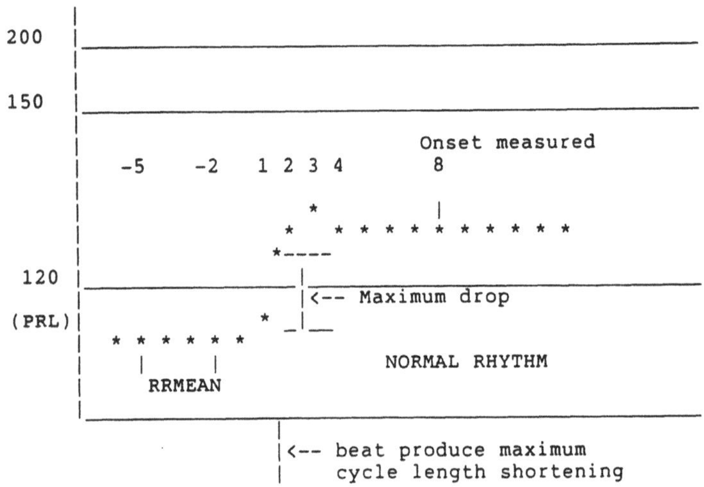

Fig. 4. The PR×algorithm of onset measurement. Although the actual calculation is done after eight fast intervals, three out of the four intervals 1–4 must be shorter than the average of intervals −2 to −5. These intervals are the ones preceding the numbered beats. The maximum drop is called the pivot interval

Stability

Examination of ventricular cycle length variability is designed to separate atrial fibrillation with a fast ventricular response from sustained monomorphic ventricular tachycardia, when these two rate ranges overlap. Should the rhythm be declared stable, an output of such an algorithm could be an average rate calculation that can be used to direct adaptive rate pacing. An additional benefit of analyzing stability is the identification of nonsustained ventricular tachycardia that is often unstable in cycle length. Since highly variable rhythms do not have a stable termination zone, antitachycardia pacing during unstable nonsustained VT has the potential to do more harm than good.

One approach to stability analysis compares each cycle length to the running four cycle length average. A cycle length that differs from the average by more than a certain % or ms is declared as unstable. A maximum number of unstable lengths is then used in order to declare an unstable rhythm. Another approach continually examines the difference between consecutive cycle lengths and categorizes the changes as a cycle length decrease, increase, or no change. If the number of cycle length increases and decreases are approximately equal and the changes are of sufficient magnitude, the rhythm is declared unstable. More cycle length decreases than increases represents acceleration, whereas more decreases than increases represents deceleration.

Post-therapy Monitoring

Different philosophies are applied when rate algorithms are designed to ascertain whether pacing or shocks were successful in arrhythmia termination. Determining success or failure of therapy is the most difficult problem in detection, since the diagnosis must be made quickly and the therapy may have changed the rhythm without actually converting it to normal.

One approach is to use the same detection scheme and parameters (with the exception of onset) as are used before therapy delivery. Another approach offers a different scheme and/or set of programmable parameters post therapy. This second approach recognizes the fact that treated rhythms do not always terminate abruptly. For instance, nonsustained polymorphic rhythms and accelerated idioventricular rhythms are not infrequently a result of defibrillating shocks. Providing a post-shock delay that ignores these rhythms for a programmable duration is a partial solution. More sophisticated algorithms examine the cycle length variability in the post-therapy condition. This offers the advantage of atrial fibrillation recognition, since atrial fibrillation induction with implantable device shocks can be a clinical problem.

Morphology Analysis

Probability density function analysis has been used in implantable defibrillators for 10 years. It's utility in arrhythmia discrimination remains controversial. It was originally designed to discriminate ventricular fibrillation from all other rhythms and was the primary detection method in the original AID defibrillator [10]. The underlying assumption was that malignant ventricular rhythms, as seen by device shocking electrodes, are sinusoidal in nature. Since the function was logically ANDed with rate, the nonfulfillment of the criteria caused inhibition of therapy delivery. The newest CPI device uses a similar function known as turning point morphology (TPM) to reduce the time to shock delivery, bypassing pacing therapy if the TPM criterion is satisfied. Both of these techniques assume that a reduction in isoelectric time is a characteristic present in malignant rhythms across the entire patient population. While often true with signals from large surface area electrodes, such as used for shocking, the designed sensitivity of these algorithms for a patient population severely limits their specificity. In addition, severe postshock distortion of the shocking lead electrogram can convert a supraventricular rhythm that does not satisfy the criterion into one that does [6]. Ability to fine-tune these algorithms for each patient has not been utilized, but is now at least possible for the newer programmable devices.

Morphologic discrimination of contacting endocardial (atrial or ventricular) electrograms has been investigated using several different techniques including frequency domain analysis, feature extraction, and template matching.

Frequency domain analysis converts the assumed periodic electrogram into a series of sine wave signals consisting of a fundamental and multiples of the fundamental, each with an amplitude and phase. Frequency domain analysis is often done by fast fourier transform, a digital computer technique that is not presently practical for implantable devices. In a study by Lin et al. only 60% of VT episodes could be distinguished from normal sinus rhythm by the technique [11]. However, Pannizzo and Furman were able to distinguish normal sinus rhythm from VT in 33 patients by passing the electrograms through a continuously tunable Butterworth filter. The filter cutoff frequency was adjusted to a value which provided the maximum NSR-VT frequency spectra difference [12]. The frequency content of normal and VT signals did not have a consistent relationship across patients, but was different in individual patients. The use of switched capacitor filters whose frequency band is controllable by a digital clock would at least be theoretically possible in an implantable device.

Feature extraction is a waveform analysis technique that identifies a particular waveform characteristic such as maximum d*V*/d*t*, peak to peak amplitude, etc., to compare two waveforms. Tomaselli et al. found a great amount of overlap between normal and abnormal canine ventricular electrograms when using this technique [13]. Although a frequency content difference existed, there was still overlap in three of eight animals studied. One feature extraction technique which has been reported to distinguish normal from abnormal ventricular depolarizations is the gradient pattern detection (GPD) algorithm, reported by Davies et al. [14]. This algorithm differentiates the electrogram and looks at its sequence of signed derivatives which can either be compared to a threshold or given an absolute number. When using thresholding, the sequence of signal derivatives is turned into a binary sequence of numbers depending upon derivative polarity. The algorithm learns the sequence of slopes pattern for the normal ventricular response assigning a value or +1, 0, or −1 to the individual slopes. Slopes less than an absolute value are assigned the zero value. This algorithm has been reported to have distinguished 10 out of 11 VT electrograms as different from normal sinus rhythm. It has also been demonstrated to separate VT from SVT with appropriate selection of derivative thresholds.

The sequence of slopes technique uses the concept of a template, whereby the device algorithm learns the normal electrogram morphology (or one or more of its characteristics) while the patient's heart rate is in the normal range. More complicated techniques require analog to digital signal conversion. A number of sequential depolarizations are then averaged to provide the template latitude in describing normal. One specific implementation is the area of difference method (Fig. 5). The template and unknown electrograms are compared by integrating both and comparing the result. Tomaselli was able to demonstrate 100% discriminatory capability in canines between NSR beats and ventricular beats with no overlap of area range [13]. The technique is sensitive to amplitude and baseline fluctuations. The sensitivity to baseline changes can be removed by subtracting the mean of the signal, producing a technique called mean area of difference [15].

Another analytical method which has achieved excellent results in separating VT from supraventricular rhythms is correlation waveform analysis [16–18]. This digital processing algorithm evaluates the shape of the electrogram. The technique is insensitive to signal amplitude or baseline changes that occur with posture or activity level. However, the technique is computationally intensive and is an unlikely candidate for

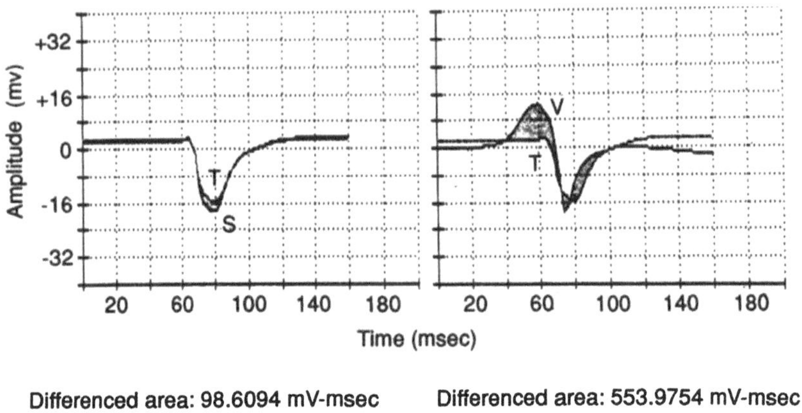

Fig. 5. Graphical representation of the area difference method of morphologic comparison. The differences between 2 waveforms and a sinus rhythm template waveform have been *shaded* and the area of these differences was calculated and shown below the graph in mV-ms. The area of difference seen with a ventricular ectopic beat (*V*) is over five times the difference seen between a sinus beat (*S*) and the template of sinus rhythm (*T*). Used by permission. (Tomaselli et al. 1988 [13])

implementation in an implantable device. Correlation waveform analysis was used as a "gold standard" by Throne et al. in a recent paper [15]. This paper investigated several new template matching techniques with the intent to make one or more of them practical for an implantable antitachycardia device.

The first of these techniques is the bin area method [15]. The number of calculations necessary for implementation is reduced because consecutive sample points in the unknown waveform and template are summed before a comparison is made. Like correlation waveform analysis, the result is independent of signal amplitude and baseline changes. By not removing the average bin value, Throne developed another new method, normalized area of difference, which is independent of amplitude but not baseline changes [15]. A third new method developed by Throne was the derivative area method [15]. This technique utilizes the derivative of the waveform (both template and unknown). The zero crossings of the template derivative are used to partition the signals, which are analyzed by comparing the area beneath the derivative in each partition.

A problem with morphology techniques is describing the range of normal depolarizations. It is well known there are amplitude and duration changes in the normal electrogram with exercise. As of this writing, the above techniques have not been extensively tested with normal exercise rhythms using chronic leads.

Atrial Sensing for Ventricular Arrhythmia Discrimination

Sensing of atrial depolarization events is more difficult than for ventricular events due to endocardial atrial signals being only about one fifth as large as ventricular signals. This causes difficulty in maintaining a good signal-to-noise ratio with implantable analog CMOS technology. In addition, reliable sensing of atrial events may have to be extended to making the distinction between antegrade and retrograde atrial depolarization. Timing algorithms, which have been proposed to separate supraventricular from ventricular rhythms, have a diagnostic problem when the ventricular rhythm is reasonably fast and there is a 1 : 1 atrial-ventricular relationship. The issue of leads is an even more difficult one, since a device designed to treat ventricular arrhythmias would presumably have three sets of leads: atrial sense/pace, ventricular sense/pace, and shocking. One way around this problem would be a floating atrial sense lead. However, reliable sensing has not been widely demonstrated with this technique. Paroxysmal atrial fibrillation is also another confounding rhythm, since reliable sensing of its presence is difficult because of the small signals involved. In those patients with chronic atrial fibrillation and ventricular tachyarrhythmia, atrial information is of little value. In spite of these problems, active work is ongoing in the use of atrial sensing to separate ventricular tachycardia from rhythms of atrial origin. Key difficulties are diagnosis of paroxysmal 1 : 1 tachycardia and separation of ventricular tachycardia from chronic atrial fibrillation with a fast ventricular response. The latter may look regular enough to overlap the irregularity of ventricular tachycardia, preventing stability analysis use.

Timing Algorithms

There has been some effort to diagnose ventricular tachycardia by observing the activation sequence of ventricular depolarization. Walsh et al. demonstrated that timing differences of 18–43 ms between right and left ventricular sites in canine myocardium could distinguish ventricular from supraventricular originated depolarizations [20]. This was also investigated by Davies et al. [21]. Because of the requirement for separate ventricular leads, this method of arrhythmia discrimination is unlikely to be a first choice among designers of implantable devices.

Summary

Since patients who are candidates for implantable devices to treat ventricular tachyarrhythmias do not frequently have electrically treatable supraventricular arrhythmias, the immediate future focus of device designers is likely to be separating ventricular arrhythmias from sinus tachycardia and atrial fibrillation. The relative success in accomplishing this task will, in large part, determine the future usefulness of implantable antitachycardia devices.

References

1. Worley SJ, Swain JL, Colavita PG, Smith WM, Ideker RE (1985) Development of an endocardial-epicardial gradient of activation rate during electrically induced, sustained ventricular fibrillation in dogs. Am J Cardiol 55:813–820
2. Winkle RA, Bach SM, Echt DS et al. (1983) The automatic implantable defibrillator: local bipolar sensing to detect ventricular tachycardia and fibrillation. Am J Cardiol 52:265–270
3. Kootsey JM, Johnson EA (1976) The origin of the electrocardiogram: relationship between transmembrane potential and electrocardiogram. In: Nelson CV, Geselowitz DB (eds) The theoretical basis of electrocardiology. Oxford University Press, New York, pp 21–43
4. Brownlee RR (1989) Toward optimizing the detection of atrial depolarization with floating bipolar electrodes. PACE 12:431–442
5. Goldreyer BN, Brueske R, Knudson MB, Cannom DS, Wyman MG (1983) Orthogonal ventricular electrogram sensing. PACE 6:761–768
6. Bach SM Jr, Shapland JS (1989) Engineering aspects of implantable defibrillators. In: Saksena S (ed) Electrical therapy for cardiac arrhythmias. Saunders, Philadelphia
7. Olson WH, Bardy GH, Lund J et al. (1988) Sensing and detection of ventricular fibrillation from human epicardial electrograms. PACE 11:485
8. Fisher JD, Goldstein M, Ostrow E et al. (1983) Maximal rate of tachycardia development: sinus tachycardia with sudden exercise vs. ventricular tachycardia. PACE 6:221–228
9. Mercando AD, Gableman G, Fisher JD (1988) Comparison of the rate of tachycardia development in patients: pathologic vs. sinus tachycardias. PACE 11:516
10. Langer AA, Heilman MS, Mower MM et al. (1976) Considerations in the development of the automatic implantable defibrillator. Med Instrum 10:163–167
11. Lin D, Dicarlo LA, Jenkins JM (1988) Identification of ventricular tachycardia using intracavitary ventricular electrograms: analysis of time and frequency domain patterns. PACE 11:1592–1606

12. Pannizzo F, Furman S (1988) Frequency spectra of ventricular tachycardia and sinus rhythm in human intracardiac electrograms-application to tachycardia detection for cardiac pacemakers. IEEE Trans Biomed Eng 35:421–425
13. Tomaselli GF, Nielsen AP, Finke WL, Singupta L, Clark JC, Griffin JC (1988) Morphologic differences of the endocardial electrogram in beats of sinus and ventricular origin. PACE 11:254–262
14. Davies DW, Wainwright RJ, Tooley MA, Lloyd D, Nathan AW, Spurrell RAJ, Camm AJ (1986) Detection of pathological tachycardia by analysis of electrogram morphology. PACE 9:200–208
15. Throne RD, Jenkins JM, Winston SA, DiCarlo LA (1990) Statistical validation of new ventricular tachycardia detection schemes. International Society of Computerized Electrocardiology, 15th Annual Conference, 1990
16. Feldman CL, Amazeen PG, Klein MD et al. (1971) Computer detection of ventricular ectopic beats. Comput Biomed Res 4:666–674
17. Arzbaecher R, Biancalana P, Stibolt T, Masek G, Dean R (1971) Computer technique for detection of cardiac dysrhythmias. J Adv Med Instrum 5:104
18. Jenkins J, Wu D, Arzbaecher R (1979) Computer diagnosis of supraventricular and ventricular arrhythmias. Circulation 5:977–987
19. Jenkins J, Bump T, Munkenbeck F, Brown J, Arzbaecher R (1984) Tachycardia detection in implantable antitachycardia devices. PACE 7:1273–1277
20. Walsh CA, Singer LP, Mercando AP, Furman S (1988) Differentiation of arrhythmias in the dog by measurement of activation sequence using an atrial and two ventricular electrodes. PACE 11:1732–1738
21. Davies DW, Nathan AW, Wainwright RJ, Large SR, Edmondson SJ, Ress GM, Camm AJ (1985) Recognition of ventricular tachycardia and fibrillation from epicardial electrogram timings. Circulation 72:III–475

Does Defibrillation Obey the Fundamental Law of Electrostimulation?

W. Irnich

Introduction

Since the introduction of external DC defibrillation, it has been common to use the energy as the defibrillation dose. This has historical reasons, as external defibrillators could not measure the voltage applied to the paddles, the current, or the duration of the pulse, as is usually done in electrostimulation. The only measurable quantity was the voltage to which the output capacitor was charged. Using the well-known formula that the stored energy is equal to half the capacitance of the charged capacitor times the voltage squared, the manufacturers were able to specify the energy of a pulse. This expedient in defining the dosage has greatly influenced the thinking of those engaged in defibrillation. Nonetheless, one has to ask whether the current practice is in accordance with the theories of electrostimulation and, if not, whether defibrillation obeys the laws of electrostimulation!

It is the intention of this article to review the theories concerning electrostimulation; to add a theory (developed by us) providing a better understanding of the stimulation effect on a cellular basis, and to critically apply this knowledge to defibrillation, thus allowing the application of engineering principles. Some of the examples presented demonstrate that nothing is as practical as a good theory.

Historical Review

Hoorweg, a physicist from Utrecht, the Netherlands, was the first to carry out quantitative investigations on electrostimulation using simple appliances with a high degree of accuracy. In 1892 [7], he found that the voltage to which a capacitor must be charged in order to initiate an excitation was a function of the capacitance of the capacitor in an inverse correlation:

$$V(C) = aR + b/C \qquad (1)$$

where $V(C)$ is the voltage as a function of capacitance C; R is the circuit resistance, and a and b are coefficients determined by the specimen.

He believed the relationship he discovered to be fundamental, though his waveform had a very specific shape; but he did not prove that other waveforms would yield the same results. From his various experiments, with different nerves and muscles, he calculated that only one specific capacitor exists, for which the threshold energy is minimum. Figure 1 demonstrates his results as published in 1892 [7]. He was not yet aware that this minimum in energy was determined by the "chronaxie time", a term which was introduced later by Lapicque. He also found that the charge needed to reach the excitation threshold was a linear function with a positive slope intersecting the y-axis above zero (Fig. 1).

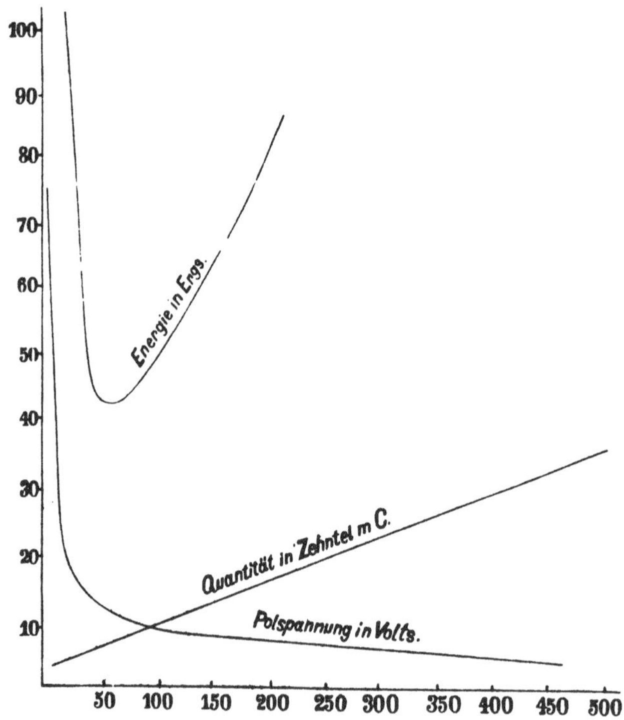

Fig. 1. Reproduction of the first quantitative analysis of stimulation phenomena published by Hoorweg in 1892 [7]. Threshold curves for capacitor discharge with the *abscissa* scaled in nF, the *energy* in erg = 0.1 μJ, the *quantity* (charge) in 0.1 μC and the *voltage* in V. The point of minimum energy is reached with 50 nF and with 4.2 μJ, 13 V and 0.7 μC

The physicist and physician Weiss, from Paris, published a paper in 1901 [22] in which he tried "to make comparable the different methods of electrostimulation." He was well aware of the work previously done by Hoorweg and generalized Hoorweg's law by finding a linear relationship between the charge needed to reach stimulation threshold and the duration of current flow and called it "formule fondamentale":

$$Q(\tau) = \int^{\tau} i \, dt = a\tau + b \tag{2}$$

where $Q(\tau)$ is the charge as a function of pulse duration τ; $i(\tau)$ is the current during pulse duration; and a and b are coefficients determined by the specimen.

He pointed out – and this makes his investigation so important for engineers – that the threshold energy varies with varying wave shape, whereas the quantity of threshold electricity remains constant.

The Parisian Lapicque performed numerous experiments on electrostimulation and was very familiar with the results and the equations of Hoorweg and Weiss [7, 22]. During the annual conference of the Society of Biology in 1909, Lapicque proposed to give the coefficients of the Weiss formula a physiological meaning [14]. Considering the Weiss formula in its hyperbolic form, he argued that, for long durations, the value a is asymptotically reached, which he called "rheobase". He recognized that, even with indefinitely long durations, there is a "fundamental threshold" which must be reached or exceeded in order to initiate excitation. He claimed that the type of excitable tissue and the surface of the active electrode in contact with the tissue would determine this minimum threshold. In addition, he found that the ratio b/a in the Weiss formula (Eq. 2) is a type of time constant which characterizes the excitable tissue for which he proposed the term "chronaxie."

$$I(\tau) = a + b/\tau = I_{\text{rheo}}(1 + t_{\text{chr}}/\tau) \tag{3}$$

where $I(\tau)$ is the current during the pulse duration τ; I_{rheo} is the rheobase current, the lowest possible current with τ going to infinity; and t_{chr} is the chronaxie time.

The chronaxie can simply be determined from the "intensity-duration-curve" in that the rheobase value is doubled. The intersection of a horizontal line of twice the rheobase value with the hyperbola then yields the chronaxie value (Fig. 2). A stimulation duration equal to the chronaxie reaches excitation with the lowest amount of energy. All other

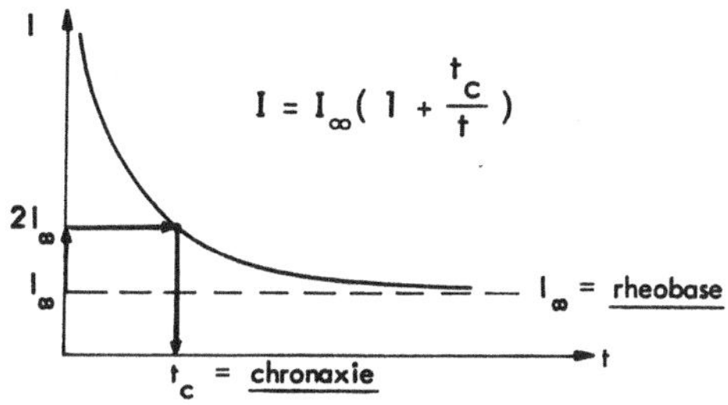

Fig. 2. Determination of the chronaxie time. The intersection of a vertical line of twice rheobase value with the hyperbola yields the chronaxie point

durations shorter or longer than chronaxie must have a higher energy level.

Though Lapicque did not find a new law of electrostimulation, his influence in electrophysiology was important for understanding and characterizing phenomena of electrostimulation.

Nernst, professor of physical chemistry in Berlin, the founder of physical chemistry, and Nobel prize winner for chemistry in 1920, was also engaged in electrostimulation studies. He developed a model of ion concentration alterations in which ions had to be moved by the stimulation current. As a result his differential equation system yielded an equation, the "square root law" which was published in 1908 [17]:

$$I(t) \cdot \sqrt{t} = c \tag{4}$$

where $I(t)$ is the current during the pulse duration t and c is the coefficient given by the specimen.

If we square Eq. (4) and multiply both sides with the resistance R of the stimulation circuit, we get by rearranging:

$$I^2 \cdot R \cdot t = R \cdot c^2 \tag{5}$$

Both Eqs. (4) and (5) suggest:

(1) The threshold expressed as energy should be constant for all durations.
(2) With the duration t approaching infinity, the current should go to zero.
(3) If both sides of Eq. (4) are multiplied by $\sqrt{t}$, we obtain the stimulation charge, which is, according to Nernst, zero when t goes to zero.

All three suggestions are not in agreement with what Lapicque and many others have worked out very clearly on the basis of Weiss' and Hoorweg's results. Though we know, for sure, that the Nernst concept of constant energy must be considered unphysiologic, it is surprising that his idea still has its thoughtless repeaters today.

Physical Interpretation of the Fundamental Law

From electrophysiology it is known that excitation of a nerve or muscle cell is initiated when the permeability of the membrane with respect to sodium is greatly increased, resulting in a breakdown of the potential profile across the membrane. This is thought to be established by a force acting on obstacles within the pores of the membrane which must be stronger than the force fixing the obstacles at or within the structure of the membrane. We developed a model [9, 10] claiming that the obstacles are not neutral electrically but either ionized or polarized. In Fig. 3 a dipole molecule is assumed to close the pore like a sluice door. Any force in an electrolytic environment can be explained by either an electric field or by a diffusion gradient. Electrostimulation, therefore, may be interpreted as the application of an exogenic field to an excitable tissue so that a change in permeability with respect to sodium occurs, resulting in a continuing excitation. The electric field seems to us to be the primary parameter. All other electric parameters, such as current or voltage (both only measurable outside the body), are derived from this field in accordance with Maxwell's laws.

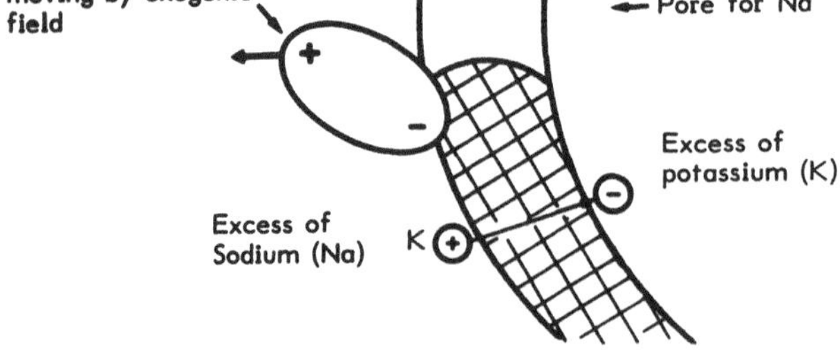

Fig. 3. Model of the membrane depicting pore obstacles susceptible to electric fields

This idea can be formulated mathematically:

$$\int^{\tau} (F_{\mathrm{exog}} - F_{\mathrm{stat}})\,\mathrm{d}t \geq I_{\mathrm{pmin}} \tag{6}$$

where F_{exog} is the exogenic force acting on the obstacles; F_{stat}, is the static force fixing the obstacle at or within the membrane; I_{pmin}, is the minimum mechanical impulse to remove the obstacles; and τ is the duration of the exogenic force.

As we assumed, the obstacles not to be neutral electrically, we can substitute the exogenic force by an exogenic electric field by the familiar relation:

$$F_{\mathrm{exog}} = q \cdot E_{\mathrm{exog}} \tag{7}$$

where q is the charge of the obstacle and E_{exog} is the exogenic electrical field strength.

Inserting Eq. (7) into Eq. (6) we get Eq. (8):

$$\int^{\tau} (E_{\mathrm{exog}} - E_{\mathrm{stat}})\,\mathrm{d}t \geq I_{\mathrm{pmin}}/q \tag{8}$$

Rearranging and dividing both sides of Eq. (8) by the pulse duration, τ, we get Eq. (9), the interpretation of which reads: the mean value of the exogenic electric field applied to an excitable membrane during the pulse duration, τ, must be equal to or larger than a minimum field strength, the "rheobase field strength", times a hyperbolic expression of the duration τ to reach excitation (Eq. 9).

$$\frac{1}{\tau}\int^{\tau} E_{\mathrm{exog}}\,\mathrm{d}t \geq \frac{I_{\mathrm{pmin}}}{q \cdot \tau} + E_{\mathrm{stat}} = E_{\mathrm{rheo}}(1 + t_{\mathrm{chr}}/\tau) \tag{9}$$

where E_{rheo} is identical with the electric field E_{stat} fixing the obstacle and t_{chr} is the chronaxie calculated from $I_{\mathrm{pmin}} : q \cdot E_{\mathrm{stat}}$.

Equation (9) is the Lapicque formula in its field version. Multiplying this equation by τ yields a similarly structured equation as the linear "formule fondamentale" found by Weiss:

$$\int^{\tau} E_{\mathrm{exog}}\,\mathrm{d}t \geq E_{\mathrm{rheo}}(\tau + t_{\mathrm{chr}}) \tag{10}$$

Equations (9) and (10) are both identical if, and only if, the amplitude of the electric field in Eq. (9) is given as a mean value.

One question raised when applying our hypothesis to reality is: How is it possible to influence the electric field of about 10^7 V/m within the membrane by an exogenic electric field of about 10^2 V/m? This paradox, published by us in 1976 [9], has never found attention among electrophysiologists.

A nonexcited cell may be regarded as a cylinder within the extracellular space [11, 18]. The cell possesses a much lower conductivity due to its insulating membrane [21] and, therefore, may be regarded as a nonconducting cell [12]. An exogenic electric field, then, is distorted in the vicinity of the cell. If we assume a homogenous electric field to be produced by large electrodes (large with respect to the length of the cell), the distortion of the electric field and the potential field can be calculated or estimated, as demonstrated by Fig. 4. It follows that the potential drop along the cross-section of a spherical cylinder is determined by the electric field strength in the extracellular space (E_{exog}) and the diameter (D) of the cylinder:

$$V = c \cdot E_{exog} \cdot D \tag{11}$$

where c is the distortion factor, with a value of 2 in Fig. 4.

The potential within the cell must be uniform, since the conductivity of the intracellular space is comparable to that of the extracellular space and is much higher than that of the membrane (this assumption is fully confirmed by calculations done by Klee and Plonsey [12]). For reasons of symmetry, it must lie in the middle of the potentials of the outside lines just touching the cell (bold vertical line in Fig. 4). This means that half the calculated potential difference drops across the membrane, yielding a membrane field strength, due to the exogenic field strength, as indicated by Eq. 12:

$$E_{mem.ex} = \tfrac{1}{2} \cdot c \cdot E_{exog} \cdot D/d \tag{12}$$

where $E_{mem.ex}$ is the membrane field strength due to an exogenic electric field E_{exog}; c is the distortion factor (= 2) for a cylinder perpendicular to the electric field; D is the diameter of the cell; and d is the thickness of the membrane.

Now, the geometry of the cell more closely resembles a rod, with a length often much greater than the diameter. We carried out a similar potential calculation for a cylindrical rod with ball-shaped ends, with a length of four diameters yielding a relatively smaller potential drop across the cell, with the distortion factor now reduced to 1.2 (see Fig. 5). The electric field in axial direction is then:

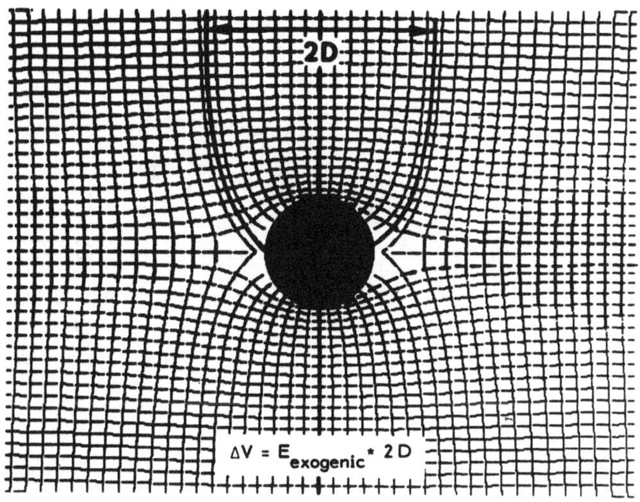

Fig. 4. Distortion of the electric field by a cylinder with an insulating membrane (seen in cross-section). Field and potential lines touching the horizontal poles of the cylinder are separated by two diameters ($2D$) in the undisturbed area. Thus, the voltage drop ΔV across the diameter D is the product of the electric field times 2D ($E_{exog} \cdot 2D$). The potential of the whole interior space is determined by the symmetry line through the center of the diameter (*bold vertical line*)

$$E_{mem.ex} = \tfrac{1}{2} \cdot c \cdot E_{exog} \cdot L/d \tag{13}$$

where $E_{mem.ex}$ is the membrane field strength due to an exogenic field strength E_{exog}; c is the distortion factor between 1 and 2 (in Fig. 5 it is 1.2); L is the length of the cell in parallel to the electric field; and d is the thickness of the membrane.

For the cell geometry assumed above (length four times greater than diameter), said to be typical of cardiac cells [3], the exogenic field can be 2.4 times lower in the longitudinal direction than in the perpendicular direction to reach excitation threshold. If the cell length is 60–100 μm [21], the ratio of radial to axial field strength increases to a value of 4.5. This simple calculation yields ratios which are well within the range published by Frazier et al. [6].

The typical structure of the excitable cell, with its high-resistance membrane insulating intracellular from extracellular space, gives rise to a transformation of the exogenic field strength which is primarily determined by the ratio of cell length (L) to membrane thickness (d). Assuming membrane thickness of a cardiac fiber to be 8 nm and cardiac fiber

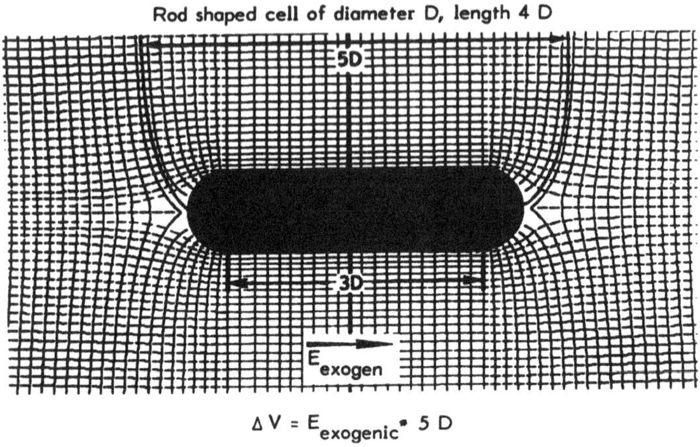

Fig. 5. Electric field lines parallel to the cell axis and the corresponding perpendicularly oriented potential lines. Potential drop V and the potential of the interior space are determined in the same way as in Fig. 4

length to be 80 µm, the geometric transformation L/d is 80 µm/8 nm $= 10 \cdot 10^3$.

Thus, the stimulation paradox can, at least partially, be explained by the geometric field transformation which increases the minimum exogenic field of 10^2 V/m outside the cell to cell membrane field strength of $6.3 \cdot 10^5$ V/m. Our theoretical results are in agreement with what has been measured so far [8].

Application of the Theory to Defibrillation

We postulate that defibrillation is governed by the same rules as all other stimulation phenomena, and there is at least one investigation, by Koning et al. [13], supporting this thesis. They reported dose-duration curves which are surprisingly similar to what Hoorweg [7] already published in 1892 (Fig. 6). Thus, we must determine if today's defibrillation practice is in accordance with theory and, further more, which improvements can be developed from it. This is especially important in a therapeutic treatment which is life-saving or, when failing, life threatening. In contrast to pacing the heart, exact measurements of defibrillation thresholds are nearly impossible [15]. Under these conditions it is highly desirable that a "trial and error" investigational system be replaced, at least partially, by theoretical considerations based on the fundamental law of electrostimulation.

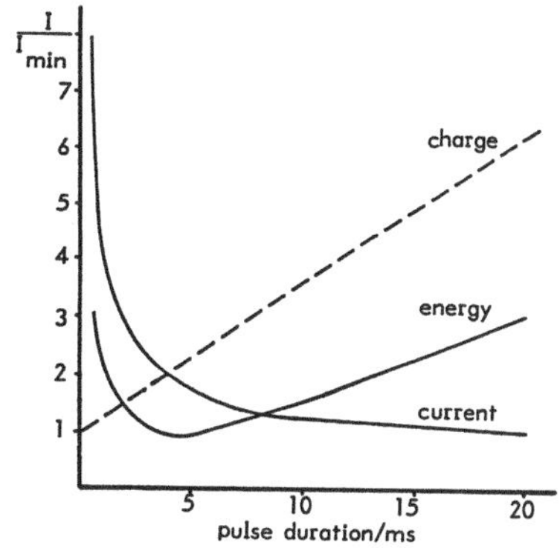

Fig. 6. Defibrillation thresholds for current, energy and charge according to Koning et al. 1975 [13]. The similarity with the Hoorweg findings in Fig. 1 is obvious. Minimum intensities I_{min} (related to heart weight): *current*, 11 mA/g; energy, 8 mJ/g; charge, 40 μC/g

The Defibrillation Hypothesis

It is frequently stated that defibrillation obeys the same rules as stimulation of nerves and muscle fibers, except that the mass of cells to be excited differs quantitatively. In both cases a "critical mass" must be influenced, which is very small in cardiac pacing but extremely large in defibrillation [1, 16]. Assuming the above hypothesis is true, we might ask which field strength is necessary to successfully defibrillate a fibrillating heart. We found that for a large area electrode (100 mm^2) and a pulse duration of 4 ms, the threshold stimulation field strength for cardiac pacing is 95 V/m [9]. Taking into account that, in this case, a stimulation of fibers parallel to the field lines of a ball-shaped electrode took place, we must consider that perpendicularly oriented fibers need a 2.5–4.5 times higher field strength to be simultaneously excited. The corresponding value of 238–428 V/m is well in agreement with what was found in the literature [2, 6, 8]. These investigators, as far as we know, were the only ones to study field strength by inserting catheters into the myocardium with spaced electrodes. Successful defibrillation was observed if the voltage across the spaced electrodes yielded a minimal field strength of 300–400 V/m. Thus, we can formulate that the basic engineering principle of defibrillation is to produce an electric field within the ventricles of 400 V/m with a pulse duration of 4–5 ms. To estimate the minimum field strength possible, a strength-duration curve must be investigated, which so far has not been done.

The Shape of the Defibrillation Pulse

Which pulse shape is best suited to reach optimum stimulation conditions is a very old question, which also initiated the work of Weiss [22].

The answer was given by him in 1901. With today's knowledge, taking into account the physical meaning of Eq. 6 in combination with Eq. 9, we can formulate: as long as the stimulation amplitude is above the rheobase value, the shape of the pulse is irrelevant. Stimulation is determined only by the time integral over the pulse duration.

The lowest possible energy is reached as the pulse approaches a rectangular shape. As applied to implantable defibrillators, this means that the output capacitor should be large in order to have the lowest possible decline during pulse. However, practical considerations demand a compromise, as the unused energy of a truncated pulse stored in the output capacitor is lost energy after successful defibrillation.

The Polarity of the Defibrillation Pulse

Which stimulation effect is produced by the cathode or the anode of a defibrillation electrode? The answer is very simple: for a homogeneous electric field, as was assumed in Figs. 4 and 5, both cathode and anode have the same effect. The cathode hypopolarizes the nearest part of the membrane, whereas the anode hypopolarizes the farthest part [6, 18]. With decreasing electrode size, however, the electric field is more radial, which will reduce the field strength with increasing distance, as is depicted in Fig. 7. In this case, the anodic threshold is higher than the cathodic one.

In defibrillation, whether intrathoracic or extrathoracic, the areas of the electrodes are always "large" so that the electric field at the site of the cardiac cells must be regarded as homogeneous. The important consequence from this is that the polarity of defibrillating electrodes plays no role in defibrillation efficiency. Technical reasons, for instance, corrosion or electrolytic effects, may limit the free polarity choice. Electrode manufacturers should indicate if such technical reasons prevail and should not suggest an electrophysiologic reason, which does not exist according to theory.

The question of whether monophasic or biphasic pulses are more efficient can also be answered with the theory outlined above. All equations formulating the fundamental law of electrostimulation are applicable only to monophasic pulses. The consideration concerning polarity, in conjunction with Figs. 4 and 5, can explain how the field strength works on cardiac cells. If we assume a rectangular biphasic wave of duration T, then the first half-wave will hypopolarize cell structures, as explained above, on one side; the second half-wave will do the same but at the opposite side of the cell. If the first half-wave fails to terminate fibrillation, it is inconceivable that the second half-wave will do it. Therefore,

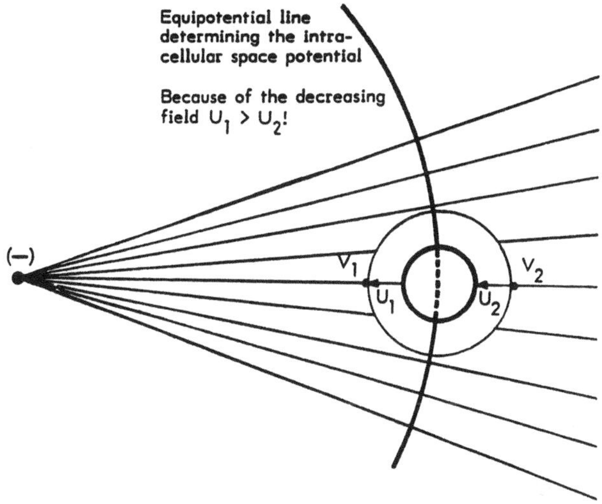

Fig. 7. Radial field of a point electrode. The potential drop across the membrane is now higher at the proximal side, thereby increasing the membrane field due to the exogenic electric field. The cathodic and anodic thresholds then are different and lower for the cathode

biphasic pulses of duration T at threshold level cannot be more effective than corresponding half-waves of duration $T/2$, which means that based on energy considerations, the half-wave is more efficient, or monophasic is better than biphasic.

Asymmetric biphasic pulses may have a lower amplitude than a monophasic pulse of the same duration. This is, however, the apparent proof that the pulse duration is longer than chronaxie. A pulse duration smaller than the biphasic one, combined with a higher amplitude, would be more efficient in saving energy.

The Stimulation Dose

Usually, as described at conferences and in publications, the defibrillation dose used is the energy, although its appropriateness has not been established. Going back to Fig. 1 it is quite clear (and has been known since 1892) that there is no general energy threshold, regardless of output capacitor and pulse duration. The threshold curves expressed as energy threshold always have a defined minimum which is determined by the chronaxie, as stated by Lapicque in 1909 [14]. The concept of constant energy, introduced by Nernst in 1908 [17], has its electrophysiological deficits, as we pointed out in discussing Eq. 5. The weakness of the energy dose may be one of the reasons why the results are so divergent.

The energy dose also has a very practical disadvantage, which physicians should be aware of: if the field strength hypothesis is accepted as true, the linear physical quantities, such as voltage and current, are closer to the field strength than to the energy. This means that if a given field strength has failed to stimulate or defibrillate, the field strength must be increased by at least 10% – 20%. Projecting this conclusion to the use of defibrillators, it is not physiologic, and could even be dangerous, if the programmable dose of an implantable defibrillator increases in steps from 20, to 22, to 24, to 27, to 30 J, corresponding to an increase in voltage of 100%, 105%, 110%, 116%, and 122%, respectively. Each physician experienced in pacing in ICU would never dare to increase an external pacemaker output with such low incremental steps. If, for technical reasons, the highest energy is limited to, let's say, 30 J, a downward scaling of 21, 14, 10, 7, 5, 2.3, 1.5, 1.0 would correspond to a decrease in field strength in steps of 20%.

We claim that a characterization of the defibrillation threshold indicating the mean output voltage and the pulse duration would drastically reduce the uncertainties of today's practice, due to the energy dose, and would probably reduce the threshold variations which make programming the output of an AICD a problem.

To reduce energy requirements, we have to apply defibrillation pulses with a duration equal to the chronaxie. This is the message derived from the fundamental law of electrostimulation. Therefore, defibrillators with variable pulse durations are needed.

Final Remarks

The work done by the investigators at the turn of this century has been admirable, as it has laid the foundation upon which engineering principles for stimulation and defibrillation can be based. We are convinced that their results, in combination with our field strength model of electrostimulation, both of which have thus far been experimentally confirmed in their practical implications, will help to reach a better understanding of electrostimulation and its associated problems. One can never derive directly the optimal engineering design from a theory alone. However, engineers dealing with electrostimulation can use theory as a guideline to determine whether their own ideas or the ideas of others, which come to their attention, have the best chance to be successful. Experimental results are so difficult to obtain, especially in defibrillation, that the trial and error procedure is too time-consuming to reach its goal or might even fail. This is especially important to those engaged in defibrillation. If defibrillation is generally accepted to be mainly ruled by the law of electrostimulation, the state of the art could take an important step forward toward on optimal engineering solution.

Is defibrillation really governed by the rules of electrostimulation? The answer is ambiguous: yes, but there are obviously additional effects which must be taken as amendments to the law. These are the prolongation of refractoriness [4, 5, 8] and the suppression of refibrillation by reduced pulses of opposite polarity at the end of a defibrillating pulse [4, 19]; neither are present in simple electrostimulation. Additionally, the field strength must be stronger to affect refractory cells [8, 20]. However, do additional effects, such as suppression of refibrillation and prolongation of refractoriness, justify the assumption that the Nernst law of constant energy (Eq. 5) will overrule Weiss' fundamental law of electrostimulation? We are of the opinion that all of the effects result from electric fields, for which strength-duration relationships exist, as formulated by Lapicque in 1909 with the two important parameters rheobase and chronaxie.

References

1. Auger PM, Bardou A, Coulombe A et al. (1989) Computer stimulation of defibrillating electric shocks: critical mass. IEEE Eng Med Biol Soc 11th Ann Int Conf, pp 75–76
2. Borman JB, Tannenbaum J, Merin B et al. (1971) External-internal defibrillation. Thorac Cardiovasc Surg 62:98–105
3. Braunwald E, Ross F, Sonnenblick EH (1967) Mechanisms of contraction of the normal and failing heart. Little, Boston
4. Chen P-S, Shibata N, Dixon EG (1986) Activation during ventricular defibrillation in open-chest dogs. J Clin Invest 77:810–823
5. Dillon SM, Wit AL (1989) Action potential prolongation by shock as a possible mechanism for electrical defibrillation. Circulation 80:II–96
6. Frazier DW, Krassowska W, Chen P-S et al. (1988) Extracellular field required for excitation in three-dimensional anisotropic canine myocardium. Circ Res 63:147–165
7. Hoorweg JL (1892) Condensatorentladung und Auseinandersetzung mit du Bois-Reymond. Pflügers Arch 52:87–108
8. Ideker RE, Krassowska W, Wharton JM et al. (1989) Experimental results pertinent to the modelling of defibrillation. IEEE Eng Med Biol Soc 11th Ann Int Conf, pp 77–78
9. Irnich W (1976) Elektrotherapie des Herzens – physiologische und biotechnische Aspekte. Schiele and Schön, Berlin
10. Irnich W (1985) The electrode myocardial interface. Clin Prog Electrophysiol Pacing 3:338–348

11. Irnich W (1989) Das Grundgesetz der Elektrostimulation. Biomed Tech (Berlin) 34:168–176
12. Klee M, Plonsey R (1976) Stimulation of spheroidal cells – the role of cell shape. IEEE Trans Biomed Eng 4:347–355
13. Koning G, Schneider H, Hoelen AJ et al. (1975) Amplitude-duration relation for direct ventricular defibrillation with rectangular current pulses. Med Biol Eng 13:388–395
14. Lapicque L (1909) Definition expérimentale de l'excitabilité. Soc Biol 77:280–283
15. McDaniel WC, Schuder JC (1985) The cardiac ventricular defibrillation threshold-inherent limitations in its interpretation. AAMI 20th Ann Meeting, Boston, May 6–8
16. Mower M, Mirowski M, Spear JF et al. (1974) Patterns of ventricular activity during catheter defibrillation. Circulation 49:858–861
17. Nernst W (1908) Zur Theorie des elektrischen Reizes. Pflügers Arch 122:275–314
18. Plonsey R, Barr RC (1986) Effect of microscopic and macroscopic discontinuities on the response of cardiac tissue to defibrillating (stimulating) currents. Med Biol Eng Comput 24:130–136
19. Schuder JC, Gold JH, Stoeckle H et al. (1983) Transthoracic ventricular defibrillation in the 100 kg calf with symmetrical one-cycle bidirectional rectangular wave stimuli. IEEE Trans Biomed Eng 30:415–422
20. Shibata N, Chen P-S, Dixon EG et al. (1988) Influence of shock strength and timing on induction of ventricular arrhythmia in dogs. Am J Physiol 255:H891–H901
21. Sommer JR (1983) Implications of structure and geometry on cardiac electrical activity. Ann Biomed Eng 11:149–157
22. Weiss G (1901) Sur la possibilité de rendre comparable entre eux les appareils servant a l'excitation électrique. Arch Ital Biol 35:413–446

Optimal Waveform Morphology for Defibrillation *

R. A. S. Cooper, R. E. Ideker, S. A. Feeser, J. P. Daubert,
J. M. Wharton

Introduction

Since the first human implant of a completely implantable cardiac defibrillator in 1980, research has focused on making the smallest, most efficient device. Currently the main size constraints of these devices are the battery and capacitor sizes [1]. If energy requirements for defibrillation could be reduced without affecting the efficacy of the device, then battery size could be decreased and/or battery life increased. Also, the capacitors used could be reduced in size. Furthermore, the reduced shock strength might lead to fewer side affects including conduction disturbances and ventricular dysfunction as well as myocardial necrosis when exposing the myocardium to high energy defibrillation shocks. Besides developing more efficient battery and capacitor systems, efforts are focusing on more efficient lead systems and defibrillation waveforms that require less energy for defibrillation [1].

Historical Perspective

Since defibrillation was first performed, multiple waveforms have been tested for clinical application. One of the first of these was transthoracically applied alternating current, which required large transformers to generate the required shock strength and therefore was not practical for implantable or portable devices [2–4]. Lown et al. [5] developed a damped sinusoidal waveform that was generated by capacitor discharge through a series inductor and a resistor which was the resistance across

---

* Supported in part by the National Institutes of Health, research grants HL-42760, HL-28429 and HL-33637, the National Science Foundation Engineering Research Center, grant CDR-8622201 and by CPI Inc. and Physio-Control Corp.

the paddles and thorax. This waveform is known as the Lown waveform and is employed in many portable defibrillators. This work demonstrated that DC shocks had fewer side affects including fewer post shock arrhythmias, less myocardial injury, as well as fewer deaths in experimental animals than AC shocks. Other waveforms tested included straight capacitor discharges as well as square wave pulses [6–9]. Straight capacitor pulses tended to have high peak currents associated with myocardial depression as well as increased post-shock arrhythmias. Furthermore, it was thought that the low voltage tail of the pulse resulted in refibrillation of the heart [8, 9]. Square wave pulses were found to be superior to the Lown and straight capacitor pulses; however, they required large capacitors and wasted energy because most of the charge remained undelivered in the capacitors at the end of the shock [10, 11]. Although impractical for implantable devices because of the large physical size of the inductor, this initial work did suggest that shorter duration waveforms required less energy than did longer pulse durations for defibrillation.

Truncated Exponential Monophasic Waveforms

The first generation ICDs use monophasic truncated exponential waveforms. Several groups have found this type of waveform to be superior to straight capacitor discharges for defibrillation [12, 13]. It was found that with truncation, the detrimental effects of the small tail of a straight capacitor discharge could be avoided. Wessale et al. [14] using a bielectrode transvenous catheter system in dogs demonstrated that peak current increased with increasing tilt and decreasing pulse duration. These studies also demonstrated that total energy increased with increasing pulse duration but was not related to tilt. Chapman et al. [15], using a transvenous catheter to subcutaneous patch system in dogs with a fixed pulse width, variable tilt, and truncated exponential monophasic waveform, showed that shorter pulse durations were associated with lower energy requirements for defibrillation. This study also demonstrated that the relationship between threshold voltage and pulse width was hyperbolic with the shortest and longest durations associated with higher threshold voltages in the middle of this spectrum. Furthermore, they found that the minimum total energy required for defibrillation was associated with the shorter pulse durations and increased with increasing pulse duration. They concluded pulse durations from approximately 5 to 15 ms with this type of electrode system were associated with the best combination of low voltage, energy, and average current for this catheter-patch electrode system.

Sequential Pulses

Wiggers in 1940 first described the application of "serial" defibrillation shocks in dog hearts, and found that three to seven AC shocks, each approximately of 1 amp and less than 1 s in duration, were as efficacious as well as less harmful to the heart than single AC shocks [16]. Orias [17] postulated that the mechanism of sequential pulses involves the first pulse depolarizing all nonrefractory cells and the second pulse depolarizing cells that were initially refractory during the first pulse. Kugelberg [18] and Resnekov et al. [19] reported that dual square-wave and trapezoidal pulses with delays between pulses from 20 to 200 ms required less energy to defibrillate than single alternating current or straight-capacitor discharge waveforms. The optimal pulse separation that was associated with the minimal successful defibrillation energy appeared to be 100 ms in both studies. However other groups [9, 20, 21] were unable to show that various types of monophasic sequential pulses required decreased energy for defibrillation. These groups [9, 20, 21] also showed that energy requirements were actually increased compared to single pulses; however, they did show that peak current was decreased. This led Geddes et al. [20] to propose that the clinical usefulness of sequential pulses could be linked to whether current or energy was thought to be the main cause of myocardial damage with large defibrillating shocks.

Bourland et al. [22] postulated the idea of temporal and spatial summation which was based on the concept that by separating pulses in time and space (i.e., different current pathways) a more uniform field would be achieved; therefore reducing defibrillation energy requirements. This theory has been supported by several groups using various monophasic waveforms with at least two different current pathways [23–27]. These experiments have been performed in dogs and pigs with nonthoracotomy lead systems, as well as in humans [28] with catheter to epicardial patch systems. In brief, all of these studies have shown significant reductions in defibrillation threshold when compared to single pulses given through the separate lead systems. Furthermore, there appears to be an optimal pulse separation from 0 to 1 ms, but the advantage of reduced defibrillation threshold is lost with separations greater than 10 ms. Several studies have also shown no distinct advantage of three or four separate current pathways compared to two pathways [29, 30]. With the continuing evolution of nonthoracotomy implantable devices, these findings suggest that the use of multiple pulses and current pathways could help reduce the size as well as shock-strength requirements of AICDs without requiring a more complex surgical implantation procedure.

Biphasic Waveforms

In the 1940s Gurvich and Markarychev first described the superiority of biphasic waveforms to monophasic waveforms for defibrillation [31]. Recently several groups have demonstrated this in a variety of experimental models as well as in humans [32–35]. Schuder et al. [32] demonstrated in calves that certain symmetric biphasic waveforms could defibrillate at lower energies and currents than monophasics of similar durations. They found that asymmetric biphasic waveforms with the second phase having a smaller amplitude than the first defibrillated at lower energies than waveforms with second phases of larger amplitude than the first phase. Dixon et al. [34] using large epicardial patches in dogs compared multiple biphasic waveforms to similar monophasic waveforms. They were able to show that biphasics in which the second phase was shorter or equal to the first phase in duration were more effective than monophasics of equal duration. They also found that, if the second phase was longer than the first phase, the defibrillation energy requirements increased (Fig. 1). Tang et al. [36] further examined the importance of phase duration with biphasics. By determining defibrillation thresholds and probability of success curves for multiple biphasic waveforms, they confirmed and extended the findings of Dixon et al. [34] for waveforms of several different durations (Figs. 2 and 3). Thus these studies demonstrate that the improved efficacy of biphasic waveforms is dependent on both the amplitudes and the durations of the two phases.

Chapman et al. [37], using a non thoracotomy canine defibrillation model with an electrode in the right ventricular apex and another as a cutaneous left chest wall patch, compared single capacitor biphasic waveforms where the leading edge voltage of the second phase was equal to the trailing edge voltage of the first phase to dual capacitor waveforms where both leading edge voltages were equal. They demonstrated that biphasic waveforms generated from a single capacitor were as effective as dual capacitor biphasics and more effective than monophasic waveforms of the same duration. Kavanagh et al. [38] used a three electrode canine model with two cathodes in the right ventricular apex and outflow tract connected in parallel and a left chest wall patch as a single anode to compare one vs two capacitor-generated biphasic waveforms with both phases 6 ms in duration. They found that the one capacitor biphasic used with this lead system required significantly less energy for defibrillation than the dual capacitor 6/6 ms biphasic or the 12 ms monophasic waveform they tested.

The limited human clinical studies to date using biphasic waveforms support the experimental findings that biphasics with a shorter second

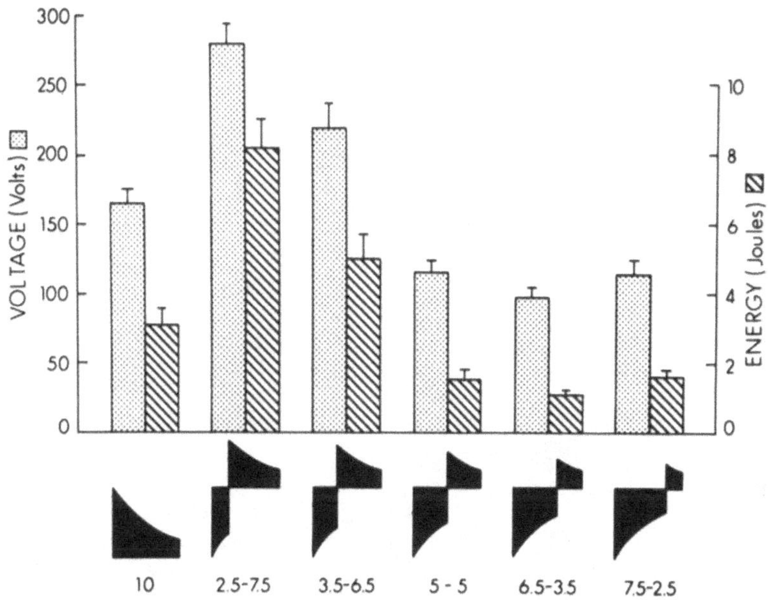

Fig. 1. Defibrillation threshold voltage and energy values for the six biphasic waveforms tested. The mean values and standard deviations are shown. Diagrams of the waveforms are shown below the bar graphs. The biphasic with an equal duration (5/5 ms) or shorter duration second phase than the first phase (6.5/3.5 and 7.5/2.5 ms) had significantly lower leading edge voltage and energy requirements than the other waveforms tested. The biphasic waveforms with shorter first phases than second phases (2.5/7.5 and 3.5/6.5 ms) had significantly higher defibrillation voltage and energy requirements than the other waveforms tested, including the 10 ms monophasic waveform. The 2.5/7.5 ms biphasic waveform had significantly higher defibrillation voltage and energy requirements than the 3.5/6.5 ms biphasic waveform. (Modified with permission from Dixon et al. 1987 [34])

phase and with a smaller amplitude than the first phase appear to be more effective [39, 40]. Furthermore, human studies appear to confirm that a single capacitor biphasic waveform is more effective than monophasics of half or equal total duration [39]. These findings suggest that effective biphasic waveforms could be generated from a single capacitor requiring less energy than the monophasic waveforms. Thus ICD size would not be increased and could possibly be decreased if less energy is required with biphasic pulses.

It has been shown that high energy shocks can cause conduction disturbances and myocardial dysfunction as well as necrosis [41–45].

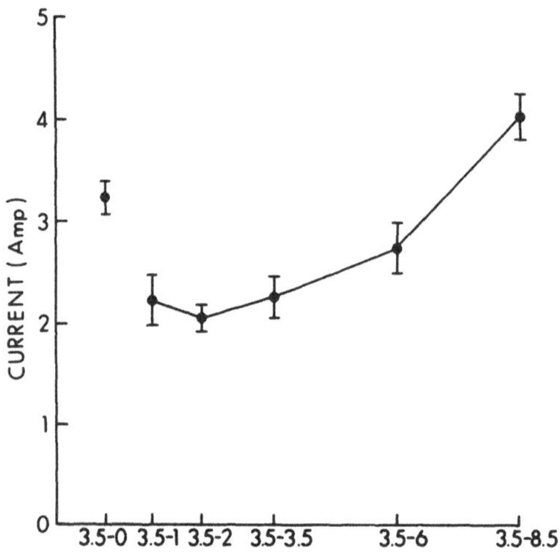

Fig. 2. Current strength (mean ± SD) at defibrillation threshold vs the duration of the second phase (T_2) of five biphasic waveforms with the first phase (T_1) of 3.5 ms. As the duration of the second phase increases, the threshold current is stable until $T_2 = T_1$, then increases sharply for $T_2 > T_1$. For comparison, the threshold current for the monophasic 3.5 ms waveform (3.5/0) is also shown. (Reproduced by permission from Tang et al. 1989 [36])

It has also been shown that for successful defibrillation, large electrical fields are produced close to the shocking electrodes. These fields are up to 20 times greater than the fields distant from the electrodes [46, 47]. Jones et al. [48] and Negovsky et al. [49] have proposed the concept of a safety factor or therapeutic index which is the ratio between the shock strength required to produce the dysfunction and that required to stimulate or defibrillate the tissue. Jones and Jones [50] using cultured chick embryo myocardial cells demonstrated that biphasic waveforms with a second phase smaller than the first were associated with shorter post-shock arrest times. They concluded that certain biphasics have a larger safety factor than the monophasic truncated or rectified waveforms they compared them with. Yabe et al. [51] found that biphasics, in which the second phase was smaller than the first, caused less conduction block and recovery was faster than comparable monophasics that created the same strength of shock field. Both Jones' [50] and Yabe's [51] groups found that polarity of the second phase was critical in that a biphasic with both phases of the same polarity produced longer post-shock arrest times and more conduction block respectively than a monophasic equal in duration to the first of the two phases. Yabe and co-workers [51] concluded that certain biphasic waveforms not only have

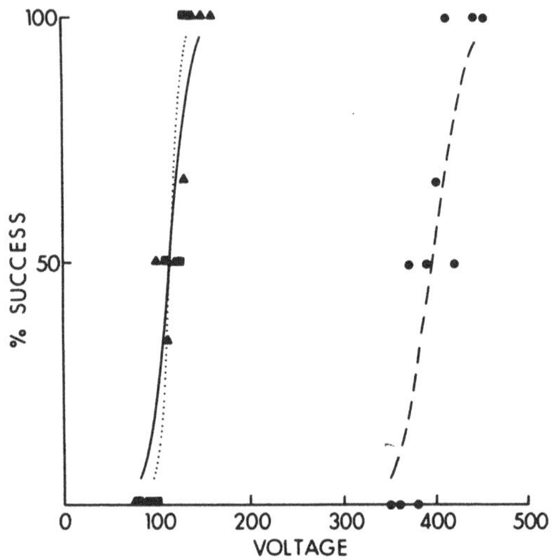

Fig. 3. Data points and dose-response defibrillation curves fitted by probit regression analysis for the three waveforms 3.5/2 ms (*triangles, solid line*), 6/6 ms (*squares, dotted line*), and 3.5/8.5 ms (*circles, dashed line*) in a representative dog. The curves for the 3.5/2 ms and the 6/6 ms waveforms are almost superimposable, but the 3.5/8.5 ms curve is shifted to the right, indicating a higher voltage requirement for defibrillation. (Reproduced by permission from Tang et al. 1989 [36])

lower energy requirements for defibrillation but that they result in less conduction block. Thus, with less block and quicker recovery times, biphasics may be associated with fewer post-shock arrhythmias as well as less myocardial dysfunction.

Proposed Mechanisms of Biphasic Waveforms

Several theories have been developed to explain the improved defibrillation efficacy of biphasic waveforms; however, the mechanism still remains unclear. Jones and coworkers [52] proposed the theory of the prepulse "conditioning" effect. They demonstrated that, compared to monophasics, biphasic pulses reduced the excitation threshold of cultured chick embryo myocardial cells [52]. It has been shown that the resting potential of the membrane is reduced to approximately −60 mV during fibrillation induced by reperfusion following ischemia [53]. Jones et al. [52] postulated that the first phase of the biphasic waveform acts

as a "conditioning" pulse, causing hyperpolarization of some portions of the heart bringing the transmembrane potentials of these portions closer to normal resting potential, thus reactivating sodium channels. The second phase then can more easily excite these portions of the heart and lower the excitation and defibrillation thresholds.

Another theory is that biphasics defibrillate better due to effects on the refractory periods of cells. As demonstrated by Cranefield and Hoffman [54], a hyperpolarizing pulse given during phase two of the action potential shortens the refractory period so that a depolarizing pulse applied afterward of a strength and timing that was ineffective if given without the hyperpolarizing pulse can now activate the cell. Thus, if one can extend this to biphasic waveforms for defibrillation, cells during the first phase that are not depolarized, but have their refractory periods shortened due to hyperpolarization of the transmembrane potential, can be excited by the second phase when the cells are less refractory.

A third proposed mechanism is that biphasic waveforms result in lower impedances across the defibrillation electrodes. However the degree in reduction in improvement of defibrillation is greater in terms of voltage and energy than the degree of reduction in impedance [36] so that biphasic waveforms result in a reduction in defibrillation current requirements which should be independent of impedance [55]. Furthermore, a reduced impedance does not explain why two biphasic waveforms of the same total duration but with different phase durations have differing defibrillation efficacies despite the same reduction in impedance. Thus, lower impedance with biphasic waveforms cannot completely account for the improved effectiveness.

Ideker et al. [56] proposed the theory that the critical point may be different for biphasic waveforms than for monophasic waveforms. Critical points occur were shock strengths of a critical value of potential gradient intersect vulnerable tissue with a critical degree of refractoriness. Rotors of leading circle reentry are formed that are centered at these critical points and reinitiate fibrillation [57–59]. This critical point theory and the fact that the potential gradient produced by a given shock decreases with distance away from the shocking electrodes may help to explain the existence of an upper limit of vulnerability (ULV) for fibrillation. The facts that shocks can defibrillate as well as cause fibrillation, and that it is possible to defibrillate with shocks larger than required to initiate fibrillation imply that there is an upper limit of shock strength that will not induce fibrillation during the vulnerable period of the cardiac cycle. The ULV has been characterized and correlates strongly with the defibrillation threshold (DFT) [41, 57, 60, 61]. The ULV hypothesis states that shocks less than the DFT stop all activation fronts of fibrillation; however, fibrillation can be reinitiated if the stimulus delivered

reaches areas of tissue that are in their vulnerable periods. Thus the probability of a successful shock depends at least partially on the probability of vulnerable myocardium being present in an area were the potential gradient created by the shock is less than the critical value even though all activation fronts were halted by the shock [62]. If there is no vulnerable tissue within these critical areas or the shock strength was sufficient to exceed the critical value in all areas, then the shock will succeed. However if vulnerable tissue is present in areas where the potential gradient spans the critical value, critical points will be established in these areas and reentry leading to fibrillation can occur.

The critical point and ULV can also help to explain the probability of success curves for defibrillation. As the amount of tissue in which the shock potential gradient equals the critical value increases, the probability of vulnerable myocardium being present increases, and thus as the shock strength is decreased the probability of successful defibrillation decreases [62]. Based on the concept of critical points and ULV, several explanations of the improved efficacy of biphasic waveform have been proposed [56]. First, the improved efficacy can be due to differences in the strength-interval curves between biphasic and monophasic waveforms [62–64]. Second, the critical points for biphasics may have different locations compared to monophasic waveforms on a strength-interval plot. Third, the characteristics of the reentrant circuits set up by biphasic waveforms may differ in duration of block as well as in conduction velocity.

Further Studies With Biphasic Waveforms

Feeser et al. [65] studied the strength-duration and probability of success curves for several biphasic waveforms and compared these to similar monophasic waveforms when the first phase of the biphasic was held constant and the second phase was increased in either amplitude or duration. They found that the strength-duration curves were not simple hyperbolas or parabolas as with monophasic waveforms. As the second phase was increased, defibrillation efficacy first improved, then declined, and then improved again (Fig. 4). Thus, the defibrillation probability of success curves were not sigmoidal. Furthermore, they demonstrated that with certain biphasic waveforms the presence of the first phase resulted in less effective defibrillation than if only the second phase had been given. Using the sodium activation theory, if the first phase reactivates sodium channels and the second phase then excites the tissue, then increasing the size of the second phase by amplitude or duration should continue to improve defibrillation efficacy. A decline in

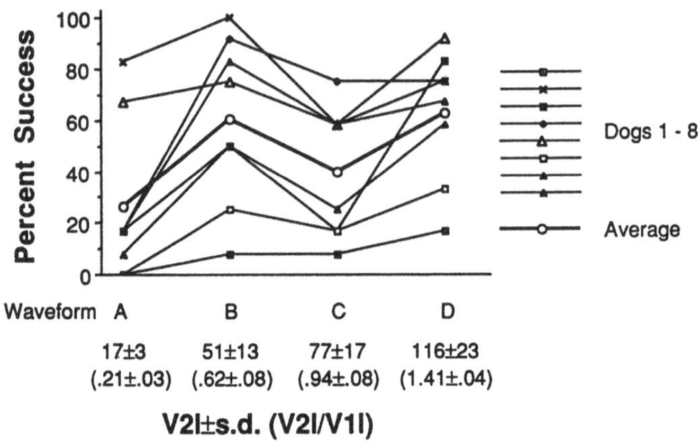

Fig. 4. Defibrillation percent success vs phase two leading edge voltage for waveform A, 6/6 ms biphasic with the leading edge voltage of phase 2 (V_{21}) 20% of the leading voltage of phase one (V_{11}). Waveform B, 6/6 ms biphasic with V_{21} approximately 60% of V_{11}. Waveform C, 6/6 ms biphasic with V_{21} approximately 90% of V_{11}. Waveform D, 6/6 ms biphasic with V_{21} approximately 140% of V_{11}. When increasing V_{21} from 21% to 141% of V_{11}, the percent success first rises ($p<0.01$), then falls ($p<0.005$), and then rises again ($p<0.02$). (Modified and reproduced with permission from Feeser et al. 1991 [65])

efficacy should only result when the second phase is so large that it results in myocardial injury. This cannot explain why for certain biphasics the defibrillation efficacy first improves, then declines, and then improves again.

These results suggest at least two mechanisms exist for the improved defibrillation efficacy of biphasic waveforms, one that is more effective for smaller second phases and another that becomes more effective as the second phase is increased. One possible explanation they offer for the dual mechanisms involves the concept of each phase of the stimulus inducing a gradation from hyperpolarization to depolarization along each myocyte [66, 67] (Fig. 5). If the first phase activates sodium channels on one half of the each myocyte and the second phase activates sodium channels on the other half of the myocyte without inactivating all the channels the first phase opened, then the biphasic pulse might be more likely to defibrillate than if only the first phase was given. However if the charge of the second phase is increased it may inactivate all the channels previously activated by the first phase and thus the positive interaction between the two phases would be cancelled. This would help explain why biphasics with larger second phases than first phases are less effective than waveforms with the first phase larger than the second

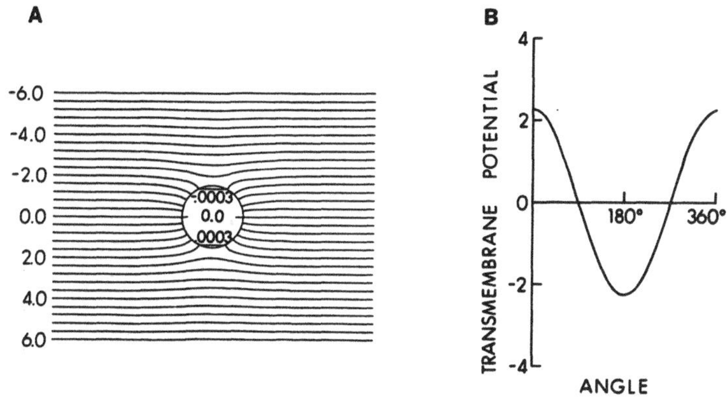

Fig. 5 A, B. Single spheroidal cell in a uniform extracellular field. **A** The cell is exposed to a uniform electrical field created by the cathode at the top and the anode at the bottom. Extracellular potentials are given in mV (*left*), with isopotential lines spaced every 0.4 mV. As indicated by the isopotential lines spaced every 0.00003 mV, the potential within the cell changes much less than the extracellular potential. **B** The transmembrane potential in mV, which is equal to the difference between the intracellular and extracellular potentials in **A**, is shown as a function of the location on the surface of the cell, as expressed by the polar angle, with 0° at the top of the cell and 180° at the bottom. The top half of the cell toward the cathode is depolarized, and the bottom half toward the anode is hyperpolarized. (Adapted from Klee and Plonsey 1976 [66])

phase. As the second phase is further increased it delivers enough energy by itself to excite the cells, thus acting like a monophasic waveform. This would help explain the improvement after the decline in defibrillation efficacy as the amplitude of the second phase is progressively increased. They also found that high tilt biphasic waveforms performed poorly as the duration of the second phase was extended producing a longer low voltage tail. This supports the idea proposed by Schuder et al. [9] that one of the reasons that exponential waveforms with long tails perform poorly was secondary to reinducing fibrillation and suggests that certain biphasic waveforms can defibrillate and refibrillate more effectively than similar monophasic waveforms.

Wharton et al. [62] examined the effects of biphasic and monophasic stimulation on various electrophysiological parameters in normal and infarcted canine hearts. They found that certain biphasic waveforms compared with equal duration monophasic pulses did not have a lower threshold for activating normal tissue during late diastole. These data suggest that the defibrillation efficacy of a particular waveform cannot be predicted by its ability to stimulate myocardium in late diastole. They

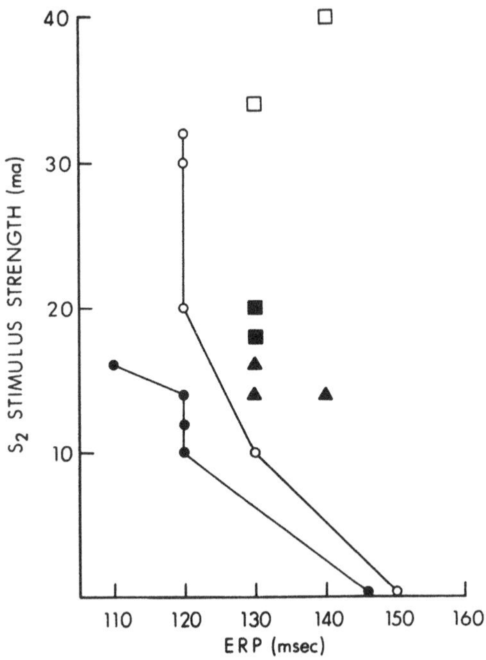

Fig. 6. Strength-interval curves for monophasic and biphasic waveforms in a non-infarcted dog. The curve for the biphasic waveform (*unfilled circles*) is shifted to the right of that for the monophasic waveform of the same total duration (*filled circles*), indicating that the biphasic waveform is less able to stimulate relatively refractory tissue. Ventricular fibrillation was induced at a lower current strength with the monophasic (*filled squares*) than with the biphasic (*unfilled squares*) stimulus. Repetitive responses were induced with the monophasic (*filled triangles*) but not with the biphasic stimulus, with stimulus strengths slightly less than the fibrillation threshold. (Reproduced with permission from Wharton et al. 1991 [62])

also found that the effective refractory period was longer and the strength-interval curve was shifted to the right for the biphasic stimuli tested compared to similar monophasic stimuli (Fig. 6). This suggests that biphasic waveforms are less able to stimulate relative refractory and thus partially depolarized tissue than monophasic stimuli with the same duration and tilt. They also found that biphasics had a higher threshold for repetitive activity and tended to have an increased fibrillation threshold. Thus it appeared biphasic stimuli were less capable of inducing ventricular arrhythmias in normal myocardium than were monophasic stimuli. Furthermore, they found that the biphasic ULV and DFT were significantly decreased in a parallel fashion compared to similar monophasic waveforms. These findings are consistent with the ULV hypothesis [61, 68] as described previously. Of note, in this study the presence of infarcted myocardium did not appear to attenuate or accentuate the improved defibrillation efficacy of biphasic waveforms. They concluded that the stimulation of fully repolarized or partially depolarized myocardium cannot be evoked as the mechanism by which biphasic waveforms have lower defibrillation thresholds than monophasic waveforms and postulated that biphasics may be more efficient for defibrillation by being less capable of reinitiating fibrillation.

Daubert et al. [69] evaluated the abilities of monophasic and biphasic shocks of equal voltage and duration to stimulate partially refractory canine myocardium. The hypothesis was tested that biphasics defibrillate at lower voltages because they can more effectively excite the relatively refractory tissue present during fibrillation. They found that a shorter biphasic (2/1 ms duration) did not excite refractory tissue as well as a similar (3 ms) monophasic waveform but that it did defibrillate better than the monophasic waveform. They also demonstrated that the shock potential gradient leading to conduction block at the directly excited border (the potential gradient at the critical point) was similar for biphasic and monophasic waveforms. The directly excited border was defined as the border between the area of tissue directly excited by the stimulus were all cells are raised above threshold and the area were the stimulus is not sufficient to raise cells above their threshold. They argue that for the shorter duration biphasics that do not stimulate tissue as well as monophasics, the relative refractory tissue adjoining the directly excited border should be less refractory for biphasic waveforms. Thus, activation fronts that spread from this border will encounter more recovered tissue and be less likely to produce reentry and refibrillation. They propose that the main determinant of successful defibrillation is not the amount of tissue directly excited by a shock but is the fate of activation fronts generated by the shock. These studies, performed with a biphasic waveform of 3 ms total duration, may not hold for longer duration biphasics. Jones et al. [52, 70] in the cultured chick embryo model have reported that longer duration (10 ms) biphasics stimulate better than monophasics of equal duration.

Triphasic Waveforms

Jones and Jones [71] demonstrated in the chick embryo myocardial model that triphasic waveforms appear to have an even greater safety factor than biphasic waveforms. They also found, as did Dixon et al. [34]

and Chapman et al. [72], that triphasic waveforms do not appear to offer any distinct advantage over biphasic waveforms in defibrillation efficacy. Jones and Jones [71] postulate that the first phase acts as the "conditioning prepulse," the second phase as the "exciting" or "defibrillating" phase, and the third phase as the "healing postpulse." Thus it is possible the triphasic waveform will cause less dysfunction at the suprathreshold shock strengths at which ICDs are likely to be set to deliver. Work with triphasic waveforms is still too limited to judge whether they will be superior to biphasic waveforms in clinical practice.

The Future

Selection of an optimal waveform for defibrillation remains empiric. Even though limited human clinical studies have been performed, it appears that the advantage of certain biphasic waveforms has carried over from the multiple animal studies. Newer generation programmable devices can utilize biphasic waveforms as well as sequential pulses [1]. However, due to the wide range of biphasics examined and the sensitivity of defibrillation threshold to phase duration, it is difficult to choose just one or several "optimal" waveforms. The data on biphasic waveforms suggest that the best waveforms are those with second phases either equal or shorter in duration to the first phase. Furthermore, the data show that equally effective biphasic waveforms can be generated from single and dual capacitor systems. Thus, with the continually expanding programmable capabilities of ICDs, there will be much greater flexibility of waveform selection which should not increase the size requirements of the devices.

Waveform selection will probably remain empirical until the mechanisms of improved efficacy of biphasic and possibly triphasic waveforms can be determined. It appears that the improved efficacy cannot be explained by any single process and involves the interaction of multiple mechanisms. Furthermore there is hope that once these mechanisms can be determined, the response of a particular patient or group of patients to a particular waveform will be predictable. If distinct characteristics of ventricular fibrillation can be determined, and the effects of defibrillation waveforms on these characteristics are known, then the optimal waveform could be employed without having to subject the patients to multiple fibrillation and defibrillation tests at the time of implantation. For example, Wharton et al. [62] found that, for the waveforms and lead system they used, the ULV represented the minimum dose almost 100% effective for defibrillation (Fig. 7). If this finding is confirmed for other waveforms and electrode configurations, it could offer a safer means for

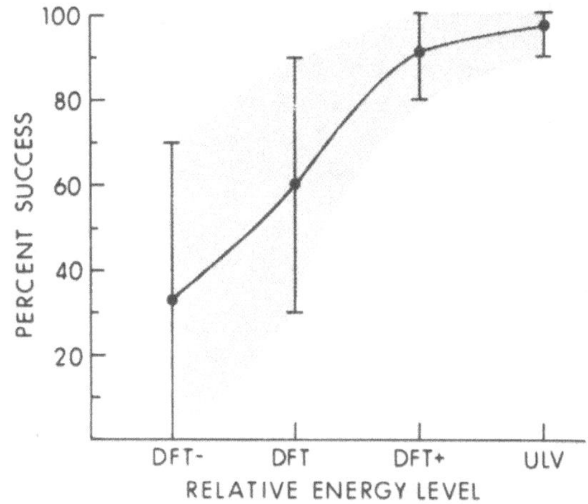

Fig. 7. Probability of defibrillation as a function of relative energy level. The mean percent success of defibrillation (*solid sigmoidal line*) is shown for 6 dogs at four different energy levels: ULV, DFT, half way between ULV and DFT (DFT+) and an equivalent distance in energy below the DFT (DFT−). The range is shown by *brackets*. The energy at the ULV was always within the 90% – 100% portion of the defibrillation probability curve. (Reproduced with permission from Wharton et al. 1991 [62])

intraoperative testing of implantable defibrillator energy output, since repeated induction of fibrillation could be avoided.

Thus, the search for the mechanisms of defibrillation continue. Although this search so far has not provided a universally accepted mechanism for defibrillation, significant advances have been made in the shock strength required for defibrillation with implantable defibrillators [1] and we hope this progress continues.

References

1. Troup PJ (1989) Implantable cardioverters and defibrillators. Curr Probl Cardiol 14:675–843
2. Hooker DR, Kouwenhoven WB, Langworthy OR (1933) The effect of alternating currents on the heart. Am J Physiol 103:444–454
3. Beck CS, Pritchard WH, Feil HS (1947) Ventricular fibrillation of long duration abolished by electric shock. JAMA 135:985–986
4. Zoll PM, Linenthal AJ, Gibson W, Paul MH, Norman LR (1956) Termination of ventricular fibrillation in man by externally applied electric countershock. N Engl J Med 254:727–732

5. Lown B, Newman J, Amarasingham R, Berkovitz BV (1962) Comparison of alternating current with direct current electroshock across the closed chest. Am J Cardiol 10:223–233
6. Gurvich NL, Yuniev GS (1939) Restoration of regular rhythm in the mammalian fibrillating heart. Bull Exp Biol Med 8:55–58
7. Pelèska B (1966) Optimal parameters of electrical impulses for defibrillation by condenser discharges. Circ Res 18:10–17
8. Geddes LA, Tacker WA (1971) Engineering and physiological considerations of direct capacitor-discharge ventricular defibrillation. Med Biol Eng 9:185–199
9. Schuder JC, Stoeckle H, Keskar PY, Gold JH, Chier MT, West JA (1970) Transthoracic ventricular defibrillation in the dog with unidirectional rectangular double pulses. Cardiovasc Res 4:497
10. Koning G, Schneider H, Hoelen AJ (1975) Amplitude-duration relation for direct ventricular defibrillation with rectangular current pulses. Med Biol Eng 13:388–395
11. Bourland JD, Tacker WA Jr, Geddes LA (1978) Strength-duration curves for trapezoidal waveforms of various tilts for transchest defibrillation in animals. Med Instrum 12:38–41
12. Schuder JC, Stoeckle H, Gold JH, West JA, Keskar PY (1970) Experimental ventricular defibrillation with an automatic and completely implanted system. Trans Am Soc Artif Intern Organs 16:207–212
13. Mirowski M, Mower MM, Reid PR, Watkins L, Langer A (1982) The automatic implantable defibrillator. PACE 5:384–401
14. Tacker WA Jr, Geddes LA (eds) (1980) The automatic implantable defibrillator (AID). In: Electrical defibrillation. CRC, Boca Raton, pp 167–178
15. Chapman PD, Wetherbee JN, Vetter JW, Troup P, Souza J (1988) Strength-duration curves of fixed pulse width variable tilt truncated exponential waveforms for nonthoracotomy internal defibrillation in dogs. PACE 11:1045–1050
16. Wiggers CJ (1940) The physiologic basis for cardiac resuscitation from ventricular fibrillation – method for serial defibrillation. Am Heart J 20:413
17. Orias O (1953) Posible mecanismo de la defibrilación miocárdica por contrachoque eléctrico. Acta Physiol Pharmacol Latinoam 3:147–150
18. Kugelberg J (1967) Ventricular defibrillation – a new aspect. Acta Chir Scand Suppl 372:1–93
19. Resnekov L, Norman J, Lord P, Sowton E (1968) Ventricular defibrillation by monophasic trapezoidal-shaped double-pulses of low electrical energy. Cardiovasc Res 3:261–264
20. Geddes LA, Tacker WA, McFarlane JR (1973) Ventricular defibrillation with single and twin pulses of half-sinusoidal current. J Appl Physiol 34:8–11
21. Moore TW, DiMeo FN, Dubin SE (1978) The effect of shock separation time on multiple-shock defibrillation. Med Instrum 12:31–33
22. Bourland JD, Tacker WA, Wessale JL, Kallok MJ, Graf JE, Geddes ME (1986) Sequential pulse defibrillation for implantable defibrillators. Med Instrum 20:138

23. Jones DL, Klein GJ, Guiraudon GM, Sharma AD, Kallok MJ, Bourland JD, Tacker WA (1986) Internal cardiac defibrillation in man: Pronounced improvement with sequential pulse delivery to two different lead orientations. Circulation 73:484–491
24. Jones DL, Klein GJ, Guiraudon GM, Sharma AD, Yee R, Kallok MJ (1988) Prediction of defibrillation success from a single defibrillation threshold measurement with sequential pulses and two current pathways in humans. Circulation 78:1144–1149
25. Bardou AL, Degonde J, Birkui PJ, Auger P, Chesnais J-M, Duriez M (1988) Reduction of energy required for defibrillation by delivering shocks in orthogonal directions in the dog. PACE 11:1990–1995
26. Jones DL, Klein GJ, Kallok MJ (1985) Improved internal defibrillation with twin pulse sequential energy delivery to different lead orientations in pigs. Am J Cardiol 55:821
27. Jones DL, Klein GJ, Rattes MF, Sohla A, Sharma AD (1988) Internal cardiac defibrillation: Single and sequential pulses and a variety of lead orientations. PACE 11:583–591
28. Jones DL, Klein GJ, Guiraudon GM, Sharma AD, Bourland JD, Tacker WA, Kallok MJ (1985) Improved internal cardiac defibrillation in man using sequential pulse countershock energy delivery. J Am Coll Cardiol 5:457 (abstr)
29. Chang MS, Inoue H, Kallok MJ, Zipes DP (1986) Double and triple sequential shocks reduce ventricular defibrillation threshold in dogs with and without myocardial infarction. J Am Coll Cardiol 8:1393
30. Kallok MJ (1987) Energy reduction for implantable defibrillation using a sequential pulse method. In: Breithardt G, Borggrefe M, Zipes DP (eds) Nonpharmacological therapy of tachyarrhythmias. Futura, Mount Kisco, pp 465–475
31. Gurvich NL, Markarychev VA (1967) Defibrillation of the heart with biphasic electrical impulses. Kardiologia 7:109–112
32. Schuder JC, McDaniel WC, Stoeckle H (1984) Defibrillation of 100-kg calves with asymmetrical, bidirectional, rectangular pulses. Cardiovasc Res 18:419–426
33. Flaker GC, Schuder JC, McDaniel WC, Stoeckle H, Dbeis M (1989) Superiority of biphasic shocks in the defibrillation of dogs by epicardial patches and catheter electrodes. Am Heart J 118:288–291
34. Dixon EG, Tang ASL, Wolf PD, Meador JT, Fine MJ, Calfee RV, Ideker RE (1987) Improved defibrillation threshold with large contoured epicardial electrodes and biphasic waveforms. Circulation 76:1176–1184
35. Chapman PD, Vetter JW, Souza JJ, Troup PJ, Wetherbee JN, Hoffmann RG (1988) Comparative efficacy of monophasic and biphasic truncated exponential shocks for nonthoracotomy internal defibrillation in dogs. J Am Coll Cardiol 12:739–745
36. Tang ASL, Yabe S, Wharton JM, Dolker M, Smith WM, Ideker RE (1989) Ventricular defibrillation using biphasic waveforms: The importance of phasic duration. J Am Coll Cardiol 13:207–214
37. Chapman PD, Vetter JW, Souza JJ, Wetherbee JN, Troup PJ (1989) Comparison of monophasic with single and dual capacitor biphasic waveforms

for nonthoracotomy canine internal defibrillation. J Am Coll Cardiol 14:242–245
38. Kavanagh KM, Tang ASL, Rollins DL, Smith WM, Ideker RE (1989) Comparison of the internal defibrillation thresholds for monophasic and double and single capacitor biphasic waveforms. J Am Coll Cardiol 14:1343–1349
39. Bardy GH, Ivey TD, Allen MD, Johnson G, Mehra R, Greene L (1989) A prospective randomized evaluation of biphasic versus monophasic waveform pulses on defibrillation efficacy in humans. J Am Coll Cardiol 14:728–733
40. Winkle RA, Mead RH, Ruder MA, Gaudiani V, Buch WS, Pless B, Sweeney M, Schmidt P (1989) Improved low energy defibrillation efficacy in man with the use of a biphasic truncated exponential waveform. Am Heart J 117:122–127
41. Lesigne C, Levy B, Saumont R, Birkui P, Bardou A, Rubin B (1976) An energy-time analysis of ventricular fibrillation and defibrillation thresholds with internal electrodes. Med Biol Eng 14:617–622
42. Jones JL, Proskauer CC, Paull WK, Lepeschkin E, Jones RE (1980) Ultrastructural injury to chick myocardial cells in vitro following "electric countershock". Circ Res 46:387–394
43. Jones JL, Lepeschkin E, Jones RE, Rush S (1978) Response of cultured myocardial cells to countershock-type electric field stimulation. Am J Physiol 235:H214–H222
44. Pansegrau DG, Abboud FM (1970) Hemodynamic effects of ventricular defibrillation. J Clin Invest 49:282–297
45. Dahl CF, Ewy GA, Warner ED, Thomas ED (1974) Myocardial necrosis from direct current countershock: effect of paddle size and time interval between discharge. Circulation 50:956–961
46. Chen P-S, Wolf PD, Claydon FJ, Dixon EG, Vidaillet HJ Jr, Danieley ND, Pilkimngton T, Ideker RE (1986) The potential gradient field created by epicardial defibrillation electrodes in dogs. Circulation 74:626–636
47. Wharton JM, Wolf PD, Ideker RE (1987) Cardiac potential gradient fields generated by single, combined, and sequential shocks during ventricular defibrillation. PACE 10:406 (abstr)
48. Jones JL, Jones RE (1983) Improved defibrillator waveform safety factor with biphasic waveforms. Am J Physiol 245:H60–H65
49. Negovsky VA, Smerdov AA, Tabak VY, Venin IV, Bogushevich MS (1980) Criteria of efficiency and safety of the defibrillating impulse. Resuscitation 8:53–67
50. Jones JL, Jones RE (1984) Decreased defibrillator-induced dysfunction with biphasic rectangular waveforms. Am J Physiol 247:H792–H796
51. Yabe S, Smith WM, Daubert JP, Wolf PD, Rollins DL, Ideker RE (1990) Conduction disturbances caused by high current density electric fields. Circ Res 66:1190–1203
52. Jones JL, Jones RE, Balasky G (1987) Improved cardiac cell excitation with symmetrical biphasic defibrillator waveforms. Am J Physiol 253: H1418–H1424
53. Akiyama T (1981) Intracellular recording of in situ ventricular cells during ventricular fibrillation. Am J Physiol 140:H465–H471

54. Cranefield PF, Hoffman BF (1958) Propagated repolarization in heart muscle. J Gen Physiol 41:633–649
55. Lerman BB, Halperin HR, Tsitlik JE, Brin K, Clark CW, Deale OC (1987) Relationship between canine transthoracic impedance and defibrillation threshold: evidence for current-based defibrillation. J Clin Invest 80: 797–803
56. Ideker RE, Tang ASL, Frazier DW, Shibata N, Chen P-S, Wharton JM (1991) Ventricular defibrillation: basic concepts. In: El-Sherif N, Samet P (eds) Cardiac pacing. Harcourt, Brace Jovanovich, Orlando (in press)
57. Shibata N, Chen P-S, Dixon EG, Wolf PD, Danieley ND, Smith WM, Ideker RE (1988) Influence of shock strength and timing on induction of ventricular arrhythmias in dogs. Am J Physiol 255:H891–H901
58. Chen P-S, Wolf PD, Dixon EG, Danieley ND, Frazier DW, Smith WM, Ideker RE (1988) Mechanism of ventricular vulnerability to single premature stimuli in open chest dogs. Circ Res 62:1191–1209
59. Frazier DW, Wolf PD, Wharton JM, Tang ASL, Smith WM, Ideker RE (1989) Stimulus-induced critical point: mechanism for the electrical initiation of reentry in normal canine myocardium. J Clin Invest 83:1039–1052
60. Fabiato A, Coumel P, Gourgon R, Saumont R (1967) Le seuil de réponse synchrone des fibres myocardiques. Application à la comparaison expérimentale de l'efficacité des différentes formes de chocs électriques de défibrillation. Arch Mal Coeur 60:527–544
61. Chen P-S, Shibata N, Dixon EG, Martin RO, Ideker RE (1986) Comparison of the defibrillation threshold and the upper limit of ventricular vulnerability. Circulation 73:1022–1028
62. Wharton JM, Richard VJ, Murry CE Jr, Dixon EG, Reimer KA, Meador J, Smith WM, Ideker RE (1990) Electrophysiologic effects in vivo of monophasic and biphasic stimuli in normal and infarcted dogs. PACE 13: 1158–1172
63. Kavanagh KM, Duff HJ, Clark R, Robinson K, Rahmberg M, Gillis AM, Mitchell LB, Wyse DG, Giles WR (1987) Decreased energy requirements for cardiac pacing using biphasic stimulation. Circulation 76:IV–242 (abstr)
64. Daubert JP, Frazier DW, Tang ASL, Hagler JA, Smith WM, Ideker RE (1988) Biphasic shocks excite refractory myocardium less effectively than monophasic shocks. PACE 11:503 (abstr)
65. Feeser SA, Tang ASL, Kavanagh KM, Rollins DL, Smith WM, Wolf PD, Ideker RE (1990) Strength-duration and probability of success curves for defibrillation with biphasic waveforms. Circulation 82:2128–2141
66. Klee M, Plonsey R (1976) Stimulation of spheroidal cells – the role of cell shape. IEEE Trans Biomed Eng 23:347–354
67. Ideker RE, Frazier DW, Krassowska W, Chen P-S, Wharton JM (1990) Physiologic effects of electrical stimulation in cardiac muscle. In: Saksena S, Goldschlager N (eds) Electrical therapy for cardiac arrhythmias: pacing, antitachycardia devices, catheter ablation. Saunders, Philadelphia, pp 357–370
68. Ideker RE, Chen P-S, Shibata N, Colavita PG, Wharton JM (1987) Current concepts of the mechanism of ventricular defibrillation. In: Breithardt G,

Borggrefe M, Zipes D (eds) Non-pharmacological therapy of tachyarrhythmias. Futura, Mount Kisco, pp 449–464
69. Daubert JP, Frazier DW, Wolf PD, Franz MR, Smith WM, Ideker RE (1991) Response of relatively refractory canine myocardium to monophasic and biphasic shock. Circulation 18:2522–2538
70. Jones JL, Sheffield C, Jones RE, Swartz J (1990) Short duration biphasic defibrillator waveforms inhibit refractory period responses. Circulation 82:III-642 (abstr)
71. Jones JL, Jones RE (1989) Improved safety factors for triphasic defibrillator waveforms. Circ Res 64:1172–1177
72. Chapman PD, Wetherbee JN, Vetter JW, Troup PJ (1988) Comparison of monophasic, biphasic, and triphasic truncated pulses for non-thoracotomy internal defibrillation. J Am Coll Cardiol 11:57A (abstr)

Prerequisites for the Safety and Efficacy of the Implantable Cardioverter Defibrillator

A. W. Nathan

The implantable cardioverter defibrillator (ICD) has been a major advance in the treatment of malignant ventricular arrhythmias. Many such devices have been implanted and the efficacy and value of these devices is now beyond dispute.

In recent times, the value of these devices has been increased because of a variety of technical advances. Defibrillators are used in patients who have syncopal ventricular fibrillation and tachycardia as well as nonsyncopal ventricular tachycardia. In addition, some patients may have bradyarrhythmias and also a variety of superventricular tachyarrhythmias. In order for the devices to function optimally, there are a number of major prerequisites. These are summarised in Table 1.

Arrhythmia Recognition

The arrhythmias that require recognition include: bradycardias, sinus tachycardias, pathological supraventricular tachycardias, ventricular tachycardias of different morphologies and rates, and ventricular fibrillation. In addition, normal sinus rhythm needs to be recognised. Different initial detection and redetection criteria are needed as different decision making processes may be necessary for the initial detection of an arrhythmia and its subsequent redetection, if therapy is not successful. Devices also need to be able to recognise and adapt to nonsus-

Table 1. ICD – Prerequisites for optimal function

- Recognition of different arrhythmias
- Appropriate therapy for each arrhythmia
- Data logging of events
- Small, long-lasting and inexpensive
- Easy and safe to implant

tained arrhythmias. Finally, some means of recognising haemodynamic collapse is important because this fundamentally alters the type of therapy delivered.

In order to recognise a rhythm, various aspects can be considered. The heart rate of course is important and this must be accurately measured and this requires sensitive sensing circuits, preferably with automatic gain control. Manipulations of heart rate have also been shown to be valuable and these include the rate of change of heart rate in order to try and detect sudden onset of tachyarrythmias, the use of rate stability in order to try and detect rhythms such as atrial fibrillation and if these are used, it is often valuable to have a "time-out" function of some sort or a sustained high rate criteria in order that prolonged arrhythmias, can eventually be treated as malign if they continue. Numerous efforts have been made to analyse electrogram sequence in various ways, including looking at atrioventricular differences or similarities in order to diagnose supraventricular from ventricular arrhythmias, but this may be problematic, particularly if ventricular tachycardia has 1 : 1 VA conduction. In addition, we have seen ventricular fibrillation coexist with atrial fibrillation and, of course, this can be extremely confusing to a device.

Various physiological sensors can be used in order to try and sense whether a tachycardia is appropriate and whether it is causing haemodynamic collapse or not. Most sensors used for rate-responsive pacemakers can be used as reverse sensors, i.e. if the rate is fast without the sensor showing any change, then pathological tachycardia, rather than sinus tachycardia can be assumed. An example would be an activity sensor and if heart rate was up, but the activity sensor showed no change in activity, this could be assumed to be pathological. This would of course misdiagnose sinus tachycardias due to stress, and could also misdiagnose pathological tachycardia occurring during exercise. In addition, these sensors are probably in general too slow and are certainly not sensitive nor specific enough to allow proper decision making processes. However, sensors such as pressure sensors have certainly been used in experimental situations and the long-term efficacy of the sensors has recently been shown. These sensors may be very valuable to look at haemodynamic collapse.

Appropriate Therapy

When considering treatment for arrhythmias, a number of different therapies may be considered. If there is a bradycardia, this may require pacing. Sinus tachycardia requires no action and supraventricular tachycardias should be treated as appropriate and of course, this may include some sort of pacing therapy for a regular supraventricular tachycardia. By and large, most ventricular tachycardias may be treated by pacing, although if they are rapid, or if pacing has been shown to be proarrhythmic or previously unsuccessful, then low energy shocks may be preferred. If the ventricular tachycardia is refractory, high energy shocks may be necessary and, of course, for ventricular fibrillation, shocks are the only therapy applicable.

Most authors consider that pacing for bradycardias should be incorporated in all modern implantable cardioverter defibrillators and indeed, this is the trend with most new models. Such pacing may be needed because the patients are frankly bradycardic, or because some patients may become bradycardic, particularly if additional drug therapy is neccessary. Some authorities have made great play of post-therapy bradycardias which may need pacing, but in fact, most of these bradycardias are very short lived and although pacing can be used it is often not necessary. There are of course problems with bradycardia pacing. The addition of bradycardia pacing and the necessity to sense asystole as well as fine ventricular fibrillation makes the decision-making processes for the device more difficult, particularly in terms of behaviour of the automatic gain control circuit. If the pacemaker is a ventricular only pacemaker, rather than dual chamber pacemaker, then the pacemaker syndrome may occur and of course, frequent or constant pacing will shorten the cell life of the device.

Diagnostic Functions

When following up patients with ICDs as much data as possible is useful in terms of making any adjustments to optimise function. It is certainly useful to know the number of interventions made, but it is even more useful to know the time and type of intervention and also the tachycardia type and rate. Some log of effective interventions is also useful and some devices are able to give us the precise timing of events, in terms of millisecond intervals, prior to intervention. Some newer devices are able to give us a "snapshot" of the electrogram when the arrhythmia is detected and one device is now able to give full electrogram retrieval for up to 2 min and this can include a variable time before and after the therapy has been given.

Physical Aspects

The size, life and cost of the devices are all important issues. The original Intec AID weighed 290 g and 162 ml, but more recent devices have weights down to 220 g and a volume of 140 ml. The life of a new unit is being projected as 5 or 6 years in comparison with the 1 or 2 years of the earlier devices and, although the costs are still relatively high in comparison with pacemakers, many more features are now available at a cost fairly similar to the cost of the simpler devices 2 or 3 years ago.

Implantation Factors

The standard implantation technique for a device requires direct access to the heart in order to place epicardial or pericardial patches. Approaches have included median sternotomy, anterior or lateral thoracotomies, subcostal approaches and a subxiphoid approach. However, the transvenous approach has been under trial for some while and recently several devices have been implanted using this approach. There have been problems. Thresholds tend to be higher and in many cases unacceptably high. Electrode stability has been a problem and some electrodes have shown major mechanical weakness and have fractured.

There is no doubt that the epicardial approaches all have a small but significant morbidity and mortality and they are expensive in terms of time, skill and hospital costs. A transvenous technique should be safer, faster and cheaper, but despite the excitement with the development of transvenous techniques, it is probable that transvenous methods will not be suitable for every case for many years to come.

There has been some concern expressed concerning the reliability of newer devices. Most new devices are much more complex and have more components and most are software based and any minor change to an algorithm can cause major errors. However, constructional techniques have improved recently and although there may be more electronic components, there may be many less discrete parts than before.

There has also been an argument that tiered therapy devices which include pacing as well as large shocks can delay the delivery of shocks which are known to be life saving and that lives may be lost because of this. Our own experience, and that of others, has not shown this to be so. It has already been mentioned that bradycardia pacing can complicate the function of the automatic gain control, but this should be soluble in most units. Finally, it must always be remembered that, in complex devices, programming by physicians or others may cause an otherwise satisfactory device to be ineffective for any given patient, and careful timing is essential.

Conclusion

Not withstanding all these limitations, this author, having used several of the new devices, has no doubt that the various advances in new devices are useful in terms of patient management, prevent patient trauma, and, if used intelligently, do not provide any danger to the patient, but instead improve patient care.

The Role of Leads and Electrodes

J. E. Shapland, D. J. Lang

Ventricular arrhythmias are the leading cause of sudden cardiac death in the western world, claiming approximately 400000 lives per year in the United States alone. In 1985, after a decade of research, development and clinical investigation, the automatic implantable cardioverter/defibrillator (AICD) was released for general clinical use. Today, the AICD has proven to be successful in treatment of ventricular tachycardias, including ventricular fibrillation [1, 2].

Since the first research efforts, much has been learned about defibrillation and the underlying tachyarrhythmias. Factors that influence the success of defibrillation shocks include the underlying physiologic substrate of the heart, the pulse waveform of the shock, and the electrode system.

The lead system and type of electrodes employed are especially critical. A uniform current distribution in excess of some minimum value is necessary for defibrillation to occur. Ideally the defibrillation electrodes are positioned so that current pathways provide a uniform voltage gradient or current density over as much of the heart as possible.

Leads not only deliver energy, but they also sense intrinsic heart activities, including the ventricular tachycardias or fibrillation. Coupled with the implantable device, they must be able to distinguish ventricular tachyarrhythmias from benign tachycardias, including discrimination of ventricular from atrial tachycardias or high rates resulting from exercise.

Sensing Electrodes

Since all present detection schemes are completely or partially based on heart rate, the fundamental requirement of device sensing is the ability to accurately count the rate of the rhythm, whether tachycardia or normal sinus. A particular challenge is that signal amplitudes can drop in order of magnitude when going from a normal rhythm to a ventricular tachycardia. The sensing leads and device must also be sensitive enough to interpret heart rate over a range of 10:1 (40–400 beats/min). For this reason, closely spaced bipolar electrodes have been found to be optimal for rate counting. Such an electrode configuration provides discrete lead sensing with relatively little far field interference. Most implanted defibrillator systems incorporate two myocardial electrodes for rate sensing. They are placed no further than 1 cm apart to form a relatively closely spaced bipolar lead. Transvenous bipolar leads, with a 1.0 cm tip to ring separation, are alternatives for rate sensing. Since signal characteristics change with electrode size, spacing and location, it is important that signals be properly matched to internal implantable cardioverter defibrillator device circuitry.

In addition to rate counting, detection criteria may require a morphological analysis. The first AICD systems used a probability density function in which signals are taken from the patch electrodes for a more global picture of the electrical activity level. Newer models have modified the probability density function but still use signals provided through the shocking electrodes. To allow other new morphological sensing, different types of electrode systems may be needed.

Future implantable cardioverter defibrillator systems will have the capability to discriminate ventricular from atrial arrhythmias. Several potential discrimination techniques involve analysis of atrial and ventricular rates and associated timing relationships [3, 4]. Such algorithms will require sensing of both atrial and ventricular chambers. Atrial sensing is more difficult due to the low signal amplitudes, especially during atrial arrhythmias such as atrial fibrillation.

Use of an atrial lead plus a ventricular lead and transvenous shocking lead may be problematic. Brownlee [5] and others [6] have investigated various designs of floating or noncontacting atrial electrode designs. Electrograms from these electrodes were of relatively short duration with high slew rates. Although chronic signal amplitudes were reported to exceed 3 mV, position sensitivity has also been reported. Reduced signal amplitudes associated with atrial arrhythmias may result in significant sensing problems.

Another potential problem involves sensing immediately after the defibrillating shock. Several researchers have demonstrated temporary cellular dysfunction following high energy shocks. Jones and Jones demonstrated that chick cell aggregates were temporarily stunned following defibrillation shocks [7]. Ideker et al. reported conduction delays in tissue receiving high energy shocks greater than 64 V/cm [8]. Thus, defibrillation may cause significant changes in electrogram amplitude and slew rates in tissue near the shocking electrodes, causing difficulties in post-shock sensing.

Defibrillation Electrodes

Early studies indicated that ventricular fibrillation conversion was achieved when shocks depolarized a critical mass of the heart [9, 10]. More recent studies reveal a uniform voltage gradient in excess of 6 V/cm in necessary for defibrillation to occur with monophasic waveforms [11]. Uniformity of current density is important since:

1) low gradient areas contribute to the continuation or reinitiation of ventricular fibrillation [12] and
2) high current areas may induce temporary damage [7, 8] that then may cause sensing difficulties, set-up areas of reinitiation of fibrillation, or even potentially cause permanent damage [13].

With two epicardial patches, the heart is between the electrodes, so most of the current goes directly into heart tissue and gives more uniform current density throughout the ventricular mass. In this case, defibrillation can occur with relatively less energy [14]. The position and size of the patches also influence energy requirements. Another way to provide uniform current distribution and lower defibrillation energy requirements is to have multiple patch electrodes on the heart.

One of the requirements of future defibrillation electrodes is that they be easy to implant, eliminating the need for thoracotomy. These transvenous lead systems can be designed in several ways. A single catheter can provide both sensing and defibrillation current. A system of separate leads could be used for sensing with other leads in the right ventricular apex, the superior vena cava, or other positions within the heart for defibrillation. Transvenous leads can also be used in conjunction with a subcutaneous patch electrode placed in the left thoracic region.

Echt et al. conducted canine studies using a special research defibrillation catheter consisting of a proximal electrode in the superior vena cava/right atrial (SVC/RA) region and a distal electrode in the right ventricular (RV) apex [15]. They compared the defibrillation thresholds (DFTs) of the lead alone to the lead plus a subcutaneous patch electrode and found a significant reduction in DFTs with the third electrode. In their testing, shocks were delivered from the RV electrode to the SVC/RA plus the subcutaneous patch electrode. Other canine studies revealed that further energy reductions could be obtained by shocking from both transvenous electrodes (RV+SVC/RA) to the subcutaneous patch [16]. However, similar studies in the pig and human have shown considerable individual variability, with no consistent decrease in energy requirements.

Initial clinical trials on a transvenous approach with the Endotak catheter from Cardiac Pacemakers, Inc. (CPI) indicate success in approximately 70% of patients with a defibrillation threshold of 15 J with monophasic waveforms. While both two and three electrode configurations were tested, the majority of patients were implanted with the three electrode system with shocks given from the RV electrode to the RVC/RA and subcutaneous patch electrodes [17].

Even though catheter systems are effective, they tend to produce large variations in current distribution. To help overcome this issue, future configurations may include multiple electrodes not only in the right ventricular apex and SVC/RA, but also in the outflow tract or the coronary sinus.

Chang et al. investigated numerous electrode configurations and reported on the importance of electrode position for defibrillation [18]. Their studies indicated that electrode position and resulting fields were more important than delivering the shocks in a temporal or sequential manner.

These multielectrode systems, catheter electrodes, patches, and combination systems provide additional current pathways and lower defibrillation energy, primarily due to more uniform fields over the ventricular mass. In other words, current is more evenly distributed, resulting in less chance of low gradient areas that can cause failed defibrillation or high gradient areas that can result in temporary dysfunction, sensing abnormalities, or even reinitiation of fibrillation.

Although multiple electrode systems tend to produce more uniform fields, each individual electrode, whether on a catheter, internal patch or external paddle [19], exhibits high current density at the edges or boundary of the electrode. Specific patch designs, i.e., size, materials, etc., can create more uniform charge transfer or current density from the electrodes, and thereby, provide more uniform current to the heart.

A new lead concept is being developed to minimize implant surgery for epicardial or intrapericardial implant. This minimally invasive lead system is inserted through a small, subxiphoid puncture. The lead would enter the pericardium where it would spiral between the pericardium and the heart to function like a patch on the left and/or right ventricles of the heart. This would provide a large surface electrode on the heart without necessitating a full thoracotomy.

Other Issues

Whether electrodes are patches or transvenous systems, they must provide chronic long-term reliability. Mechanically, they must be reliable to last many years because defibrillators are implanted in a much younger patient population than are pacemakers. The ability to remove the leads, whether due to infection, lead failure, or other reasons, must also be considered.

Epicardial patches, whatever their size, have the potential to abrade the epicardial coronary vessels, which is why some surgeons are now implanting patches on the outside of the pericardium. Also, large patch electrodes could be difficult to place on diseased hearts that are enlarged or that have aneurysms or vascular grafts. Large patches that cover the majority of the heart become an insulator or shield around the heart, making external defibrillation difficult.

Implantable cardioverter defibrillators with back-up pacing capability are now being implanted. High energy shocks not only cause post-shock sensing abnormalities, but also transient increases in local pacing threshold [20, 21]. Therefore, lead position and pacing outputs will have to be adjusted to prevent associated problems.

Future Systems

While the implantable cardioverter defibrillator has proven successful, future lead systems will provide improved arrhythmia detection and discrimination and more efficient defibrillation. Needs for future development of lead systems are predictable. A future lead system must have dedicated sensing electrodes and multiple shocking electrodes and allow transvenous implantation.

There is a need for a bipolar myocardial electrode for obtaining discrete localized sensing of rate counting, thus alleviating the requirement of two myocardial leads commonly used during present implants.

Also, in the future, shocking leads as well as rate sensing leads may be used to obtain additional morphological analysis to discriminate ventricular rhythms from atrial tachycardias or to sense atrial tachyrhythmias and normal sinus rhythm in the atrium.

New lead designs will overcome potential sensing problems associated with temporary, localized tissue damage due to high current density around the shocking electrodes. These same designs will also positively influence post-shock pacing thresholds.

In addition, hemodynamic sensors will be added to the lead systems. These could be monitors for continuous pressure, volume or other hemodynamic sensors, such as continuous stroke volume monitoring by intracardiac impedance for discriminating unstable from stable ventricular tachycardias. The resulting data would be used to direct appropriate therapy for unstable or stable tachycardias:

1) Patients with unstable tachycardia could be treated aggressively with a high energy shock and

2) stable patients could be treated less aggressively, for example with antitachycardia pacing.

In the future, new electrode designs and position will optimize current distribution. Radically different subcutaneous electrodes will be designed to enhance defibrillation. Present electrode materials are either titanium or platinum. New electrode materials and designs will aid in charge transfer and be more efficient electrodes. There may be areas with a surface activation material to increase surface area or certain material that can effectively transfer the high currents associated with defibrillation [22].

Advances in lead systems will result in patients receiving more reliable arrhythmia discrimination and appropriate therapy. Significantly lower defibrillation energy requirements, based on new leads/electrodes, will decrease device size, extend device longevity and reduce patient discomfort. Implantation will be simplified due to transvenous lead systems and smaller devices. These changes will result in wider therapy acceptance, thus fulfilling the true lifesaving potential of the implantable cardioverter defibrillator.

References

1. Mirowski M, Mower MM, Reid PR, Watkins L, Langer A (1982) The automatic defibrillator: new modality for treatment of life-threatening ventricular arrhythmias. PACE 5:384–401
2. Mirowski M, Reid PR, Winkle RA, Mower MM, Watkins L Jr, Stinson EB, Griffith LSC, Kallman CH, Weisfeldt ML (1983) Mortality in patients with implanted automatic defibrillators. Ann Intern Med 98:585–588
3. Arzbaecher R, Bump TE, Jenkins J, Glick K, Munkenbeck F, Brown J, Nandhakumar N (1984) Automatic tachycardia recognition. PACE 7:541–547
4. Camm AJ, Davies DW, Ward DE (1987) Tachycardia recognition by implantable electronic devices. PACE 7:1175–1190
5. Brownlee RR (1989) Toward optimizing the detection of atrial depolarization with floating bipolar electrodes. PACE 12:431–442
6. Goldreyer BN, Shapland E, Cannom DS, Wyman MG (1983) A new lead for improved atrial sensing in DDD pacing. Circulation 68:III–379
7. Jones JL, Jones RE (1984) Decreased defibrillator-induced dysfunction with biphasic rectangular waveforms. Am J Physiol 247:H792
8. Yabe S, Daubert JP, Wolf PD, Rollins DL, Smith WM, Ideker RE (1988) Effect of strong shock fields on activation propagation heart defibrillation electrodes. Circulation 78:II–154
9. Mower MM, Mirowski M, Spear JF, Moore EN (1974) Patterns of ventricular activity during catheter defibrillation. Circulation 49:858–861

10. Zipes DP (1975) Electrophysiological mechanisms involved in ventricular fibrillation. Circulation 52:III – 120
11. Warton JM, Wolf PD, Chen PS, Bowling SD, Clayton FJ, Pilkington TC, Ideker RE (1986) Is an absolute minimum potential gradient required for ventricular defibrillation? Circulation 74:342
12. Chen P-S, Wolf PD, Claydon FJ, Dixon EG, Vidaillet HJ Jr, Danieley ND, Pilkington TC, Ideker RE (1986) The potential gradient field created by epicardial defibrillation electrodes in dogs. Circulation 74:626 – 636
13. Dahl CF, Ewy GA, Warner ED, Thomas ED (1974) Myocardial necrosis from direct current countershock: effect of paddle electrode size and time interval between discharges. Circulation 50:950 – 961
14. Troup PJ, Chapman PD, Olinger GN, Kleinman LH (1985) The implanted defibrillator: relation of defibrillating lead configuration and clinical variables to defibrillation threshold. J Am Coll Cardiol 6:1315
15. Echt DS, Sepulveda NG, Wikswo JP Jr (1986) Development of a mathematical model of defibrillation current distributions. Circulation 74:II – 341
16. Shapland JE, Dawson AK, Bach SB Jr, Lang DJ (1987) Improved defibrillation efficacy in the dog with an equipotential transvenous electrode configuration. Circulation 76:IV – 462
17. Bach SM Jr, Barstad J, Harper N, Mayer D, Moser S, Smutka M, Theis R, Wollins J (1989) Initial clinical experience: ENDOTAK™ – implantable transvenous defibrillator system. J Am Coll Cardiol 13:65 A
18. Chang MS, Inoue H, Kallock MJ, Zipes DP (1986) Double and triple sequential shocks reduce ventricular defibrillation threshold in dogs with or without myocardial infarction. J Am Cardiol 8:1339 – 1405
19. Kim Y, Fahy JB, Tupper BJ (1986) Optimal electrode design for electrosurgery, defibrillation, and external cardiac pacing. IEEE Trans Biomed Eng MBE 33:845 – 853
20. Rubin L, Hudson P, Driller J, Parsonnet V (1976) Pacing thresholds immediately after defibrillation. Circulation 54::II – 168
21. Yee R, Jones DL, Klein GJ (1984) Pacing threshold changes after transvenous catheter countershock. Am J Cardiol 53:503
22. Alt E, Theres H, Heinz M, Albrecht K, Georg H, Bloemer H (1991) A new approach towards defibrillation electrodes: Highly conductive isotropic carbon fibers. PACE 14:1923 – 1928

PART IV

The Role of the Automatic Implantable Cardioverter Defibrillator in the Treatment of Ventricular Tachyarrhythmia

Long-Term Clinical Results with the Implantable Defibrillator

E. Veltri, L. S. C. Griffith, G. Tomaselli, R. Lewis,
J. Juanteguy, L. Watkins, T. Guarnieri

Introduction

Sudden cardiac death is the leading cause of cardiac mortality in patients with heart disease. Approximately 400000 such deaths occur in the United States alone each year [1]. It has been established that the vast majority of sudden cardiac deaths are due to ventricular tachyarrhythmias, with only approximately 20% of such cases due to identifiable etiology such as acute myocardial infarction [2, 3]. Tragically, when out-of-hospital cardiac arrest occurs, only one of five individuals will survive to hospital discharge. Those patients at high risk for sudden cardiac death are survivors of out-of-hospital cardiac arrest without identifiable causes and patients with recurrent ventricular tachycardia with underlying heart disease, particularly those with remote myocardial infarction with associated poor left ventricular function and those with cardiomyopathy. In such patients, the automatic implantable cardioverter defibrillator (AICD) has been the landmark breakthrough in therapy [4].

The objective of this paper is to review our long-term clinical results with the AICD in the treatment of patients with high risk of recurrent life-threatening ventricular tachyarrhythmias.

Historical Perspective

The concept of an automatic implantable device that would monitor cardiac rhythm continuously and automatically deliver an electrical discharge across the heart to terminate life-threatening ventricular tachyarrhythmias was first conceived by Dr. Michel Mirowski in the late 1960s. In 1968, Dr. Mirowski immigrated from Israel to Baltimore, assuming the position as Director, Coronary Care Unit at Sinai Hospital. Assisted by Dr. Morton Mower and others, the first model of the automatic implantable defibrillator was developed in 1969 [5]. The device was first successfully tested in a canine model [6] and following more than a decade of further testing and development, the first device was implanted in a human at The Johns Hopkins Hospital in 1980 [7]. After 5 years of subsequent clinical testing and further refinements, experience had demonstrated a significant reduction in expected mortality due to sudden cardiac death in high risk patients [8], leading to widespread use of the device following the approval of the United States Food and Drug Administration in 1985 [9].

Patient Selection

Although the criteria for implantation of the AICD has evolved over the last decade, certain indications and contraindications have remained constant in our patient selection experience.

Indications for AICD implantation include all of the following:

1) at least one previous documented episode of out-of-hospital hypotensive sustained ventricular tachycardia or ventricular fibrillation,
2) absence of identifiable, correctable cause of sustained ventricular tachyarrhythmias (such as acute myocardial infarction, electrolyte imbalance, or drug toxicity),
3) refractoriness to antiarrhythmic drug therapy as assessed by Holter monitoring and electrophysiologic testing, and
4) absence of other noncardiac medical illnesses limiting expected life span to less than 6 months.

In some instances, patients presenting with recurrent syncope of undocumented origin and refractory inducible sustained ventricular tachycardia or patients at high risk for sudden cardiac death awaiting heart transplantation in the not immediate future have undergone AICD implantation.

Contraindications to device implantation have included:

1) incessant ventricular tachyarrhythmias, and
2) patients with New York Heart Association class IV heart failure.

Preimplantation Evaluation

Prior to device implantation, virtually all patients have undergone cardiac diagnostic procedures to assess underlying cardiac substrate (coronary disease, cardiomyopathy, valvular disease, etc.) to exclude concomitant ischemic or valvular dysfunction which should be corrected and to assess the cardiac impulse initiation and conduction system.

Such testing at minimum should include:

1) 12-lead electrocardiogram,
2) echocardiography or radionuclide imaging of valvular and ventricular function,
3) exercise stress testing,
4) Holter monitoring,
5) coronary angiography, and
6) electrophysiologic testing.

Patient Population

From February 1980 through September 1990, 403 patients underwent automatic implantable defibrillator or AICD implantation at The Johns Hopkins Hospital and Sinai Hospital of Baltimore. Table 1 depicts the characteristics of our patient population.

There were 283 males and 120 females; the mean age was 59 years. Coronary artery disease was found in 73%, cardiomyopathy in 19% (including hypertrophic and sarcoid disease in three patients each), mitral valve prolapse or primary electrical disease in 6%. The mean left ventricular ejection fraction was moderately depressed at 35%. There were 296 patients (73%) who had experienced a previous cardiac arrest,

Table 1. Patient population

Total	403
Male/female	283/120
Age (years)	59 ± 13
Cardiac disease	
Coronary	295 (73%)
Cardiomyopathy	77 (19%)
Mitral prolapse	11 (3%)
Primary electrical	11 (3%)
Long QT	4 (<1%)
Valvular	3 (<1%)
Spasm	2 (<1%)
Ejection fraction (%)	35 ± 17
Previous drugs failed	3.3 ± 1.9
Prior sudden deaths	1.5 ± 1.0

with a mean of 1.5 prior sudden cardiac deaths with resuscitation per patient.

At baseline electrophysiologic heart catheterization, sustained ventricular tachycardia or fibrillation was induced in 69%, nonsustained ventricular tachycardia ($\geq$5 beats, <30 s duration, and self-terminating) in 11%, and no inducible ventricular tachyarrhythmias in 20%. Our programmed ventricular stimulation protocol has previously been reported [10]. Patients had failed mean 3.3 serial antiarrhythmic drug trials in an effort to suppress spontaneous and inducible ventricular tachyarrhythmias.

Operative Approach

There are presently four conventional approaches for AICD implantation [11]. Patients requiring concomitant cardiac surgery (coronary bypass, aneurysmectomy, valvular replacement or repair) undergo a median sternotomy. Patients with a history of previous cardiac surgery, pericarditis, or enlarged hearts undergo anterior thoracotomy. Other patients may either undergo a subcostal or subxiphoidal approach.

In our patient population 169 patients (42%) had anterior thoracotomy, 108 patients (27%) had median sternotomy, 101 patients (25%) had subxiphoid, and 25 patients (6%) had subcostal approaches.

AICD implantation was the sole operative procedure in 305 patients (76%). Concomitant cardiac surgery was performed in 24%. Coronary artery bypass grafting was performed in 52 patients (13%), coronary artery bypass grafting plus subendocardial resection and aneurysmectomy in 23 patients (6%), coronary artery bypass grafting and aneurysmectomy in 7 patients (2%), subendocardial resection and aneurysmectomy in 12 patients (3%), coronary artery bypass grafting and mitral valve replacement in 2 patients, and mitral valve replacement in 2 patients.

There were 17 patients (4.2%) who died within 30 days postoperatively, never leaving the hospital. Operative deaths were due to incessant ventricular tachyarrhythmias in 9, congestive heart failure in 3, acute myocardial infarction in 1, and noncardiac death in 4.

Clinical Outcome

Following a mean 23 day hospitalization, 386 patients were discharged. Of these, 20% were discharged on class I antiarrhythmic drugs, 30% were discharged on no specific antiarrhythmic drugs, 30% were discharged on amiodarone (70% of whom were on amiodarone alone and 30% on amiodarone plus class I drugs), and 20% were discharged on a blinded placebo vs amiodarone protocol.

At 29±25 months (mean±standard deviation) follow-up, 230 patients (60%) had experienced at least one appropriate AICD discharge (i.e., associated with premonitory symptoms of presyncope, syncope, cardiac arrest, or electrocardiographic documentation of sustained ventricular tachyarrhythmia). Approximately 30% of patients experienced at least one asymptomatic or indeterminant AICD discharge. At follow-up,

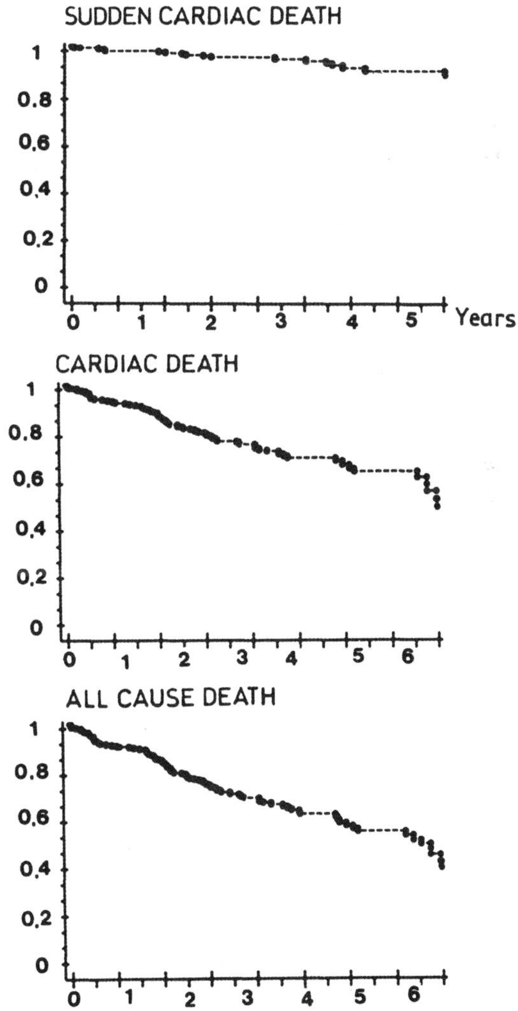

Fig. 1. The actuarial incidence of sudden cardiac death, cardiac death, and deaths from all causes

Table 2. Actuarial mortality

	1 Year	2 Year	3 Year	4 Year	5 Year
Sudden	1.7%	4.1%	5.5%	9.8%	10.6%
Cardiac	7.4%	17.2%	24.0%	30.5%	32.2%
Total	10.2%	21.2%	30.1%	36.5%	42.7%

284 patients were alive, 102 patients (26%) were dead. Cardiac deaths were congestive heart failure in 32, sudden cardiac death in 18, nonsudden arrhythmic (in-hospital from uncontrolled ventricular tachyarrhythmias following out-of-hospital AICD rescue) in 20, and acute myocardial infarction in 8. There were 24 patients who died from noncardiac cause.

Figure 1 and Table 2 depict the actuarial incidence of sudden cardiac death, cardiac death, and all causes of death. Sudden cardiac death was 1.7%, 5.5%, and 10.6% at 1, 3, and 5 years, respectively. Cardiac deaths were 7.4%, 24%, and 32.2% at 1, 3, and 5 years, respectively. Total deaths were 10.2%, 30.1%, and 42.7% at 1, 3, and 5 years, respectively.

Comparison to Other Therapies

The treatment of ventricular tachyarrhythmias includes antiarrhythmic drugs, surgical ablation of substrate, and device therapy. Certainly, empirical drug therapy would not be advised given the serious consequences of tachyarrhythmic recurrence. Previous historical control studies have revealed a 30%–45% recurrence of cardiac arrest in such patients [2, 3]. Overall, pharmacologic therapy as assessed by either noninvasive (Holter monitoring) or invasive (electrophysiologic testing) has not been shown to be highly effective in patients presenting with cardiac arrest, hemodynamically unstable sustained ventricular tachycardia, and moderate to severe left ventricular dysfunction [12, 13]. Furthermore, side effects from antiarrhythmic drugs are numerous and include aggravation of arrhythmias, i.e., proarrhythmia.

Surgical therapy includes heart transplantation (for those patients with class IV heart failure) and electrophysiologic map-guided endocardial resection. The latter surgical approach has a 12% operative mortality and approximate 20% arrhythmia recurrence at 2 years [14]. Notwithstanding, patients with noninducible ventricular tachycardia, cardiomyopathy, and those with poor left ventricular function are not optimal candidates for surgical resection.

The impressive reduction of expected sudden cardiac death incidence by the AICD in high risk patients from our present experience and others [15] has led investigators to propose the AICD as the "gold standard" therapy for cardiac arrest survivors [16].

We would propose that AICD implantation should be the therapy of first choice in:

1) patients with documented cardiac arrest, noninducible arrhythmia and poor left ventricular function (ejection fraction $<30\%$ or class II–III heart failure),
2) patients with hemodynamically compromising sustained ventricular tachycardia and poor left ventricular function, perhaps irrespective of response to electrophysiologic-guided drug therapy,
3) patients with sustained ventricular tachyarrhythmias and associated nonischemic cardiomyopathy, and
4) those patients in whom antiarrhythmic drug efficacy cannot be adequately assessed or in whom patient compliance with such therapy may be questionable.

Future Directions

A decade has now passed since the first human implant of the AICD. This device which delivers a high energy shock to automatically terminate life-threatening ventricular tachyarrhythmias has revolutionized therapy for patients at high risk for sudden cardiac death. As growing numbers of patients at risk are being identified and increasing numbers of hospital centers are developing clinical arrhythmia services with electrophysiologic testing facilities, AICD implantation will become the major treatment modality.

Research goals continue to include early identification of patients at high risk for sudden cardiac death and continued technological development of devices with multiple functions which will be able to prescribe a tiered approach for delivery of electrical treatment options. With improvement in technology and the competitive marketplace for industry, the cost of such therapy will also decrease, as will the cost per life-year saved [17].

Acknowledgement. We thank Ms. Linda Schenker for assistance in the preparation of this manuscript.

References

1. Kuller L (1969) Sudden death in arteriosclerotic heart disease: the case for preventive medicine. Am J Cardiol 24:617–642
2. Liberthson RR, Nagel EL, Hirshman JC (1975) Prehospital ventricular defibrillation. Prognosis and follow-up course. N Engl J Med 29:317
3. Shaffer WA, Cobb LA (1974) Recurrent ventricular fibrillation and modes of death in survivors of out-of-hospital ventricular fibrillation. N Engl J Med 293:259
4. Mirowski M (1985) The automatic implantable cardioverter-defibrillator: an overview. J Am Coll Cardiol 6:461–466
5. Mirowski M, Mower MM, Staewen WS et al. (1970) Standby automatic implantable defibrillator: an approach to prevention of sudden coronary death. Arch Intern Med 126:158–161
6. Mirowski M, Mower MM, Langer A et al. (1978) A chronically implanted system for automatic defibrillation in active to conscious dogs: experimental model for treatment of sudden death from ventricular fibrillation. Circulation 58:90–94
7. Mirowski M, Reid P, Mower MM et al. (1980) Termination of malignant ventricular arrhythmias with an implanted automatic defibrillator in human beings. N Engl J Med 303:322–324
8. Echt DS, Armstrong K, Schmidt P et al. (1985) Clinical experience, complications, and survival in 70 patients with the automatic implantable cardioverter-defibrillator. Circulation 71:289–296
9. Department of Health and Human Services (1986) Health Care Financing Administration. Section 35–85. Implantation of automatic defibrillators, January, 1986
10. Veltri EP, Mower MM, Mirowski M et al. (1989) Followup of patients with ventricular tachyarrhythmia treated with the automatic implantable cardioverter-defibrillator: programmed electrical stimulation results do not predict clinical outcome. J Electrophysiol 3:467–476
11. Watkins L, Guarnieri T, Griffith LSC et al. (1986) Implantation of the automatic defibrillator: current surgical techniques. Clin Prog Electrophysiol Pacing 4:286–291
12. Lampert S, Lown B, Graboys TB et al. (1988) Determinants of survival in patients with malignant arrhythmia associated with coronary artery disease. Am J Cardiol 71:791–797
13. Wilber DJ, Garan H, Finklestein D et al. (1988) Out-of-hospital cardiac arrest: use of electrophysiologic testing in the prediction of long-term outcome. N Engl J Med 318:19–24
14. Borggrefe M, Podczeck A, Ostermeyer J et al. (1987) Long-term results of electrophysiologically guided antitachycardia surgery in ventricular tachyarrhythmias: a collaborative report on 665 patients. In: Breithardt G, Borggrefe M (eds) Nonpharmacological therapy of tachyarrhythmias. Futura, Mount Kisco, chap 7, pp 109–125

15. Winkle RA, Mead RH, Ruder MA et al. (1989) Long-term outcome with the automatic implantable cardioverter-defibrillator. J Am Coll Cardiol 13:1353–1361
16. Lehman MH, Steinman RT, Schuger CD et al. (1988) The automatic implantable cardioverter defibrillator as antiarrhythmic treatment modality of choice for survivors of cardiac arrest unrelated to acute myocardial infarction. Am J Cardiol 62:803–805
17. Kuppermann M, Luce B, McGovern B et al. (1990) An analysis of the cost effectiveness of the implantable defibrillator. Circulation 81:91–100

Clinical Results with the Implanted Cardioverter Defibrillator

J.C. Griffin

Introduction

Since its inception, investigators have been eager to explore the question "What is the impact of the automatic implanted cardioverter defibrillator, (ICD), on the management of patients with life threatening ventricular arrhythmias?" Several questions have been posed including:

1) Does the device reduce the incidence of sudden out-of-hospital death?
2) Does the device improve survival?
3) How does it compare to pharmacologic, ablative, and other surgical therapies?

It also must be kept in mind that each of these questions must be asked and answered separately for every indication for the device. As an example, results may be very different in the population surviving an episode of sudden death compared to those patients thought only to be at risk for sudden death. To date, indications and the reported clinical experience are limited almost exclusively to patients who have survived at least one episode of ventricular fibrillation or hemodynamically significant ventricular tachycardia. Therefore, the current body of experience speaks only to that particular indication.

Several methods are available to assess the efficacy of a therapy (Table 1). All but one have been used to provide data regarding the implanted cardioverter defibrillator. Rigidly controlled, prospectively randomized studies have not yet been performed.

Reports Based on a Single Clinical Experience

When one compares the survival rates of patients receiving the ICD to those resulting from other forms of therapy, the device appears efficacious [1–11]. A finding common to these studies is a very low risk of recurrent out-of-hospital sudden death. Winkle and colleagues in a

Table 1. Methods available to assess the efficacy of a therapy

– Report of a clinical experience with no control group
– Comparison of a clinical experience to historical controls
– Comparison of real to hypothetical events ("appropriate shock")
– Retrospective comparison of nonrandomized, unmatched cohorts
– Comparison of retrospectively matched cohorts
– Comparison of prospectively randomized cohorts

report [3] involving the largest number of patients from a single center ($n = 270$) found 8% and 26% mortality at 1 and 5 years. The incidence of sudden death, however, was only 1% and 4% at 1 and 5 years. As in most reports these patients typically were victims of a previous cardiac arrest, suffered from coronary artery disease and had decreased left ventricular function (mean ejection fraction 34%). This compares favorably with previously published reports of the fate of such patients [12–14]. A large multicenter registry [15] with nearly 1400 patients experienced a lower survival rate, 86.9% and 61.6% at 1 and 4 years. The reason for the disparity between these two reports is not known, but most likely it involves differences in patient selection.

Unfortunately comparisons of a new therapy and a previously published one have proved misleading when used in other areas of cardiovascular medicine [16]. Subsequent prospective trials have either shown no differences or smaller differences than predicted between the tested therapy and the control therapy. Most often this occurs because the patient populations are different prior to initiation of the trial or results with the control therapy have improved with time. The use of drug selection by programmed stimulation, amiodarone, vasodilators, and thrombolysis may have a significant impact on survival rates in the population of patients who are now candidates for the ICD (Table 2). Generally, patients involved in clinical trials also tend to do better than expected. This may be due in part to the extra attention they tend to receive. In many reports from which historical control data are taken the patient population was not part of a prospective clinical trial and thus may not have received extra attention. In a recent report [17] of patients having a cardiac arrest between 1980 and 1987, the recurrence rate was 24.4% at 4 years. For those patients whose inducible VT was suppressed by drugs the recurrence rate was only 9.5%, and for those not suppressed the risk was 40.9%. These data also show that the risk is not constant over time and is highest early after the index event. If referral for a therapy causes a delay in receiving the tested therapy (and initiation of follow-up) compared to that of a control population receiving therapy in the primary

Table 2. Potential reasons for different risks in two unmatched study populations

Different selection/eligibility criteria were used
The pretreatment risk was different
Primary vs tertiary population
Only one group constituted a "clinical trial"
The study populations were not concurrent:
– Empiric selection of therapy vs inducibility testing by PES
– Greater empirical use of IA drugs vs empirical amiodarone
– Less use of vasodilator for treatment of heart failure
– Greater use of thrombolysis, CABG, and PTCA in CAD
– Generally declining death rates from coronary disease

care setting, the study group will appear to do better. Some of the high risk patients will die during the process of referral and assessment, causing the final study population to be at lower risk.

Comparison of Real with Hypothetical Events ("Appropriate Shock")

Other reports have compared actual survival rates of patients receiving the ICD to those calculated from the same patients after equating the first "appropriate" ICD shock to death [18–20]. Tchou et al. [19] reported their results in 77 patients and found an actual 2 year survival of 93.4% compared to an estimated survival of only 60.3%. Though the authors felt the patient population and their estimated survival were representative of historical controls, only 25 of 77 patients had ejection fractions less than 30%.

This approach tends to overstate the efficacy of the device. First there is the difficulty of defining an "appropriate" shock. Once defined it may still be difficult to get an accurate description of the event from the patient. Finally there is the problem of equating a shock, even an "appropriate" one to an out-of-hospital sudden death. Many shocks, though preceded by symptoms, are not truly lifesaving (slower VT, longer runs of what would have otherwise been non-sustained VT, symptomatic SVT, etc.). Earlier nonprogrammable devices with low detect rates and short delay times may have been particularly susceptible to discharging during such rhythms. The presence of the ICD may also appropriately modulate the use of other antiarrhythmic therapies. Drug therapy can frequently be reduced, altered in favor of less potent agents, or omitted altogether once an ICD is implanted. Tachycardia recurrence may be more likely, and if it occurs it may occur earlier than if maximal medical therapy were pursued.

Retrospective Comparison of Nonrandomized, Matched, and Unmatched Cohorts

Attempts have been made to derive more concurrent control populations with which to compare the results of patients receiving the ICD [21, 22]. These studies have also shown a beneficial impact of the device on patient survival. Fogoros et al. [21] developed a treatment algorithm for patients with ventricular arrhythmias consisting of both amiodarone and the ICD if their presentation included loss of consciousness (group A) and amiodarone alone if not (group C). During a part of their study the ICD was not available, producing a third group (B), those with loss of consciousness treated with amiodarone alone. The actuarial risk for sudden death in group B was 31% (95% confidence interval, 11%–51%) at 1 and 2 years ($p<0.003$ vs group A which had no sudden deaths).

Hargrove et al. [22] compared their results with the ICD to those with subendocardial resection. These patients groups were obviously different and the authors did not attempt to compare them. At 4 years the mortality rates were equal at approximately 40%. Early results were different due largely to the operative mortality of 15% for subendocardial resection.

Tordjman Fuchs et al. [23] evaluated the results of therapy in 285 patients with out-of-hospital sudden death and documented ventricular arrhythmias. By Cox analysis they were able to identify three factors associated with improved survival: implantation of an AICD, use of beta blocker therapy, and coronary revascularization.

In an attempt to provide a suitable control population from which to judge the efficacy of the ICD we turned to a case-control design (D. Newman, M.J. Sauve, J. Herre, J. Langberg, M.A. Lee, C. Titus, J. Franklin, M.M. Scheinman, J.C. Griffin, unpublished data). We compared the actuarial survival of 60 consecutive recipients of the ICD with 120 retrospectively matched control patients. All patients, both cases and controls, presented initially with sustained ventricular tachycardia or ventricular fibrillation. We matched controls to patients using five clinical variables: age, left ventricular ejection fraction, arrhythmia at presentation, underlying heart disease, and drug therapy status. Drug therapy status corrected for the reasons patients received devices in our institution and for amiodarone usage. Ages were 58 and 59 years in cases and controls, and the ejection fractions were 36% and 35%. Coronary artery disease was present in 75% and 79%, respectively. During follow-up sudden deaths were fewer in ICD recipients compared to controls (5% vs 10%; $p<0.01$). At 1 and 3 years, actuarial survival was 0.89 vs 0.72 and 0.65 vs 0.49 for ICD recipients and controls. The 5 year actuarial survival curves were significantly different by the Cox proportional hazards model ($p<0.05$).

The problem with unmatched, and to a lesser extent retrospectively matched control groups, is that uncontrolled population biases can persist. Subgroup survivals in most reports of outcomes of patients at increased risk for sudden death show large differences when the subjects are stratified by elements of known risk such as ejection fraction. While one can remove some bias by matching for known risk factors, one cannot remove similar bias due to unknown factors. If they exist, such factors can produce significant differences between treated subjects and controls.

Conclusion

The implanted defibrillator (ICD) is an important tool for the management of patients with life threatening ventricular arrhythmias. The device appears to lower significantly the subsequent risk of sudden death in survivors of such events. Whether implantation of the device improves overall patient survival is less clear but existing data from reports using nonrandomized trial designs suggest it does. Randomized trials in patients surviving cardiac arrest are underway and should help to resolve this question.

References

1. Mirowski M (1985) The automatic implantable cardioverter-defibrillator: an overview. J Am Coll Cardiol 6:461–466
2. Echt DS, Armstrong K, Schmidt P, Oyer P, Stinson EB, Winkle RA (1985) Clinical experience, complications, and survival in 70 patients with the automatic implantable cardioverter-defibrillator. Circulation 71:289–296
3. Winkle RA, Mead RH, Ruder MA, Gaudiani VA, Smith NA, Buch WS, Schmidt P, Shipman T (1989) Long-term outcome with the automatic implantable cardioverter-defibrillator. J Am Coll Cardiol 13:1353–1361
4. Gabry MD, Brodman R, Johnston D, Frame R, Kim SG, Waspe LE, Fisher JD, Furman S (1987) Automatic implantable cardioverter-defibrillator: patient survival, battery longevity and shock delivery analysis. J Am Coll Cardiol 9:1349–1356

5. Holt PM, Crick JC, Sowton E (1987) Experience with an automatic implantable cardioverter-defibrillator. Lancet i:551 – 552
6. Kelly PA, CannomS, Garan S, Mirabal GS, Harthorne W, Hurvitz RJ, Vlahakes GJ, Jacobs ML, Ilvento JP, Buckley MJ, Ruskin JN (1988) The automatic implantable cardioverter-defibrillator: Efficacy, complications and survival in patients with malignant ventricular arrhythmias. J Am Coll Cardiol 11:1278 – 1286
7. Borbola J, Denes P, Ezri MD, Hauser RG, Serry C, Goldin MD (1988) The automatic implantable cardioverter-defibrillator. Clinical experience, complications, and follow-up in 25 patients. Arch Intern Med 148:70 – 76
8. Jordaens L, Waleffe A, Derom F, Rodriguez LM, Clement DL, Kulbertus H (1988) Experience with the automatic implantable defibrillator. Acta Clin Belg 43:209 – 218
9. Manolis AS, Wilson TD, Lee MA, Rastegar H, Haffajee CI, Huang SKS, Estes NAM III (1989) Clinical experience in seventy-seven patients with the automatic implantable cardioverter defibrillator. Am Heart J 118:445 – 450
10. Slater AD, Singer I, Stavens CS, Zee-Cheng C, Ganzel BL, Kupersmith J, Mavroudis C, Gray LA Jr (1989) Treatment of malignant ventricular arrhythmias with the automatic implantable cardioverter defibrillator. Ann Surg 209:635 – 641
11. Paull DL, Fellows CL, Guyton SW, Anderson RP (1989) Early experience with the automatic implantable cardioverter defibrillator in sudden death survivors. Am J Surg 157:516 – 518
12. Liberthson RR, Nagle EL, Hirschman JC, Nussenfeld SR (1974) Prehospital ventricular defibrillation. N Engl J Med 291:317 – 321
13. Baum RS, Alvarez H, Cobb LA (1974) Survival after resuscitation from out-of-hospital ventricular fibrillation. Circulation 50:1231 – 1235
14. Schaffer WA, Cobb LA (1975) Recurrent ventricular fibrillation and modes of death in survivors of out-of-hospital ventricular fibrillation. N Engl J Med 293:259 – 262
15. Song SL (1991) Performance of implantable cardiac rhythm management devices (Bilitch Report). PACE 14:1198 – 1200
16. Chalmers TC (1972) Randomization and coronary artery surgery. Ann Thorac Surg 14:323 – 327
17. Furukawa T, Rozanski JJ, Nogami A, Moroe K, Gosselin AJ, Lister JW (1989) Time-dependent risk of and predictors for cardiac arrest recurrence in survivors of out-of-hospital cardiac arrest with chronic coronary artery disease. Circulation 80:599 – 608
18. Mirowski M, Reid PR, Winkle RA, Mower MM, Watkins L Jr, Stinson EB, Griffith LSC, Kallman CH, Weisfeldt ML (1983) Mortality in patients with implanted automatic defibrillators. Ann Intern Med 98:585 – 588
19. Tchou PJ, Kadri N, Anderson J, Caceres JA, Jazayeri M, Akhtar M (1988) Automatic implantable cardioverter defibrillators and survival of patients with left ventricular dysfunction and malignant ventricular arrhythmias. Ann Intern Med 109:529 – 534

20. Myerburg RJ, Luceri RM, Thurer R, Cooper DK, Zaman L, Interian A, Fernandez P, Cox M, Glicksman F, Castellanos A (1989) Time to first shock and clinical outcome in patients receiving an automatic implantable cardioverter-defibrillator. J Am Coll Cardiol 14:508–514
21. Fogoros RN, Fiedler SB, Elson JJ (1987) The automatic implantable cardioverter-defibrillator in drug-refractory ventricular tachyarrhythmias. Ann Intern Med 107:635–641
22. Hargrove WC III, Josephson ME, Marchlinski FE, Miller JM (1989) Surgical decisions in the management of sudden cardiac death and malignant ventricular arrhythmias. Subendocardial resection, the automatic internal defibrillator or both. J Thorac Cardiovasc Surg 97:923–928
23. (1989) Out-of-hospital cardiac arrest: improved long-term outcome in patients with automatic implantable cardioverter defibrillator (AICD). Circulation 80:II–121 (abstr)

Combining Drugs with the Implantable Cardioverter Defibrillator: Clinical Implications

D. S. Echt

The majority of patients with implantable cardioverter defibrillator (ICD) devices receive antiarrhythmic drugs [1]. A major advantage of using drugs in an ancillary role is that less toxic drugs and lower drug doses can be utilized. The rationale for concomitant antiarrhythmic drug therapy includes:

1) suppression of frequent sustained and unsustained ventricular tachycardia,
2) suppression of supraventricular tachycardia,
3) slowing the maximal sinus rate to below the ventricular tachycardia rate, and
4) slowing the rate of ventricular tachycardia to avoid syncope prior to device discharge.

ICD devices and antiarrhythmic drugs can interact in several ways. They can affect arrhythmia occurrence, arrhythmia detection, and arrhythmia termination.

With regard to arrhythmia occurrence, the interactions between ICD devices and antiarrhythmic drugs are generally favorable, the drugs suppressing clinical arrhythmias and the device successfully converting drug-induced arrhythmias. Since the energy required to defibrillate ventricular fibrillation is usually higher than the energy required to cardiovert ventricular tachycardia, it would be ideal for a drug to prevent ventricular fibrillation. Class III antiarrhythmic agents may have this potential. In the example in Fig. 1, taken during intraoperative testing, ventricular fibrillation was easily induced with AC current of antiarrhythmic drugs. After oral sotalol, AC current was no longer capable of inducing sustained ventricular fibrillation. Figure 2a is an example of the other extreme of drug-induced arrhythmia occurrence, or proarrhythmia. These are ECG recordings obtained from a patient with an ICD who was receiving amiodarone. She was treated for CHF as an outpatient, became hypokalemic, and developed drug-induced long QT intervals and torsade de pointes. Some episodes were self-terminating and

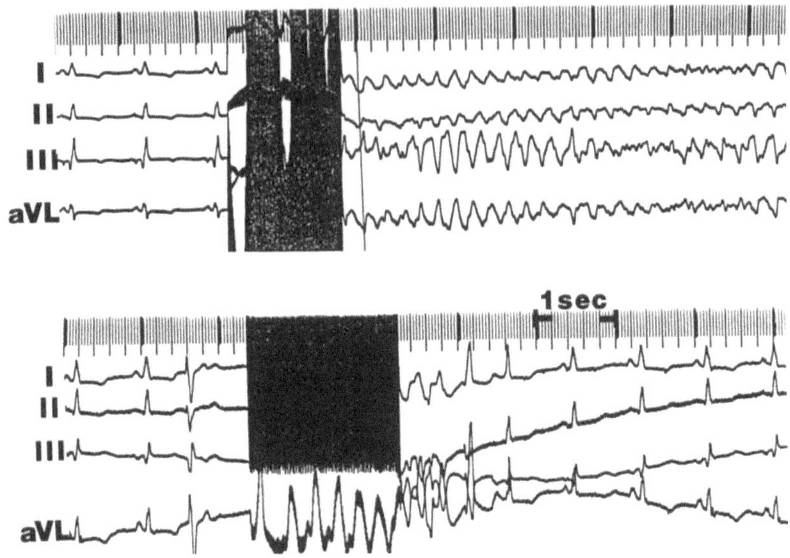

Fig. 1. Surface electrograms obtained during testing for implantation of an ICD device in a patient. In the *top panel*, ventricular fibrillation is readily induced with AC current during intraoperative testing when the patient was not receiving antiarrhythmic drug therapy. In the *lower panel*, ventricular fibrillation was unable to be induced with AC current during a postoperative electrophysiology study when the patient was receiving oral sotalol

resulted in synchronous shocks during sinus rhythm. However, as illustrated in Fig. 2b, most of the episodes were sustained and degenerated into ventricular fibrillation. Therefore, the interaction between the ICD and drugs can be positive, whether the drugs suppress or induce ventricular tachyarrhythmias.

Devices and antiarrhythmic drugs can interact by altering arrhythmia detection of either rate or morphology. The effects of commonly used antiarrhythmic drugs on slowing ventricular tachycardia rate are listed in Table 1. In general, beta-blockers, class Ib agents (mexiletine, tocainide), and class III agents (sotalol) have only a minor effect on ventricular tachycardia rate. Class Ia drugs (quinidine, procainamide, disopyramide) have a moderate effect, and class Ic drugs (encainide, flecainide, and propafenone) and amiodarone (class I, II, III, IV) have major effects. More importantly, there is marked individual variation in the response of drugs on ventricular tachycardia rate, and the effects are concentration-dependent. Antiarrhythmic drug effects on rate and probability density function (PDF) morphology can have complex interactions. The

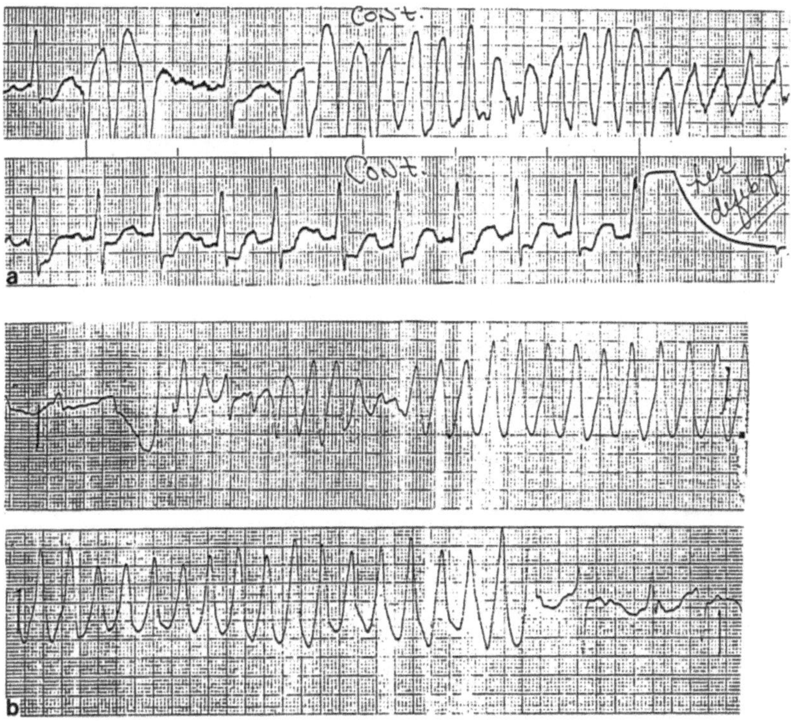

Fig. 2a, b. Rhythm strips from a patient on amiodarone who became hypokalemic and demonstrated drug-induced long QT intervals with typical torsades de pointes arrhythmia. **a** The polymorphic ventricular tachycardia self-terminated but the ICD device was committed to discharge. **b** Most episodes, however, were sustained

Table 1. Slowing of ventricular tachycardia rate by antiarrhythmic drugs

Minor	Moderate	Major
Propranolol	Quinidine	Encainide
Mexiletine	Procainamide	Flecainide
Tocainide	Disopyramide	Propafenone
Sotalol		Amiodarone

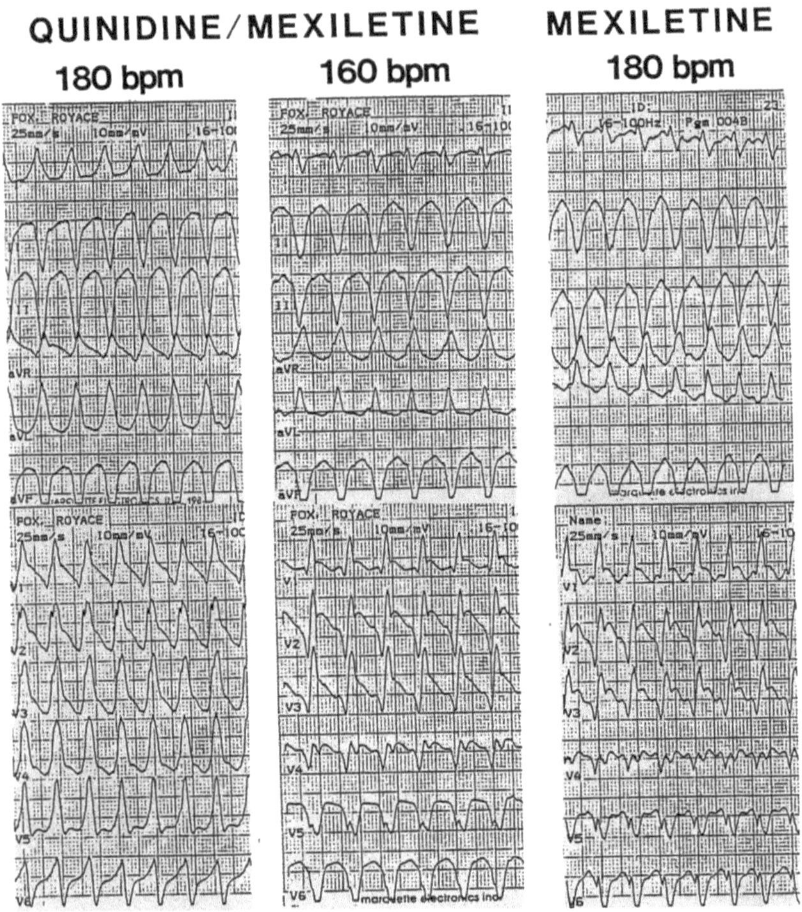

Fig. 3. Twelve lead electrocardiograms of ventricular tachycardia induced in a patient with programmed stimulation. The patient had a previously implanted non-programmable AICD device (CPI, St. Paul, MN) with rate detection set at 153 bpm and probability density function (PDF) morphology detection. On the combination of quinidine and mexiletine therapy, ventricular tachycardias of two different morphologies were induced. The ventricular tachycardia in the *left panel* satisfied both rate and PDF. The ventricular tachycardia in the *middle panel* satisfied rate but was not detected by PDF. However, after discontinuing quinidine (*right panel*), the rate of the ventricular tachycardia that previously did not satisfy PDF increased from 160 to 180 bpm and PDF was satisfied

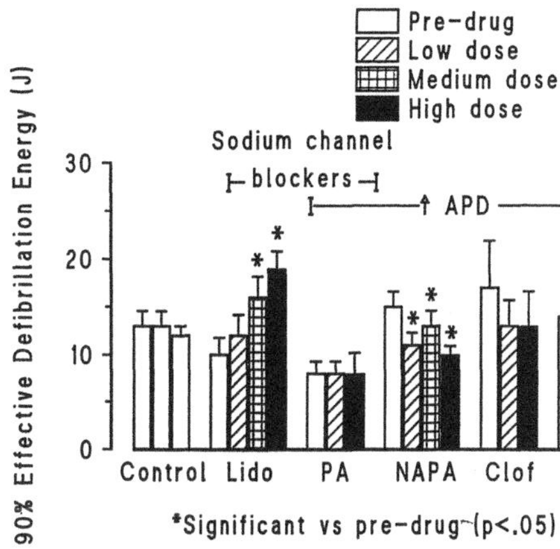

Fig. 4. Effects of lidocaine, procainamide (*PA*), *N*-acetyl procainamide (*NAPA*), clofilium (*Clof*), and cesium (*Cs*) on the mean 90% effective defibrillation energy (*J*). Lidocaine is a sodium channel blocking agent; *NAPA*, clofilium, and cesium prolong action potential duration (APD) probably by blocking potassium channel; and procainamide both blocks sodium channels and prolongs action potential duration. The defibrillation energy requirements were increased with lidocaine administration, unchanged in control experiments and with procainamide administration, and decreased with *NAPA*, clofilium, and cesium administration. (Adapted from Echt et al. 1985 [2])

electrocardiograms in Fig. 3 are from a patient with an automatic implantable cardioverter defibrillator device (AICD; CPI, St. Paul, MN) with a nonprogrammable rate cutoff of 153 bpm. On the combination of quinidine and mexiletine, two ventricular tachycardias were induced with programmed stimulation. The ventricular tachycardia at 180 bpm was detected by both PDF and rate, the ventricular tachycardia at 160 bpm was detected by rate but not morphology. After discontinuing quinidine, the second ventricular tachycardia was again induced at the faster rate of 180 bpm, and PDF was satisfied.

The third and probably the most important type of device-drug interactions are effects on arrhythmia termination. Antiarrhythmic drugs may affect the energy required to defibrillate or cardiovert. Results from canine experiments in our laboratory assessing the 90% effective defibrillation energy dose (ED90), an index of defibrillation energy requirements derived from logistic regression curves, are shown in Fig. 4 [2]. In addition to control studies, we evaluated antiarrhythmic drugs at multiple plasma concentrations: lidocaine, procainamide, the active metabolite *N*-acetyl procainamide (NAPA), clofilium, and the metal cesium. We found that lidocaine, which is a relatively pure sodium chan-

Table 2. Drug effects on defibrillation energy requirements in canine experiments

Class	Increase	Mixed	Decrease
I	Lidocaine Phenytoin Encainide Flecainide Recainam	Procainamide Quinidine	
II	Propranolol		
III		Bretylium Amiodarone	NAPA *d*-Sotalol Clofilium
IV	Verapamil		

nel blocking agent, increased defibrillation energy requirements, while the drugs NAPA and clofilium and the metal cesium, which are pure action potential-prolonging agents (by blocking potassium currents), decreased defibrillation energy requirements. Procainamide, having effects on sodium and potassium ionic channels, had little overall effect possibly due to cancellation of opposing effects on defibrillation energy requirements (Table 2).

We performed additional experiments to support the idea that lidocaine's effect on defibrillation energy requirements is due to its sodium channel blocking properties [3]. Lidocaine demonstrates pH-dependent effects upon sodium currents because it is a weak base. Lidocaine is present in both cationic and neutral forms at physiologic pH. Small changes in pH can result in substantial changes in the ratio of charged to uncharged drug which accounts for its effects. At low pH, sodium channel block is enhanced by lidocaine, and at high pH it is reduced. We demonstrated that lidocaine has pH-dependent effects on defibrillation energy requirements. We first evaluated acidosis alone with intravenous hydrochloric acid infusion (Fig. 5). We found that lowering arterial pH to 7.18 had no significant effect on ED90. However, we found that acidosis during lidocaine infusion significantly enhanced the increase in ED90 caused by lidocaine alone. Note that the effect was marked despite a mid-therapeutic lidocaine concentration. We then evaluated the effects of alkalosis (Fig. 6). We found that alkalosis alone (pH 7.6) produced by mechanical hyperventilation significantly lowered the ED90. Alkalosis during lidocaine infusion more than reversed the increase in ED90

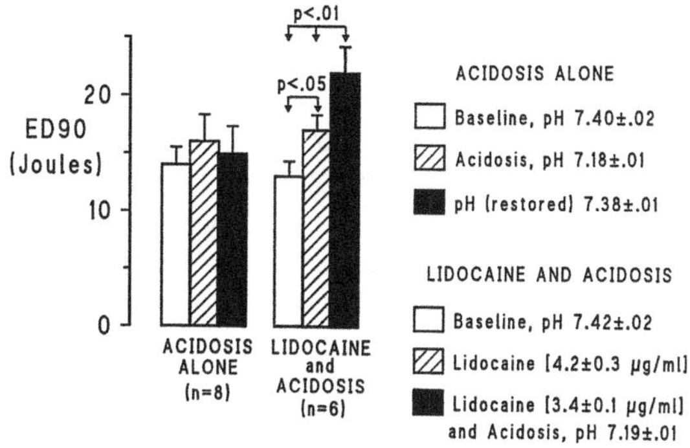

Fig. 5. Effects of acidosis and lidocaine on ED90 (90% effective defibrillation energy dose) in canine experiments. The effect of acidosis alone was evaluated in the bar graphs on the *left*, and the effects of acidosis in the presence of lidocaine in the bar graphs on the *right*

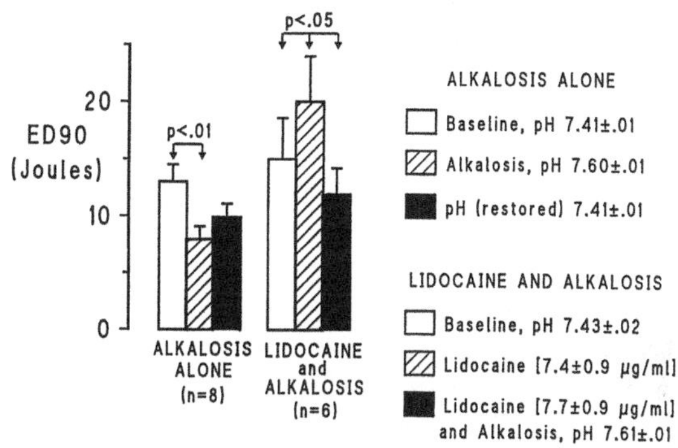

Fig. 6. Effects of alkalosis and lidocaine on ED90 in canine experiments. The effects of alkalosis alone were evaluated in the bar graphs on the *left*, and the effects of alkalosis in the presence of lidocaine in the bar graphs on the *right*

caused by lidocaine. We believe this reflects a partial reversal of lidocaine effect by alkalosis as well as an independent effect of alkalosis alone. Note that the defibrillation energy requirements are reduced to below baseline despite achieving supratherapeutic lidocaine plasma concentrations of >7 μg/ml. Moreover, the results of the pH experiments may have significant clinical implications to patients receiving transthoracic ventricular defibrillation during cardiopulmonary resuscitation. For patients in whom electrical defibrillation is initially unsuccessful, hyperventilation causing alkalosis may be helpful, and acidosis in combination with lidocaine infusion may be detrimental.

We speculated that the calcium entry blocker verapamil might lower defibrillation energy requirements by preventing intracellular calcium overload, but we found that intravenous verapamil increased the ED90 even at low therapeutic plasma concentrations [4]. Moreover, the extent of change in ED90 was not closely correlated with hemodynamic alterations or standard electrophysiologic measurements.

To summarize the results in canine experiments from our laboratory and others: it appears that relatively pure sodium channel blockers in the class Ib and Ic categories (lidocaine [2], phenytoin [5], encainide [6], flecainide [7], recainam [8]) increase defibrillation energy, as do class II (propanolol [9]) and IV (verapamil [4]) agents, and class III (*d*-sotalol [10], clofilium [2, 11], NAPA [2]) agents decrease defibrillation energy. Drugs which affect more than one ionic channel (quinidine [12, 13], procainamide [2]) or have complex ancillary actions (bretylium [11, 12], amiodarone [14, 15]) have mixed effects on defibrillation energy.

Do these animal data have any relevance in patients? In a number of reports, encainide, flexainide, amiodarone, and mexiletine have been associated with inability to cardiovert or defibrillate [16–18]. We recently began testing in patients undergoing AICD implant before and during lidocaine infusion [19]. We first validated our human testing protocol from results in canine studies. The testing protocol we used identifies a defribrillation energy in the upper portion of the defibrillation energy dose response curve and requires only five to six ventricular fibrillation inductions, far fewer than our animal experiments [20]. The results from seven patients in whom testing was performed at baseline and during lidocaine concentration <5 μg/ml were compared to seven patients in whom the lidocaine plasma concentration exceeded 5 μg/ml. We found that lidocaine increased defibrillation energy in patients with a mean plasma lidocaine concentration of 6 μg/ml, but not in patients with a lower mean plasma concentration of 4 μg/ml. This is consistent with our findings in dog experiments in Fig. 4 in which the increase in defibrillation energy requirement was significant at 6 but not 3 μg/ml [2].

Pacing threshold is increased immediately post-shock and there is experimental evidence supporting a further increase in post-shock pacing threshold by class 1c agents [21]. However, in general, antiarrhythmic drugs enhance the efficacy of antitachycardia pacing and low energy cardioversion modalities. Antiarrhythmic drugs increase the success of ventricular tachycardia termination using either pacing or low energy cardioversion techniques by prolonging ventricular tachycardia cycle length [22, 23]. Antiarrhythmic drugs do not affect the incidence of ventricular tachycardia acceleration [23].

Newer ICD devices have implications for antiarrhythmic drug use. Programmability allows for greater flexibility in adding drugs or changing drug regimens post implant. The overall influence of programmability may be to decrease drug usage. For instance, the detection delay feature may obviate the need for drugs in some patients with frequent nonsustained ventricular tachycardia. Low energy cardioversion and antitachycardia pacing will definitely result in an increased use of drugs to slow ventricular tachycardia rate. Nonthoracotomy systems, being less efficient, may encourage the development of drugs that lower defibrillation energy requirements or are antifibrillatory.

In conclusion, drugs continue to have a role in patients with ICD devices. Drugs that increase defibrillation energy requirements should be avoided, if possible, since the devices have a limited output. Since drugs can affect arrhythmia occurrence, detection, and termination, always retest the ICD in a patient when adding or changing drugs or dosage.

References

1. Echt DS, Armstrong K, Caltagerone P, Oyer PE, Stinson EB, Winkle RA (1985) Clinical experience, complications and survival in 70 patients with the automatic implantable cardioverter/defibrillator. Circulation 71:291–296
2. Echt DS, Black JB, Barbey JT, Coxe DR, Cato E (1989) Evaluation of antiarrhythmic drugs on defibrillation energy requirements in dogs: sodium channel block and action potential prolongation. Circulation 79:1106–1117
3. Echt DS, Cato EL, Coxe DR (1989) pH-dependent effects of lidocaine on defibrillation energy requirements in dogs. Circulation 80:1003–1009
4. Schräder R, Brooks M, Echt DS (1990) Verapamil increases the internal defibrillation energy requirements in anesthetized dogs. A Am Coll Cardiol 15:73A
5. Babbs CF, Yim GKW, Whistler SJ, Tacker WA, Geddes LA (1979) Elevation of ventricular defibrillation threshold in dogs by antiarrhythmic drugs. Am Heart J 98(3):345–350
6. Fain ES, Dorian P, Davy JM, Kates RE, Winkle RA (1986) Effects of encainide and its metabolites on energy requirements for defibrillation. Circulation 73(6):1334–1341
7. Hernandez R, Mann DE, Breckinridge S, Williams GR, Reiter MJ (1989) Effects of flecainide on defibrillation thresholds in the anesthetized dog. J Am Coll Cardiol 14(3):777–781
8. Frame LH, Sheldon JH (1988) Effect of recainam on the energy required for ventricular defibrillation in dogs as assessed with implanted electrodes. J Am Coll Cardiol 12(3):746–752
9. Ruffy R, Schechtman K, Monje E (1985) β-adrenergic modulation of direct defibrillation energy in anesthetized dog heart. Am J Physiol 248: H674–H677

10. Wang M, Dorian P (1989) DL and D sotalol decrease defibrillation energy requirements. PACE 12:1522–1529
11. Tacker WA, Niebauer MJ, Babbs CF, Combs WJ, Hahn BM, Barker MA, Siepel JF, Bourland JD, Geddes LA (1980) The effect of newer antiarrhythmic drugs on defibrillation threshold. Crit Care Med 8(3):177–180
12. Dorian P, Fain ES, Davy JM, Winkle RA (1986) Effect of quinidine and bretylium on defibrillation energy requirements. Am Heart J 112(1):19–25
13. Woolfolk DI, Chaffee WR, Cohen W, Neville JF, Abildskov JA (1966) The effect of quinidine on electrical energy required for ventricular defibrillation. Am Heart J 72(5):659–663
14. Frame LH (1989) The effect of chronic oral and acute intravenous amiodarone administration on ventricular defibrillation threshold using implanted electrodes in dogs. PACE 12:339–346
15. Fain ES, Lee JT, Winkle RA (1987) Effects of acute intravenous and chronic oral amiodarone on defibrillation energy requirements. Am Heart J 114:8–17
16. Fogoros RN (1984) Amiodarone-induced refractoriness to cardioversion. Ann Intern Med 100(5):699–700
17. Winkle RA, Mason JW, Griffin JC, Ross D (1981) Malignant ventricular tachyarrhythmias associated with the use of encainide. Am Heart J 102(5):857–864
18. Marinchak RA, Friehling TD, Kline RA, Stohler J, Kowey PR (1988) Effect of antiarrhythmic drugs on defibrillation threshold: case report of an adverse effect of mexiletine and review of the literature. PACE 11:7–12
19. Echt DS, Lee JT, Roden DM, Crawford DM, Horrell KD, Frist WH, Hammon JW (1989) Effects of lidocaine on defibrillation energy requirements in patients. Circulation 80:II–224
20. Lang DJ, Cato DL, Echt DS (1989) Protocol for evaluation of internal defribrillation safety margins. J Am Coll Cardiol 13:111A
21. Guarnieri T, Datorre SD, Bondke H, Brinker J, Myers S, Levine JH (1988) Increased pacing threshold after an automatic defibrillator shock in dogs: effects of Class I and Class II antiarrhythmic drugs. PACE 11:1324–1330
22. Ciccone JM, Saksena S, Shah Y, Pantopoulos D (1985) A prospective randomized study of the clinical efficacy and safety of transvenous cardioversion for termination of ventricular tachycardia. Circulation 71(3):571–578
23. Naccarelli GV, Zipes DP, Rahilly GT, Heger JJ, Prystowsky EN (1983) Influence of tachycardia cycle length and antiarrhythmic drugs on pacing termination and acceleration of ventricular tachycardia. Am Heart J 105(1):1–5

Antitachycardia Pacing, Cardioversion, and Defibrillation: From the Past to the Future

J. D. Fisher, S. Furman, S. G. Kim, K. J. Ferrick, J. A. Roth, J. Gross, R. F. Brodman

Introduction

Nearly three decades ago, it was known that ventricular tachycardias in the presence of bradycardia could be prevented by pacing at physiologic rates [1–10]. Temporary and implanted pacers have long been used to prevent tachycardias by rate support or suppressing ventricular premature complexes (VPCs) and to terminate tachycardias using competitive stimulation. In the 1970s, implantable antitachycardia pacemakers became commercially available. That decade saw many new antitachycardia applications and an increased understanding of the mechanisms involved in tachycardia termination. It appeared that pacers would play a major role in the treatment of tachycardias. Pacing failed, however, to reach projections for many reasons: physicians often fail to recognize the benefits of temporary as well as permanent antitachycardia pacing; implanted units require frequent reprogramming, rapid ventricular responses can occur if atrial fibrillation is provoked; younger patients balked because of the "image" of pacing as a treatment for the elderly. The danger of accelerating ventricular tachycardia (VT) into ventricular fibrillation (VF) produced great reluctance to implant pacemakers for VT termination. The implantable cardioverter defibrillator (ICD) further relegated pacing for VT to the background. Pacing for VT will enjoy much wider application in the 1990s in devices that combine cardioverter, defibrillator, and antitachycardia pacing modalities. In contrast, there has been some erosion of the potential growth of pacing for SVT as antitachycardia surgery and catheter ablation have become increasingly prevalent.

Pacing for Tachycardia Prevention

Rate support [1–4, 11] (Fig. 1 A) can prevent bradycardia-related tachycardias. Pacing at rates slightly higher than the spontaneous rhythm

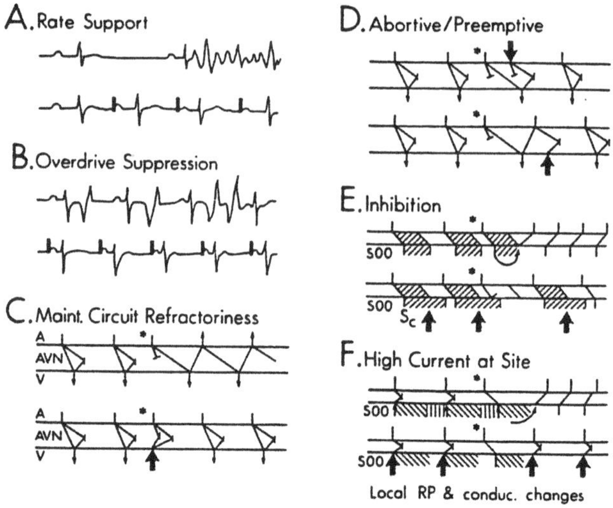

Fig. 1A–F. Tachycardia prevention. **A, B, C, E,** and **F** Tachycardia initiation in the *upper lines* and prevention in the *lower lines* of each panel. **D** Prevention is shown in both *upper* and *lower lines. Asterisk* (*), spontaneous extrasystole that would initiate tachycardia. **E, F** *500* indicates the site of origin of the tachycardia; **E** S_c represents a conditioning stimulus. The larger, bolder stimulus artifacts in the *bottom line* of **F** indicate high current stimulation. See text for details. (From Fisher et al. 1991 [249] by permission)

(overdrive suppression) [5–21] (Fig. 1B) suppresses tachycardias by reducing premature beats that can cause tachycardia. This has been well demonstrated using VVI pacing [19]. Atrial or dual chamber pacing may be even more effective for a variety of arrhythmias, including prevention of atrial fibrillation (AF) [11, 20, 21]. Automatic overdrive pacemakers increase their rates automatically until VPCs are suppressed [22, 23]. Homogenization of refractoriness by pacing at physiologic rates may prevent tachycardias in patients with prolonged QT interval syndromes [12, 24–26].

Programmed extrastimuli [27–30] or short slow pacing bursts [27] in response to spontaneous extrasystoles may prevent sustained tachycardia. AV nodal reentry tachycardia can often be prevented by maintaining circuit refractoriness if the initiating atrial premature beat is followed immediately by a ventricular stimulus (or, vice versa, DDT mode) [31–34] (Fig. 1C). In other instances of this arrhythmia, prevention can be accomplished by preemptive atrial or ventricular stimulation coupled to the spontaneous beat [28–30, 35] (Fig. 1D) delivered as a single extrastimulus [28–30, 35] or a train of ultra-rapid stimulation [28, 35].

Single or train stimulation delivered during the effective refractory period (ERP) as a conditioning stimulus may produce inhibition [36] (Fig. 1 E), preventing activation in the same area by a subsequent wavefront that would otherwise have been well beyond the ERP.

Some VTs can be prevented by high current strength pacing at the mapped site of origin (Fig. 1 F) [37].

Role of Preventive Pacing

Pacing for bradycardia-related tachycardias and for torsades de pointes is well established for both acute and chronic therapy. Overdrive suppression of extrasystoles may be more effective with temporary pacing. A permanent pacemaker should not be implanted for overdrive suppression without convincing evidence from several Holter monitors that it is effective. The more exotic stimulation techniques used for prevention of tachycardias have been used primarily on a temporary basis.

Pacing for Hemodynamic Support During Continuing Tachycardias

Under certain circumstances, such as a proarrhythmic effect of antiarrhythmic drugs, patients may develop a virtually incessant tachycardia. The patient is said to be "stuck in tachycardia". Such tachycardias may abate when the problem is reversed, but the ongoing tachycardia may create a clinical crisis situation.

The ventricular rate during SVT may be slowed by pacing the atrium to produce 2:1 block [38–45] (Fig. 2A). This can be accomplished by rapid atrial pacing [38–41], or by coupled atrial pacing [42–45], i.e. a programmed atrial extrastimulus so early that conduction to the ventricle is impossible. Slowing the ventricular rate may produce a narrower QRS if rate-related bundle branch block exists during SVT [45]. The benefits of a narrower QRS complex may also be seen in some VT cases [46]: in slow VTs, atrial pacing at a somewhat faster rate may be conducted to the ventricle with improvement in blood pressure even though the rate is faster than the VT (Fig. 2B). Ventricular pacing at comparable rates usually causes further hemodynamic deterioration. Occasionally pacing simultaneously at several ventricular sites produces a narrower QRS complex and a gain in blood pressure.

Additional gains in blood pressure during VT may be realized by atrial pacing synchronized to sensed ventricular depolarizations (AVT mode) [38, 46, 47] to produce an "atrial kick" (Fig. 2C). The effective ven-

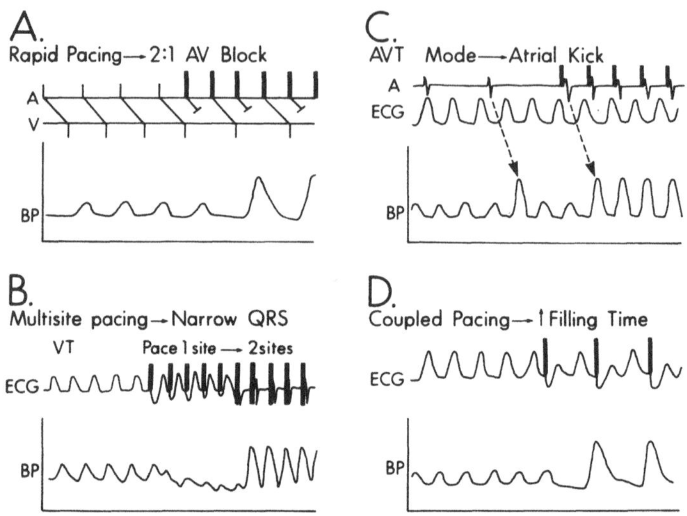

Fig. 2A–D. Pacing for hemodynamic support during continuing tachycardias. See text for details. (From Fisher et al. 1991 [249] by permission)

tricular rate can also be reduced by "coupled pacing" [38, 45, 46] with a programmed ventricular extrastimulus delivered before there is sufficient ventricular filling for opening of the aortic valve (Fig. 2D). However, coupled pacing often produces negative results in patients with ischemia and stimulation during the potential vulnerable period of ventricular tachycardia may cause acceleration.

These techniques are almost exclusively reserved for temporary use though occasional patients have benefited from implanted pacers designed to provide long-term rapid atrial pacing.

Pacers for "Noninvasive Programmed Stimulation"

Years ago implantation of a pacemaker capable of performing noninvasive programmed stimulation was suggested for patients undergoing surgical ablation of VT [48]. This may be even more applicable to patients whose arrhythmogenic substrate has not been ablated and who are dependent on medications for protection [45].

Patients with SVT or VT who require pacing should have a device that is capable of noninvasive programmed stimulation [45, 46]. Routine noninvasive programmed stimulation can be performed in the properly prepared Pacemaker Center as an outpatient procedure. Many of the newer implantable cardioverter defibrillators (ICDs) are also capable of noninvasive programmed stimulation.

Pacers for Termination of Tachycardias

General Principles

Most organized tachycardias are assumed to be reentrant. Pacer termination of a reentrant tachycardia occurs when a stimulated wavefront reaches the circuit so that anterograde propagation is not possible due to refractoriness and retrograde propagation collides with the tachycardia wavefront, extinguishing it (Fig. 3). Multiple extrastimuli or rapid

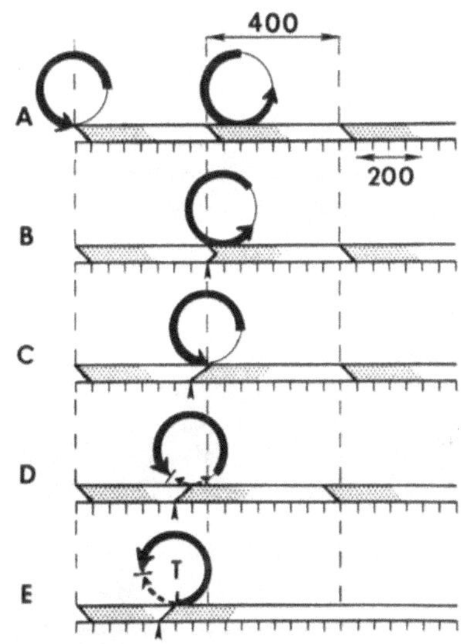

Fig. 3 A–E. Termination of reentrant tachycardia by a single programmed extrastimulus. *T*, termination; *dashed vertical lines*, basic tachycardia cycle length of 400 ms. The circuit is represented by a *circle* with the refractory period equivalent to the *heavy line* following the *arrowhead* and occupying 3/4 of the *circle*. Beneath the *circle* are *two lines*, the *upper* representing the myocardium at the site of origin of the tachycardia and the *lower* the site of stimulation. The *shaded area* represents the refractory period of the intervening myocardium. **A–E**, Successively earlier extrastimuli are delivered, with termination occurring in **E** where anterograde conduction in the circuit is impossible and retrograde conduction collides with the tachycardia wavefront, extinguishing both. In this example, as in clinical examples, the termination zone begins at the end of refractoriness int he myocardium. See Text for details. (Reproduced with permission from Fisher et al. 1984 [52])

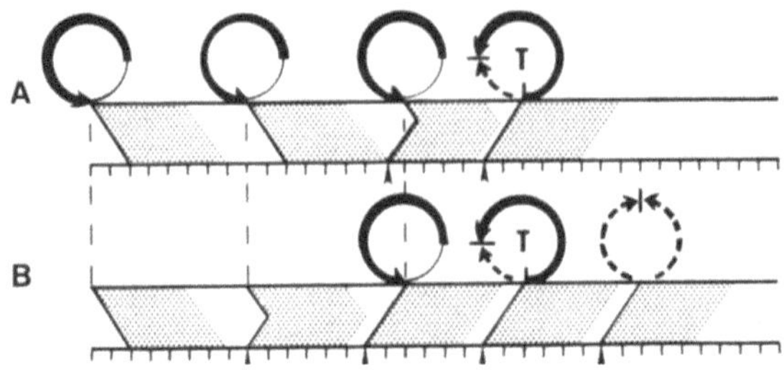

Fig. 4 A, B. Termination of tachycardia by multiple extrastimuli and by rapid pacing. Conventions as for Fig. 3. See text for details. **A** Even an early extrastimulus fails to terminate the tachycardia because of a relatively longer (physical or physiologic) distance between the site of stimulation and the tachycardia circuit. However, a second extrastimulus introduced immediately after the refractory period of the first successfully terminates the arrhythmia. **B** A burst of 4 rapid pacing stimuli similarly terminates the arrhythmia. (Reproduced with permission from Fisher et al. 1984 [52])

pacing may be necessary to "peel back" refractoriness in the myocardium between the site of stimulation and the reentrant circuit (Fig. 4). Determinants of reentrant tachycardia termination by pacing include:

1) the circuit must be accessible;
2) there must be an excitable gap;
3) the refractory period of the anterograde limb in the tachycardia circuit must be longer than that of the intervening myocardium;
4) reproducibility of pacer termination requires stable electrophysiology. Extensive reviews [50–53] have examined these concepts in more detail.

Pacing at higher amplitudes than the conventional two to four times diastolic threshold enhances the likelihood of termination [54].

In most instances where single capture termination of tachycardia is possible, the termination zone is contiguous with the end of the effective refractory period of the myocardium at the site of stimulation (Figs. 3 and 4) [46, 50–53, 55]. This holds true even if the actual duration of the ERP changes. The implication is that the most efficient termination method is to initiate ultra-rapid train stimulation during the ERP and continue it long enough to cause only a single capture [55, 56].

Single Capture Termination Techniques

Properly timed single extrastimuli can terminate reentrant tachycardias if other conditions are met. Competitive pacing at rates slower than the

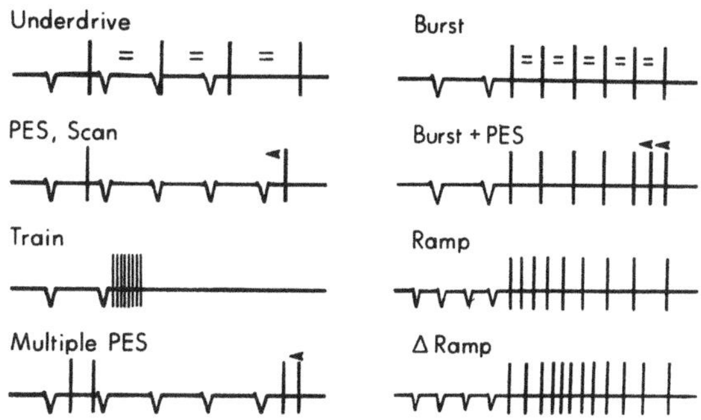

Fig. 5. Basic stimulation patterns for tachycardia termination. In this, and in Figs. 6, 9 and 10, spontaneous ventricular or atrial depolarizations are represented by a V-like deflection from the baseline. *Small arrowheads* at the top of the pacer stimulation lines represent the direction of changes in timing of successive stimuli. Tachycardia depolarizations are omitted after termination has occurred or when they might obscure this stimulation pattern. See text. *PES*, programmed extrastimulus. (Reproduced with permission from Fisher et al. 1986, 1988 [78, 46])

tachycardia (underdrive pacing) may terminate tachycardias with a wide termination zone and is simple enough to attempt using virtually any pacing system [14, 46]. "Dual demand" pacers are available for automatic underdrive pacing [58–60]. Scanning or programmed extrastimulus techniques [61] are somewhat more efficient, since they introduce extrastimuli in an orderly fashion. Some devices remember the timing of the extrastimulus that terminated the tachycardia, though this is less successful than hoped, because posture, activity, and metabolic status may alter the timing of the termination zone (Fig. 5).

Multiple Capture Techniques for Termination of Tachycardia

More than one stimulus may be required to peel back the refractoriness and allow the stimulated wavefront to reach the tachycardia circuit during the termination zone. Double and triple programmed extrastimuli [42, 62, 63] (Fig. 5) are relatively inefficient.

Simple Rapid Pacing Techniques

Burst pacing is the standard [64]. Pacing is initiated at a rate faster than the tachycardia, and a burst at a constant rate is delivered for 5–15 cap-

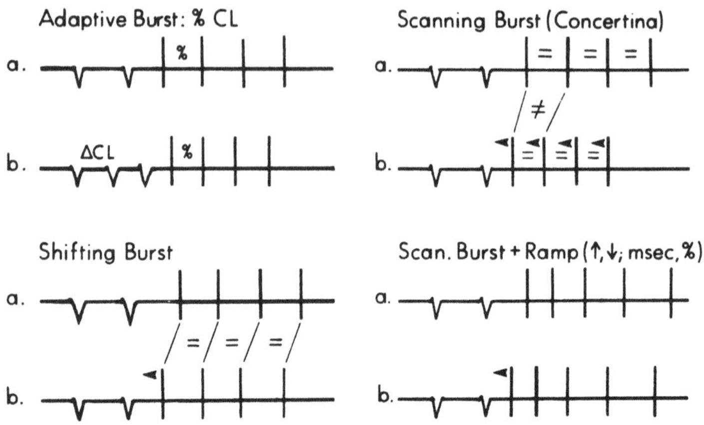

Fig. 6. Additional stimulation patterns. All of these are available in implantable antitachycardia pacemakers. Conventions as for Fig. 5. *CL*, cycle length. (Modified with permission from Fisher et al. 1986, 1988 [78, 46])

Fig. 7 A–F. Transient entrainment. **A** The major portion of the myocardium (*large box*) is depolarized by a sinus or paced wavefront entering from the top. This wavefront encounters an area of impaired conduction (*small box*) which is depolarized from two directions, preventing tachycardia under these conditions. Two recording electrograms in the myocardium (*EG1* and *EG2*) record a "normal" sequence of conduction from top to bottom and the schematic ECG represents a normal complex. **B** A tachycardia exists, depolarizing the major portion of myocardium in an abnormal direction represented by shading of the *large box*. Both the electrogram sequence and the ECG are also abnormal. *X* represents the tachycardia cycle responsible for the recordings. **C** During relatively slow pacing the last wavefront (*X*) to use the tachycardia circuit now fills the bottom (*shaded*) half of the *large box*, with the upper half being depolarized by the next paced beat (*X+1*). This results in an EG sequence in which two different cycles (*X* and *X+1*) contribute to fusion of the ECG. **D** During pacing at a moderately faster rate, more of the *large box* is depolarized in the normal direction. Since conduction is in the impaired area remains slow, EG 2 now depolarizes somewhat later than EG 1, and the electrogram at EG 2 is also fused. If pacing is stopped at this point, as in **E**, the last paced beat (*X+1*) will continue through the impaired area and produce an EG and ECG sequence and morphology identical to the tachycardia (i.e., there is entrainment but no fusion with the last paced beat). **F** With faster pacing there is anterograde block in the circuit so that the paced beat (*X+1*) cannot propagate if pacing is stopped, and the tachycardia is now terminated. Demonstration of the third criterion of entrainment (activation of the site of block from a different direction with a shorter conduction period) would not be demonstrated by **F**. Rather, block would have to be shown at the bottom of the area of impaired conduction, and another EG recording at just that point would fulfill criterion 3. Not all criteria can be demonstrated for every tachycardia, and **F** represents an alternative. (From Fisher et al. 1991 [249] by permission)

tures. With each attempt, the rate is increased until termination or acceleration occurs. Many pacemakers allow the burst rate to be determined in increments of rate or decrements of cycle length; or as a decremental percentage of the tachycardia cycle length on sequential attempts ("adaptive burst pacing"). Another technique adds one or more programmed extrastimuli to the end of a burst [65, 66] (Fig. 6).

Transient Entrainment

Entrainment is not a technique, but a phenomenon sometimes observed when moderately rapid pacing is continued for longer periods of time than described for burst pacing (Fig. 7) [67–78]. Incremental rates are used in sequential termination attempts. Four criteria (Table 1) have been used to characterize the phenomenon of transient entrainment, based on an additional number of observations. Any one of the criteria are sufficient to demonstrate entrainment, but entrainment may exist even if none of the criteria are satisfied [73, 75].

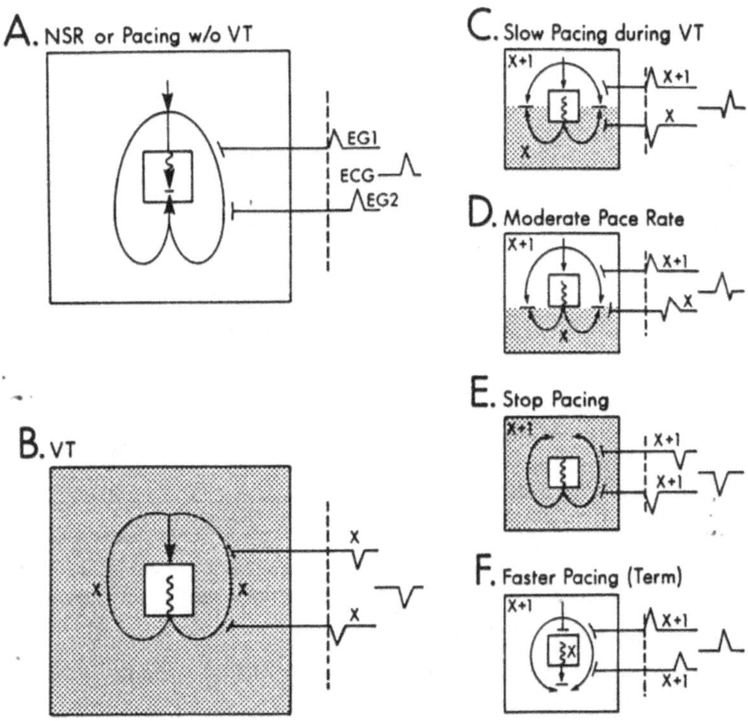

Table 1. Transient entrainment: four criteria

1) Constant fusion beats in the ECG during pacing at a constant rate which is faster than the tachycardia, except for the last captured beat which is entrained but not fused.
2) Progressive fusion in the ECG during pacing in steps of progressively faster constant rates. At each step the fusion remains constant.
3) Interruption of the tachycardia associated with localized conduction block for one beat, with the next paced beat causing activation of the site of block from a different direction with a shorter conduction time.
4) A change in conduction time to a recording site associated with a change in the bipolar electrogram morphology at that site during pacing from a single site at two different constant rates.

From Brugada and Wellens 1984 [72], Okumura et al. 1985 [73]

The phenomenon of transient entrainment is dependent on the presence of several determinants:

1) a wide excitable gap in the tachycardia circuit;
2) a relatively short effective refractory period in the circuit;
3) slow conduction in the anterograde limb;
4) relative sites of stimulation and circuit (direction of approach of stimulated wavefront) [76, 77].

Complex Pacing Patterns

To improve hemodynamic toleration of prolonged pacing, one method initiates pacing at rates well in excess of the tachycardia and then gradually decreases the rate (rate decremental ramp pacing or "tune down") [53, 78] (Fig. 8). In some cases ramping up relatively rapidly and then ramping down again may be less "jolting" than simple burst pacing. Autodecremental pacing [79] (Figs. 8, 9), in which cycle length decremental ramp pacing is used with an additional stimulus added for each attempt until a minimum cycle length, after which additional stimuli plateau (no additional decrement); "universal" pacing [80, 81] (Figs. 8, 10) in which a rapid cycle length decremental ramp is followed by an early plateau have been compared to burst pacing and have received favorable reports. Other stimulation patterns have been described (Figs. 5–10). Among them are changing ramps [38, 46], shifting bursts, scanning bursts (concertina/accordion) [62], and centrifugal scan [63, 82]. More exotic techniques include subthreshold extrastimulus or burst pacing [83–85].

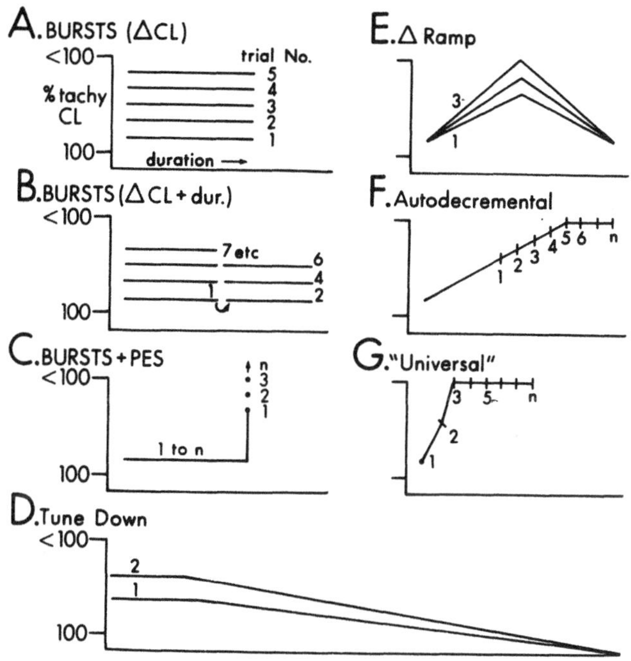

Fig. 8. Graphic representations of pacing for tachycardia termination. *Trial numbers* indicate successive attempts at termination. In ΔCL+ duration (second from top, left), trial 2 indicates a pacing duration twice as long as trial 1, but at the same rate

Acceleration

The most serious complication of antitachycardia pacing is acceleration of a tolerated rhythm into one that causes collapse. Acceleration of SVT into AF is usually not catastrophic except in cases of very enhanced AV nodal conduction or WPW. Acceleration of VT may well be catastrophic. With temporary pacing it occurs in about 4% of episodes, but at least once in more than a third of patients who have several episodes treated with antitachycardia pacing [64].

Several factors may account for acceleration [50, 51]: (1) multiple potential circuits; (2) 2:1 exit block converted to 1:1; (3) a short ERP in the tachycardia circuit allowing two wavefronts to coexist in the circuit; (4) unmasking of a potential "short circuit" within a larger circuit.

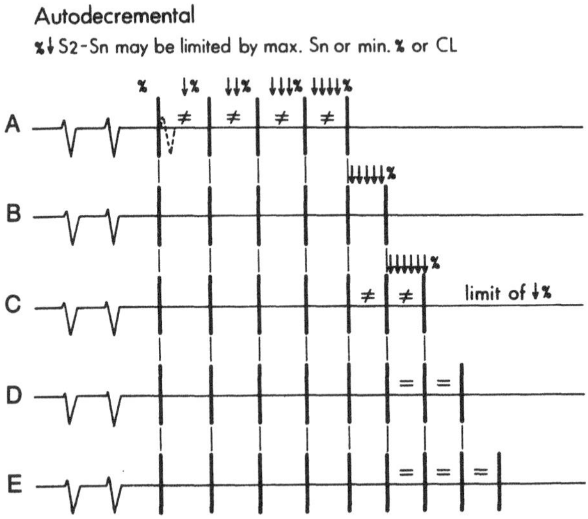

Fig. 9 A–E. Autodecremental pacing. The sequence begins in **A** in this case with 5 stimuli with progressively shorter cycle lengths; **B, C** additional stimuli are added, again with progressively shorter cycle lengths; **D, E** additional stimuli are added, but there is no further decrement in cycle length. (From Fisher et al. 1991 [249] by permission)

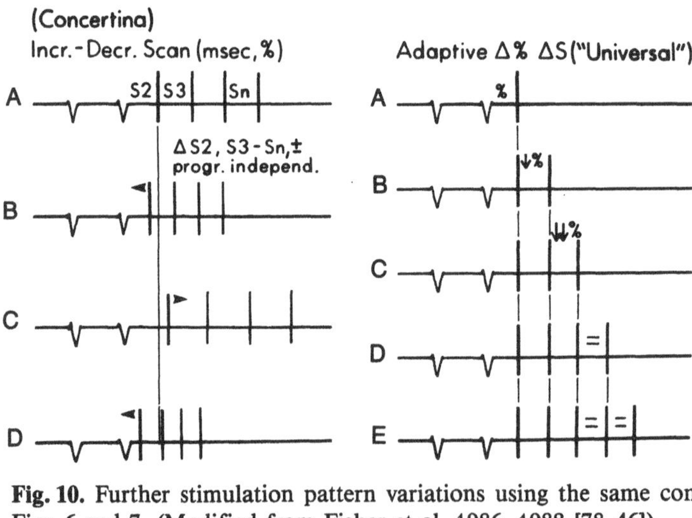

Fig. 10. Further stimulation pattern variations using the same conventions as Figs. 6 and 7. (Modified from Fisher et al. 1986, 1988 [78, 46])

Concurrent Medications

Antiarrhythmic medications can have a salutory effect on pacer termination of tachycardias [86–88]. Although some subjects do well without medications, continued treatment (often at a lower and well-tolerated dose) may reduce the incidence of recurrences and improve the chances of pacer termination [45, 46].

Temporary Antitachycardia Pacing [89–96]

Antitachycardia pacing remains underutilized. Pacing is a mainstay during electrophysiologic studies. Success rates are lower in acutely ill patients with VT [64], but pacing is still preferable to DC shocks. We recommend temporary pacemakers in patients with acute myocardial infarctions who have had two episodes of tachycardia requiring termination by chemical or electrical methods.

Antitachycardia pacing, including esophageal [91, 92] or transcutaneous [93–95] pacing can be very useful in the emergency room. Such pacers require special stimulators capable of high amplitude/long pulse duration stimuli, together with special electrode systems. After following open-heart surgery, atrial arrhythmias often respond to pacing used for prevention, hemodynamic support, or termination [96].

Implanted Antitachycardia Pacemakers

Prevention

Atrial pacing for patients with atrial arrhythmias can be helpful in some subjects, as can atrial or ventricular pacing for patients with ventricular tachycardia, especially torsades de pointes/long QT syndromes; atrioventricular (DDT) or nearly-simultaneous pacing may aid some patients with AV node reentry tachycardia [1–36, 45].

Longitudinal Follow-up

Antitachycardia therapy based on electrophysiologic studies conventionally requires another invasive study to confirm continuing therapeutic efficacy. Pacers capable of performing noninvasive programmed stimulation obviate the need for invasive studies, help to assess continuing efficacy of the chosen therapy, and can he helpful in predicting need for major changes in therapy. This should be recognized as an indication for implantation of a permanent pacemaker in certain individuals [45, 46, 48, 49].

Automatic and Manually Activated Antitachycardia Pacers and Detection Algorithms

The patient is responsible for initial detection with manually activated systems. Because some patients may initiate therapy inappropriately [39], transtelephone monitoring is helpful to confirm the presence of tachycardia.

All the automatic detection algorithms have limitations. Rapid rate [58, 61, 62, 97, 98] may not distinguish sinus tachycardia from pathologic tachycardias. Sudden onset [99–102] or constancy of cycle length [102] may not distinguish SVT from VT, or AF from other rhythms. Overlap can occur in endocardial signal amplitude, slew rate, morphology, frequency content or sequence [39, 103–110]. The probability density function [109, 110] detects fibrillation better than regular tachycardia. Diagnostic responses to extrastimuli [111, 112] are known for a few varieties of tachycardias. Timing of termination zones may change spontaneously [55, 113] or with changes in posture or activity [114], limiting the effectiveness of the therapy "remembered" by the pacer. Multiple programmable types of detection algorithms are needed.

Antitachycardia pacemakers are wide ranging in sophistication and capabilities [46]. Many bradycardia pacers also have antitachycardia capability [57, 115–117]. Some can perform programmed stimulation or bursts using special programmers [115]. Others have specific modes, such as DDT, which allow noninvasive programmed stimulation and antitachycardia pacing [117].

Successful antitachycardia pacing may require antiarrhythmic drugs [45, 86–88]. Because doses may be smaller, these drugs may cause fewer adverse effects as adjuvant rather than primary therapy [45, 46].

Candidates for Pacers for Tachycardia Termination

Selection is critical and often complex. Alternative therapy should be used whenever possible for patients with Wolff-Parkinson-White (WPW) syndrome and VT (unless used with ICD backup).

General criteria are:

1) recurrent but not incessant tachycardia;
2) drug therapy insufficient or not tolerated;

Table 2. Implanted pacers for SVT termination[a]

	Outcome				
	Total	Excellent	Good	Poor	Unstated
Number of patients	471	371	49	18	33
Patients (%)	100	79	10	4	7

[a] See Appendix Table A for details of studies and references.

3) surgical or catheter ablation not advisable or refused;
4) demonstrated success in scores of trials with variations in posture, activity, and drug levels [38, 45, 46].

Termination of Supraventricular Tachycardia

There is extensive worldwide experience in antitachycardia pacing for SVT. The long-term efficacy of pacing for SVT is only fair (93% at 1 year, 86% at 2–4 years, and 68% by 8 years), due to the development of chronic atrial fibrillation, or precipitation of atrial fibrillation during pacing for termination of SVT (Table 2 and Appendix Table A).

Pacers for Termination of Ventricular Tachycardia

There has always been great concern over the risk of acceleration to ventricular fibrillation. The use of antitachycardia pacers backed up by separate implantable cardioverter defibrillators addresses this, though inefficiently [158, 160]. Newer devices with both pacing and shock capabilities, in tiered sequences (see a later section), will lead to a resurgence of pacing for VT. Occasional patients with slow and well-tolerated tachycardias are candidates for manually activated pacers [45] (Table 3 and Appendix Table B).

Implantable Cardioverter Defibrillators (ICDs)

After initial skepticism [163] during the developmental period [164–166] the ICD became widely appreciated soon after its clinical introduction. After a decade of clinical use, we have passed the overshoot period of enthusiasm, and the value of the ICD can now be seen in better perspective.

Table 3. Implanted pacers for VT termination[a]

	Outcome			
	Total	Good to excellent	Poor	Unstated
Number of patients	228	150	9	69
Patients (%)	100	66	4	30

[a] See Appendix Table B for details of studies and references.

The advantages of ICDs are:

1) Compliance with therapy requires periodic checkups rather than multiple daily drug doses.
2) Countershock may remain effective to extremes of metabolic imbalances.
3) The patient may derive psychologic confidence in automatic rescue [167–169] (guardian angel factor).
4) ICD implant is less risky than surgical ablation.
5) Implant is possible at less specialized centers.

The disadvantages and problems of ICDs are:

1) They offer rescue rather than preventive therapy.
2) They may result in unpleasant shocks.
3) Certain patient activities such as automobile driving are limited.
4) Antiarrhythmic drugs can adversely affect defibrillation thresholds [169–173].
5) The ICD may be misled by pacemaker stimuli [174, 175] and it may fail to detect VF under certain circumstances [175, 178].
6) ICDs may not be activated by relatively slow VT (chest wall stimulation can [178] "trick" a nonprogrammable ICD into discharging).
7) Inappropriate ICD shocks may occur due to imperfect rhythm discrimination algorithms [174].
8) The immediate surgical and infection risks are higher than the immediate drug therapy risks, and replacement operations are needed periodically.
9) ICD patches may interfere with external defibrillation [181]. The ICD nevertheless represents a significant advance in the prevention of sudden arrhythmic death.

Development Challenges: Nonthoracotomy Implants and Waveform and Electrode Configurations

Early work included transvenous systems [164, 165], but other approaches seemed more reliable. Animal studies have shown that transvenous cardioversion of VT is possible with very low energy levels [182]. Clinical studies have demonstrated that synchronized low energy (less than 5 J) transvenous cardioversion of VT is similar to antitachycardia pacing in both termination and acceleration [183–187]. However, transvenous cardioversion is more painful and may produce atrial fibrillation [184–186]. Properly synchronized, transvenous shocks can be used to manage SVTs [187, 188].

A transvenous lead delivering truncated expotential shocks between the right ventricular apex and the superior vena cava or right atrium does not provide reliable defibrillation [184]. Other monophasic waveforms have been proposed, but some are not easily adaptable for technical reasons (Fig. 11).

Efficacy appears to be increased by sequential or unipolar or biphasic shocks delivered using conventional spring-patch, or patch-patch leads, or between several different sites [189]. Biphasic shocks seem more effective than sequential shocks; more than two shocking poles may also reduce the defibrillation threshold. Until recently, some form of thoracotomy has been required for implantation of current defibrillators [206–211]; development of a nonthoracotomy approach increases the acceptability of ICDs (Fig. 12).

Improved ICDs

Among the improvements [212] are:

1) antitachycardia and antibradycardia pacing in the same unit [213];
2) tiered therapy to avoid countershock when pacing is effective;
3) nonthoracotomy implantation;
4) improved shock characteristics to increase successes at reduced energies;
5) increased device longevity;
6) multiprogrammability;
7) Holter-like event reporting (Table 4).

In the absence of skillful programming, some patients might not benefit from the advanced features incorporated in the newer devices, while others would suffer if the ICD were programmed inappropriately.

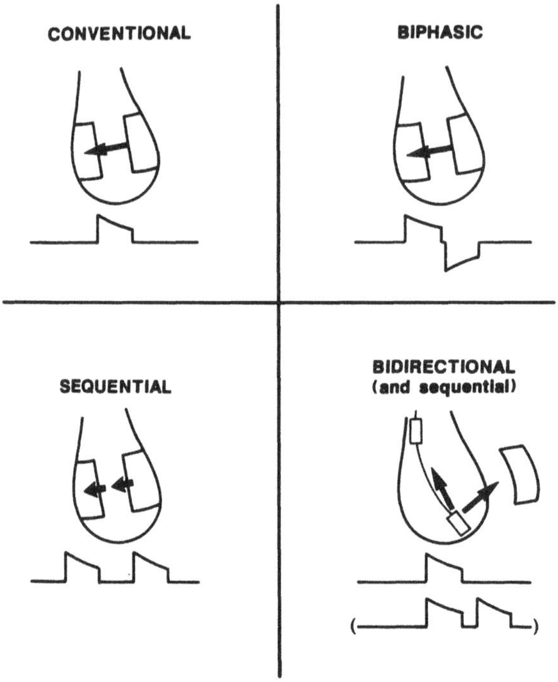

Fig. 11. ICD shock waveforms and configurations. *Upper left*, the now-conventional patch-patch system with a monophasic shock waveform; *lower left*, similar but closely sequential shocks are delivered. *Upper right*, a single biphasic shock is employed; *lower right*, a transvenous electrode with two poles is used in conjunction with an extrathoracic patch. *Bottom* of each panel, the upper waveform represents a single monophasic shock delivered simultaneously from the apex to both the right atrial pole and extrathoracic patch; the lower waveform e.g. (*lower right*) represents sequential monophasic shocks delivered, e.g., to the right atrium followed quickly by the extrathoracic patch. (From Fisher et al. 1991 [249] by permission)

Judging the Efficacy of ICDs

The ICD has been revolutionary. The 1 year sudden death rate for patients with an ICD is often reported to be under 2% [213, 215–221], compared with 2%–15% for patients with electrophysiologic or Holter-guided medical therapy [222–224], 15%–24% for patients treated with amiodarone [225, 226] and 20%–50% for patients receiving empirical drug therapy [222–224, 227, 228]. Antitachycardia surgery may be effective but initial operative mortality averages 12% and can be higher [229–231].

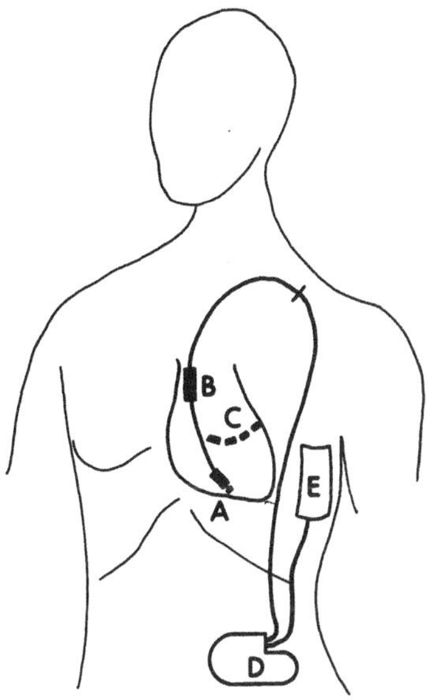

Fig. 12. ICD electrode configurations for nonthoracotomy implants. Most systems involve some form of: (1) transvenous electrode system with active poles in any of several locations, e.g., right ventricular apex (*A*); right atrium or superior vena cava (*B*); coronary sinus (C), (2) an extrathoracic patch electrode (*E*); or (3) others, such as the pulse generator itself, (*D*). These systems can be used for multidirectional or biphasic shocks as well as more conventional shocks between any two poles. (From Fisher et al. 1991 [249] by permission)

Table 4. ICD-anti tachycardia pacer combinations: devices and features

Trials in progress or late planning stages:
PRx (CPI), Guardian (Telectronics), ResQ (Intermedics), PCD (Medtronic), Cadence (Ventritex), Sie-Cure (Siemens/Pacesetters)
All feature
Brady and ATP (ATP in later model Guardians)
Tiered or graded responses to VT/VF (ATP. . . shock)
Programmable shock outputs
Some feature
Transvenous approach; later likely for all
Sequential/biphasic/bidirectional shocks

Sudden death and other cardiac deaths nevertheless remain frequent in ICD patients [232–237, 248]. The overall survival of 60% at 60 months [235–238, 248] is comparable to survival with other therapies used in nonrandomized studies [235, 238]. There is need to standardize the nomenclature used in survival analysis [235, 239]. ICDs are essentially inert (nonprotective) prior to delivery of a rescue shock, and after the first shock may be poor.

Not all appropriate shocks actually prevent sudden death. Patient selection may play a key role in outcome: when ICDs are implanted in patients after failure of one to three drug trials, survival is similar for patients who do and do not receive appropriate shocks. In contrast, when ICDs are implanted in patients who have failed exhaustive drug trials delivery of an appropriate shock may signal a dire outcome: in one series [234], the 5 year survival of patients who did not receive a shock was 94%, vs only 8% for patients who did receive an appropriate shock. Even in its worst-case presentation and even if previously overrated [240], the ICD is clearly of immense clinical value.

Criteria for Implantation of an Automatic Implantable Cardioverter Defibrillator

A triage situation has been created by the high cost of the ICD, uncertain reimbursement and low availability of more capable devices. The ICD is clearly indicated after one or more cardiac arrests not related to acute myocardial infarction or remediable drug or metabolic disturbances, especially with inducible arrhythmias after drug trials. Guidelines for other indications are being developed on multiple levels, including by professional organizations [241–243].

An ICD can supplement other forms of therapy. Patients receiving an ICD may be kept on the most effective drug regimen. Some centers implant the ICD in most postoperative VT patients whether or not the VT remains inducible [244]. Implantation of an ICD may become the "conservative" approach [46] for patients without other convincing protection.

Prophylactic ICDs

Patients who survive an initial cardiac arrest are few compared to the 400,000 people who die suddenly each year in the United States. Efforts are now being made to use risk stratification in patients with known heart disease. Medical prophylaxis has far been disappointing, e.g., the CAST study showing significantly greater mortality in the treated group. Prophylactic ICDs in VT patients following CABG or endocardial resection are nearly routine in some institutions [244, 245]. Studies are now being initiated to determine whether high risk patients can benefit from implantation of an ICD prophylactically. Some of these studies have catchy names such as CABG-patch, First AID, MUSTT (Multicenter Un-Sustained Tachycardia Trial), and others.

Substantially smaller devices for prophylactic use may be developed, with battery power to provide only a few shocks, insuring patient survival long enough to reach the hospital.

Conclusions

After a very long gestation period, the success of ICDs has led to a rebirth of interest in antitachycardia devices in general. Temporary pacing for tachycardia control remains underutilized. More pacers capable of noninvasive programmed stimulation are needed for follow-up of patients with serious arrhythmias. The benefits of the ICD are recognized worldwide, with the Soviets also pursuing development of an ICD/pacer [246]. The combination ICD-antitachycardia pacers, implanted without thoracotomy, are an important step in the evolution of therapy for malignant arrhythmias.

Acknowledgements

The authors acknowledge the assistance of Ms. Stephanie Olsen and of many other members of the arrhythmia, pacer, and cardiothoracic groups.

Appendix

The following tables provide additional information regarding studies cited in the text and in Tables 2 and 3.

Table A: SVT termination by implanted pacers

First author	Reference	Patients (n)	Pacer model	Pacer type	Pre-implant tests (n)	Post-implant tests (n)	Drugs	Duration of follow-up (months)	Results: Excellent (n)	Results: Good (n)	Results: Poor (n)	Comments
Bertholet et al. 1985	[118]	13	PASAR 4151, Medt SPO 500	Auto, scan, PES, manual, extrastimuli, bursts	At least 100	Q 1 month x3 then Q 3 months	5	5–30	7	3	3	
Spurrell et al. 1984	[62]	21	PASAR 4151, 4171	Auto, shift, scan, bursts	NS	NS	8	2–40	16			Sudden deaths (2), deactivated and surg Rx (3)
Luck et al. 1988	[93]	1	Cordis Orthocor	Manual, scan, bursts	"Extensive evaluation"	NS	No	3	1			
Sowton 1984	[82]	16	Siemens Elema Tachylog	Auto, scan, PES, bursts	NS	NS	3	5–19	14			Surg Rx for WPW with rapid AF (2)
Zipes et al. 1984	[119]	21	Medt Symblos 7008	Auto, scan, PES, bursts	NS	NS	NS	NS	21			
Moss and Rivers 1974	[14]	2	Medt 5842 1317A	Manual, magnet	NS	NS	No	2–7	2			
Goyal et al. 1975	[120]	1	Medt 5998RF	Manual, burst	NS	NS	Yes	8	1			

Wyndham et al. 1978	[121]	1	Medt 5998	Manual, burst	NS	NS	Yes	21	1		Some problems with AF
Arbel et al. 1978	[128]	1	Cordis Atricor	Auto, coupled	NS	NS	NS	up to 48	1		CHF and cardio-megaly resolved 4 months after implant
Fahraeus et al. 1984	[114]	8	PASAR 4151	Auto, scan	NS	NS*	2	NS	4		Sinus tachy-cardia/SVT rate overlap caused inappropriate stimulation
Lüderitz et al. 1982	[129]	9	Intermed Cybertach	Auto, manual underdrive, burst	NS	NS	Yes	NS	5	4	
Nilsson and Ringqvist 1982	[130]	1	CPI Micro Lith	Auto, synchronous V pacing	NS	NS	Yes	NS			
Preston et al. 1979	[40]	1	Medt 5998 RF	Auto	NS	NS	Yes	5 1/2	1		Rapid A pacing with 2:1 or 4:1 conduction
Mandel et al. 1976	[131]	1	Am. Opt custom	Manual ramp	NS	NS	NS	7	1		Ramp pacing to 300 beats/min
Saksena et al. 1986	[132]	2	Cordis Ortho 234 A	Manual burst	>10	"Multi"	No	20	2		
Solti et al. 1982	[122]	1	Medt 5998 RF	Manual, burst	NS	NS	NS	>11	1		

* One patient had exercise test.

Table A (continued)

First author	Reference	Patients (n)	Pacer model	Pacer type	Pre-implant tests (n)	Post-implant tests (n)	Drugs	Duration of follow-up (months)	Results: Excellent (n)	Good (n)	Poor (n)	Comments
Peters et al. 1985	[123]	10	Medt 5998 RF	Manual, burst	"At least 50"		4	24 – 60	6	1	3	
O'Keefe et al. 1981	[124]	1	Telct. 150B (custom device)	Auto, underdrive	NS	NS	Yes	6	1			
den Dulk et al. 1984	[125]	12	Medt SPO 500	Manual, PES	NS	NS	8	3 – 26	8	4		
Portillo et al. 1982	[126]	8	Medt DVI-M	Auto	NS	NS	2	4 – 20	5			No SVT after implant (3)
Spurrell and Sowton 1976	[33]	1	Devices 4271	Auto, VAT	NS	NS	Yes	10	1			
Abinader 1976	[127]	1	Manual, magnet	NS	NS	Yes	>16		(1)			SVT became unresponsive after 16 months
Krikler et al. 1979	[58]	2	Ela Stanium	Auto, VVT or AAT	NS	NS	1	18	2	0		
Fisher et al. 1987	[45]	16	Misc	Misc	100	100	Yes	6 – 177	12	4		Not all patients had 100 pre- and postimplant trials
Kahn et al. 1976 (multicenter)	[133]	12	Medt 5998 RF	Manual, burst	NS	NS	8	15 – 36	10			Explant (1), Chr pericarditis (2), died CVA (1)

Griffin and Sweeny 1987 (multicenter)	[134]	91	Intermed Cybertach	Auto, burst	NS	NS	NS	>21	75%			Eight pacers explanted due to inadequate sensing
Rothman and Keefe 1984 (multicenter)	[135]	16	Cordis Orthocor	Manual, burst	NS	NS	NS	1–40	14%			
Palakurthy and Slater 1988	[136]	5	Telec. PASAR	Auto, scan	NS	NS	4/80	4–25 (12)	2	2	1	Of 5 pacers, 4 needed reprogramming, all >2x
Kappenberger et al. 1989	[137]	63	Siemens tachylog	PES, bursts	NS	NS	31/49	2–100 (30)	53	9	4	
Occhetta et al. 1989	[138]	7	Cordis Orthocor II	Bursts	10	>30	5/71	2–30 (20)	7	0	0	
Moller et al. 1989	[139]	13	Telec PASAR 4171	Scan (2–7 stim)	>10	NS	8/61	4–53 (20)	12	0	1	
Moreira et al. 1989	[140]	1	Medt. 5998 RF then 2434	Continuous rapid	–	–	1/100	48	0	1	0	
Schnittger et al. 1989	[141]	11	Intermed C'tach 60	Bursts	NS	50	4/36	54–108/84	6	4	1	
Nürnberg et al. 1989	[142]	1	Medt. 7008	Bursts	NS	NS	NS	8	0	0	1	
Van Hemel and Bakema 1979	[143]	2	Biotr IDP 64SD	Bursts	NS	NS	2	?–9	1	1	0	
Waxman et al. 1979	[144]	9	Medtr. 5998 RF	Bursts	50–100	NS	6/67	12–72	9	0	0	
Todo et al. 1979	[145]	19	Sokki Atricon RF	Bursts	NS	NS		<9 years	(19)			

Table A (continued)

First author	Reference	Patients (*n*)	Pacer model	Pacer type	Pre-implant tests (*n*)	Post-implant tests (*n*)	Drugs	Duration of follow-up (months)	Results			
									Excellent (*n*)	Good (*n*)	Poor (*n*)	Comments
Pistolese et al. 1979	[146]	4		RV burst and undeveloped	NS	NS	NS	4–20	4	0	0	
Simonsen and Fabricius 1986	[147]	1	Telec PASAR 4151	RV PES	NS	NS	1	12	1	0	0	
Critelli et al. 1979	[148]	4	Medt. Devices RF	RV PES	NS	NS	NS	<12	4	0	0	
Krikler et al. 1976	[149]	2	ELA dual demand	RV and RA underdrive	NS	NS	1	NS	2	0	0	
Case et al. 1990	[150]	1	Intermed Intertach	Auto, RA burst	NS	NS	No	48	1	0	0	
Li et al. 1990	[151]	17	Intermed Intertach	Auto, RA stim	NS	NS	9	15 ± 8	13	4	0	Major point is socioeconomic
den Dulk et al. 1990	[152]	40	Misc.	Auto, manual	NS	NS	17	38	30?	10	?	10 from RV

Modified and expanded with permission from PACE [78]

AF, atrial fibrillation; *CHF*, congestive heart failure; *chr*, chronic; *CVA*, cardiovascular accident; *expl*, explanted; *NS*, not significant; *PES*, programmed extrastimuli; *RF*, radiofrequency; *SVT*, supraventricular tachycardia; *Surg*, surgical; *WPW*, Wolf-Parkinson-White Syndrome

Table B. Ventricular tachycardia termination by implanted pacers

First author	Reference	Patients (n)	Pacer model	Pacer type	Pre-implant tests (n)	Post-implant tests (n)	Drugs	Duration of follow-up (months)	Results			
									Excellent	Good	Poor	Comments
Reddy et al. 1984	[153]	1	PASAR 4151	Auto, scanning PES	"Many"	"Several"	Yes	6	1			
Bertholet et al. 1985	[118]	3	Medt SPO 5000	Manual, scanning, or burst	"At least 100"	NS	Yes	17–30	3			
Spurrell et al. 1984	[62]	1	PASAR 4151	Auto, shifting	NS	NS	NS	NS	1			Unit explanted after patient free of VT
Sowton 1984	[82]	9	Siemens Elema Tachylog	Auto, scanning, PES, or burst	NS	NS	3	6–14	5			
den Dulk et al. 1984	[125]	6	Medt SPO 500	Manual, variable modes	NS	NS	5	6–20	4	2		
Moss and Rivers 1974	[14]	1	Medt 5842	Manual via magnet	NS	NS	?	6	1			No VT after pacer rate increased
Hartzler 1979	[154]	2	Medt 5998	Manual RF	>30–100	>50–70	Yes	1–11	1			Death at 4 weeks due to VT (1)
Ruskin et al. 1980	[155]	3	Medt 5998	Manual RF	>100	100 each	Yes	Mean 13.6	3			Lung cancer (1)

Table B (continued)

First author	Reference	Patients (*n*)	Pacer model	Pacer type	Pre-implant tests (*n*)	Post-implant tests (*n*)	Drugs	Duration of follow-up (months)	Results			
									Excellent	Good	Poor	Comments
Herre et al. 1985	[156]	28	Medt 5998	Manual RF	NS	125 EP studies	18	1–25	97% success in 9 patients			No spont VT in 19 patients, sudden death (1)
Peters et al. 1985	[123]	6	Medt	Manual RF	NS	NS	Yes	3–36	1	5		accelerated (2), refractory (3)
Strassberg et al. 1982	[48]	2	Medt 5998	Manual RF	NS	NS	NS	–	–		–	No recurrence (1), one recurrence (1)
Tanabe et al. 1985	[115]	1	Medt Spect	Manual	NS	NS	NS	–	–		–	
Higgins et al. 1985	[157]	1	PASAR 4151	Auto, scan, burst, or PES	NS	NS	No	16	–	1	–	
Lüderitz et al. 1982	[129]	3	2 Magnet 1 Cordis Orthocor 234A	Manual, underdrive Manual, burst	NS	NS	NS	Yes	NS	2	1	
Saksena et al. 1986	[132]	11	Cordis Ortho 234A	Manual, burst	NS	NS	10	(0–28)	Not certain; see comments			VT term (4); others mostly for PES (7)

Fisher et al. 1987	[45]	20	Misc	Misc	>100	>100	Yes	2–92	16	2	2	explant at 1 month (1), disarmed at 1 month (4), 4 sudden, no pacer-related deaths
Griffin and Sweeney 1987 (multicenter)	[134]	52	Inter-Medics Cybert	Auto, burst	NS	NS	NS	12	30			Nontachycardia deaths (14), sudden deaths (4)
Rothman and Keefe 1984 (multicenter)	[135]	53	Cordis Orthocor	Manual, burst, etc.	NS	NS	NS	1–41	45			Sudden deaths (3), documented VT/VF deaths (3)
Palakurthy and Slater 1988	[136]	1	Telec PASAR 4171	Auto, scan, 2 PES	NS	NS	1	23	1	0	0	
Occhetta et al. 1989	[138]	1	Cordis Orthocor	Bursts	10	>30	1	21	1*	0	0	Finally failed, AICD

Table B (continued)

First author	Reference	Patients (*n*)	Pacer model	Pacer type	Pre-implant tests (*n*)	Post-implant tests (*n*)	Drugs	Duration of follow-up (months)	Results			
									Excellent	Good	Poor	Comments
Moller et al. 1989	[139]	2	Telec PASAR 4171	Bursts			2	26.5	2	0	0	
Newman et al. 1989	[158]	11	Intermed Intertach	ADP	>20	>20	10	2–29 (12)	11	0	0	AICD in 8
Fromer et al. 1987	[159]	1	Intermed Intertach	2 PES, scan	>25	NS	1	12	1	0	0	
Manz et al. 1986	[160]	5	Siemens Tachylog	Burst	NS	NS	5	3–8 (5.4)	2	2	1	AICD in all 5, most term w/ATP; AICD in 3
Falkoff et al. 1986	[161]	2	Intermed C'tach	Burst	Many	Many	2	7 and 64	2	0	0	Pacer syndrome (1)
Greene et al. 1982	[162]	2	Cordis Orthocor	2 PES	Multiple	Multiple	4.9	2	0	0	0	Never used (1)

Modified and expanded with permission from PACE [78]. EP, electrophysiologic; NS, not significant, miscellaneous; PES, programmed extrastimuli; RF, radiofrequency; spont, spontaneous; VF, ventricular fibrillation; VT, ventricular tachycardia

References

1. Schwedel JB, Furman S, Escher DJW (1960) Use of an intracardiac pacemaker in the treatment of Stokes-Adams seizures. Prog Cardiovasc Dis 3:170–177
2. Zoll PM, Linenthal AJ (1963) External and internal cardiac pacemakers. Circulation 28:455–466
3. Sowton E, Leathman A, Carson P (1964) The suppression of arrhythmias by artificial pacing. Lancet ii:1098–1100
4. Escher DJW (1969) The treatment of tachyarrhythmias by artificial pacing. Am Heart J 78:829–832
5. Heiman DF, Helwig J Jr (1966) Suppression of ventricular arrhythmias by transvenous intracardiac pacing. JAMA 195:172–175
6. Lew HT, March HW (1967) Control of recurrent ventricular fibrillation by transvenous pacing in the absence of heart block. Am Heart J 73:794–797
7. Zipes DP, Festoff B, Schaal SF, Cox C, Sealy WC, Wallace AG (1968) Treatment of ventricular arrhythmia by permanent atrial pacemaker and cardiac sympathectomy. Ann Intern Med 68:591–597
8. DeFrancis NA, Giordano RP (1968) Permanent epicardial atrial pacing in the treatment of refractory ventricular tachycardia. Am J Cardiol 22:742–745
9. DeSanctis RW, Kastor JA (1968) Rapid intracardiac pacing for treatment of recurrent ventricular tachyarrhythmias in the absence of heart block. Am Heart J 76:168–172
10. Friedberg CK, Lyon LJ, Donoso E (1970) Suppression of refractory recurrent ventricular tachycardia by transvenous rapid pacing and antiarrhythmic drugs. Am Heart J 79:44–50
11. Silka MJ, Manwill JR, Kron J, McAnulty JH (1990) Bradycardia-mediated tachyarrhythmias in congenital heart disease and responses to chronic pacing at physiologic rates. Am J Cardiol 65:483–493
12. Lichstein E, Chadda K, Fenig S (1972) Atrial pacing in the treatment of refractory ventricular tachycardia associated with hypokalemia. Am J Cardiol 30:550–553
13. Johnson RA, Hutter AM, DeSanctis RW, Yurchak PM, Leinback RC, Harthorne JW (1974) Chronic overdrive pacing in the control of refractory ventricular arrhythmias. Ann Intern Med 80:380–383
14. Moss AJ, Rivers RJ (1974) Termination and inhibition of recurrent tachycardias by implanted pervenous pacemakers. Circulation 50:942–947
15. Dreifus LS, Berkovits BV, Kimibiris D et al. (1975) Use of atrial and bifocal cardiac pacemakers for treating resistant dysrhythmias. Eur J Cardiol 3:257–266
16. Cooper TB, Maclean WAH, Waldo A (1978) Overdrive pacing for supraventricular tachycardias: a review of theoretical implications and therapeutic techniques. PACE 1:196–221
17. Ector H, Brabandt HV, DeGeest H (1984) Treatment of life-threatening ventricular arrhythmias by a combination of antiarrhythmic drugs and right ventricular pacing. PACE 7:622–627

18. Crick JCP, Way B, Sowton E (1984) Successful treatment of ventricular tachycardia by physiological pacing. PACE 7:949–951
19. Fisher JD, Teichman S, Ferrick A, Kim SG, Waspe LE, Martinez MR (1987) Antiarrhythmic effects of VVI pacing at physiologic rates: a crossover controlled evaluation. PACE 10:822–830
20. Attuel P, Pellerin D, Mugica J, Coumel PH (1988) DDD pacing: an effective treatment modality for recurrent atrial arrhythmias. PACE 11:1647–1654
21. Feuer JM, Shandling AH, Messenger JC, Castellanet CD, Thomas LA (1990) Influence of cardiac pacing mode on the long-term development of atrial fibrillation. Am J Cardiol 64:1376–1379
22. Zacouto F, Juillard A, Gerbaux A (1982) Prevention of ventricular tachycardias by automatic rate pacing. Reanim Artif Organ 8:3–11
23. Behrenbeck DW, Winter UJ, Hoher M, Brill TH, Ebeling H, Hirche HJ, Hilger HH (1985) Dynamic overdrive pacing for suppression of ventricular ectopic activity. In: Proceedings of the International Symposium on Invasive Cardiovascular Therapy: recent advances and future developments, Cologna, pp 47–47A
24. Han J, Millet D, Chizzonitti B, Moe GK (1966) Temporal dispension of recovery of excitability in atrium and ventricle as a function of heart rate. Am Heart J 71:481–487
25. Khan MM, Logan KR, McComb JM, Adgey AAJ (1981) Management of recurrent ventricular tachyarrhythmias associated with Q-T prolongation. Am J Cardiol 47:1301–1308
26. Bhandari AK, Scheinman MM, Morady F, Svinarich J, Mason J, Winkle R (1984) Efficacy of left cardiac sympathectomy in the treatment of patients with the long QT syndrome. Circulation 70:1018–1023
27. Gurtner HP, Gertsch M, Zacouto F (1975) Orthorhythmischer Herzschrittmacher und salvenförmige Herzstimulation. Schweiz Med Wochenschr 105:33–38
28. Kuck KH, Kunze KP, Schluter M, Bleifeld W (1984) Tachycardia prevention by programmed stimulation. Am J Cardiol 54:550–554
29. Davies DW, Butrous GS, Spurrell RAJ, Camm AJ (1987) Pacing techniques in the prophylaxis of junctional reentry tachycardia. PACE 10:519–532
30. Begemann MJS, Bennekers JH, Kingma JH, Lie KI (1987) Prevention of Tachycardia Initiation by Programmed Stimulation. J Electrophysiol 4:350–356
31. Sung RJ, Styperek JL, Castellanos A (1980) Complete abolition of the reentrant SVT zone using a new modality of cardiac pacing with simultaneous atrioventricular stimulation. Am J Cardiol 45:72–78
32. Akhtar M, Gilbert CJ, Al-Nouri M, Schmidt DH (1979) Electrophysiologic mechanisms for modification and abolition of atrioventricular junctional tachycardia with simultaneous and sequential atrial and ventricular pacing. Circulation 60:1443–1453
33. Spurrell RAJ, Sowton E (1976) An implanted atrial synchronous pacemaker with a short atrioventricular delay for the prevention of paroxysmal supraventricular tachycardias. J Electrocardiol 9:89–96

34. Mehra R, Gough WB, Zeiler R, El-Sherif N (1984) Dual ventricular stimulation for prevention of reentrant ventricular arrhythmias. J Am Coll Cardiol 3:472 (abstr)
35. Schluter M, Kunze KP, Kuck KH (1987) Train stimulation at the atria for prevention of atrioventricular tachycardia: dependence on accessory pathway location. J Am Coll Cardiol 9:1288–1293
36. Prystowsky EN, Zipes D (1983) Inhibition in the human heart. Circulation 68:707–713
37. Marchlinski FE, Buxton AE, Miller JM, Josephson ME (1987) Prevention of ventricular tachycardia induction during right ventricular programmed stimulation by high current strength pacing at the site of origin. Circulation 76:332–342
38. Fisher JD, Kim SG, Furman S, Matos JA (1982) Role of implantable pacemakers in control of recurrent ventricular tachycardia. Am J Cardiol 49:194–206
39. Furman S (1973) Therapeutic uses of atrial pacing. Am Heart J 86:835–840
40. Preston TA, Haynes RE, Gavin WA, Hessel EA (1979) Permanent rapid atrial pacing to control supraventricular tachycardia. PACE 2:331–334
41. Waldo AL, MacLean WAH, Karp RB, Kouchoukos NT, James TN (1976) Continuous rapid atrial pacing to control recurrent or sustained supraventricular tachycardias following open heart surgery. Circulation 54: 245–250
42. Arbel ER, Cohen HC, Langendorf R, Glick G (1978) Successful treatment of drug-resistant atrial tachycardia and intractable congestive heart failure with permanent coupled atrial pacing. Am J Cardiol 41:336–340
43. Langendorf R, Pick A (1965) Observations on the clinical use of paired electrical stimulation of the heart. Bull NY Acad Med 41:535–540
44. Waldo AL, Krongrad E, Kupersmith J, Levine OR, Bowman FO Jr, Hoffman BF (1976) Ventricular paired pacing to control rapid ventricular heart rate following open heart surgery. Circulation 53:177–181
45. Fisher JD, Johnston DR, Furman S, Waspe LE, Kim SG (1987) Long-term efficacy of antitachycardia devices. Am J Cardiol 60:1311–1316
46. Fisher JD, Kim SG, Mercando AD (1988) Electrical devices for the treatment of arrhythmias. Am J Cardiol 61:45A–57A
47. Hamer AW, Zaher CA, Rubin SA, Peter T, Mandel WJ (1985) Hemodynamic benefits of synchronized 1:1 atrial pacing during sustained ventricular tachycardia with severely depressed ventricular function in coronary heart disease. Am J Cardiol 55:990–994
48. Strassberg B, Fetter J, Palileo E, Levitsky S, Rosen KM (1982) Post-operative electrophysiological studies with a modified radio-frequency system. Technical aspects and clinical usefulness. PACE 5:688–693
49. Fisher JD, Furman S, Kim SG, Matos JA, Waspe LA (1984) DDD/DDT pacemakers in the treatment of ventricular tachycardia. PACE 7:173–178
50. Fisher JD, Kim SG, Waspe LE, Matos JA (1983) Mechanisms for the success and failure of pacing for termination of ventricular tachycardia: clinical and hypothetical considerations. PACE 6:1094–1105

51. Fisher JD, Kim SG, Matos JA, Waspe LE (1985) Pacing for tachycardias: clinical translations. In: Zipes D, Jalife J (eds) Electrophysiology and arrhythmias. Grune and Stratton, Orlando, pp 507–511
52. Fisher JD, Kim SG, Matos JA, Waspe LE (1984) Pacing for ventricular tachycardia. PACE 7:1278–1290
53. Fisher JD (1986) Electrical devices for the treatment of tachyarrhythmias. Cardiol Clin 4:527–542
54. Waxman HL, Cain ME, Greenspan AM, Josephson ME (1982) Termination of ventricular tachycardia with ventricular stimulation: salutary effect of increased current strength. Circulation 65:800–804
55. Fisher JD, Ostrow E, Kim SG, Matos JA (1983) Ultrarapid single-capture train stimulation for termination of ventricular tachycardia. Am J Cardiol 51:1334–1338
56. Spurrell RAJ, Sowton E (1975) Pacing techniques in the management of supraventricular tachycardia. J Electrocardiol 8:287–295
57. Barold SS, Ryan GF, Goldstein S (1989) The first implanted tachycardia-terminating pacemaker. PACE 12:870–874
58. Krikler DM, Curry PVL, Buffet J (1979) Dual-demand pacing for reciprocating atrioventricular tachycardia. Br Med J 1:1114–1117
59. Fisher JD, Furman S (1978) Automatic termination of tachycardia by an implanted "upside down" demand pacemaker. Clin Res 26:231 a (abstr)
60. Fisher JD, Kim SG, Matos JA, Ostrow E (1983) Comparative effectiveness of pacing techniques for termination of well-tolerated sustained ventricular tachycardia. PACE 6:915–922
61. Nathan AW, Camm AJ, Bexton RS, Hellestrand KJ, Spurrell RAJ (1982) Initial experience with a fully implantable, programmable, scanning, extrastimulus pacemaker for tachycardia termination. Clin Cardiol 5:22–26
62. Spurrell RAJ, Nathan AW, Camm AJ (1984) Clinical experience with implantable scanning tachycardia reversion pacemakers. PACE 7:1296–1300
63. Holt P, Crick JCP, Sowton E (1986) Antitachycardia pacing: a comparison of burst overdrive, self-searching and adaptive table scanning programs. PACE 9:490–497
64. Fisher JD, Mehra R, Furman S (1978) Termination of ventricular tachycardia with bursts of ventricular pacing. Am J Cardiol 41:94–102
65. Gardner MJ, Waxman HL, Buxton AE, Cain ME, Josephson ME (1982) Termination of tachycardia: evaluation of a new pacing method. Am J Cardiol 50:1338–1345
66. Jantzer JH, Hoffman RM (1984) Acceleration of ventricular tachycardia by rapid overdrive pacing combined with extrastimuli. PACE 7:922–924
67. Waldo AL, Henthorn RW, Plumb VJ, MacLean WAH (1984) Demonstration of the mechanism of transient entrainment and interruption of ventricular tachycardia with rapid atrial pacing. J Am Coll Cardiol 3:422–430
68. MacLean WAH, Plumb VJ, Waldo AL (1981) Transient entrainment and interruption of ventricular tachycardia. PACE 4:358–366
69. Waldo AL, Plumb VJ, Arciniegas JG, MacLean WAH et al. (1982) Transient entrainment and interruption of A-V bypass pathway type paroxysmal atrial

tachycardia. A model for understanding and identifying reentrant arrhythmias in man. Circulation 67:73–83
70. Waldo AL, MacLean WAH, Karp RB, Kouchoukos NT, James TN (1977) Entrainment and interruption of atrial flutter with atrial pacing. Studies in man following open heart surgery. Circulation 56:737–745
71. Anderson KP, Swerdlow CD, Mason JW (1983) Entrainment of ventricular tachycardia. Am J Cardiol 53:335–340
72. Brugada P, Wellens HJJ (1984) Entrainment as an electrophysiologic phenomenon. J Am Coll Cardiol 3:451–454
73. Okumura K, Henthorn RW, Epstein AE, Plumb VJ, Waldo AL (1985) Further observations on transient entrainment: importance of pacing site and properties of the components of the reentry circuit. Circulation 72:1293–1307
74. Henthorn RW, Okumura K, Olshansky B, Plumb VJ, Hess PG, Waldo AL (1988) A fourth criterion for transient entrainment: the electrogram equivalent of progressive fusion. Circulation 77:1003–1012
75. Waldo AL, Plumb VJ, Arciniegas JG, MacLean WAH, Cooper TB, Priest MF, James TN (1983) Transient entrainment and interruption of the atrioventricular bypass pathway type of paroxysmal atrial tachycardia. A model for understanding and identifying reentrant arrhythmias. Circulation 67:73–83
76. Mann DE, Lawrie GM, Luck JC, Griffin JC, Magro SA, Wyndham CRC (1985) Importance of pacing site in entrainment of ventricular tachycardia. J Am Coll Cardiol 5:781–787
77. Plumb VJ, Henthorn RW, Waldo AL (1984) Characteristics of the transient entrainment of ventricular tachycardia by ventricular pacing. PACE 7:463 A
78. Fisher JD, Johnston DR, Kim SG, Furman S, Mercando AM (1986) Implantable pacers for tachycardia termination: Stimulation techniques and long-term efficacy. PACE 9:1325–1333
79. Charos GS, Haffajee CI, Gold RL, Bishop RL, Berkovits BV, Alpert JS (1986) A theoretically and practically more effective method for interruption of ventricular tachycardia: self-adapting autodecremental overdrive pacing. Circulation 73:309–315
80. den Dulk K, Bertholet M, Brugada P, Bar FW, Richards D, Demoulin JC, Waleffee A, Bakels N, Lindemans FW, Bourgeois I, Kulbertus HE, Wellens HJJ (1986) A versatile pacemaker system for termination of tachycardias. Am J Cardiol 57:950–955
81. den Dulk K, Kersschot IE, Brugada P, Wellens HJJ (1986) Is there a universal antitachycardia pacing mode? Am J Cardiol 57:950–955
82. Sowton E (1984) Clinical results with the tachylog antitachycardia pacemaker. PACE 7:1313–1317
83. Von Leitner R, Linderer T (1984) Subthreshold burst pacing: A new method for termination of ventricular and subventricular tachycardia. J Am Coll Cardiol 3:472
84. Gang ES, Peter T, Nalos PC, Meesmann M, Karagueuzian HS, Mandel WJ, Oseran DS, Myers MR (1988) Subthreshold atrial pacing in patients with a

left-sided accessory pathway: an effective new method for terminating reciprocating tachycardia. J Am Coll Cardiol 11:515–521

85. Shenasa M, Cardinal R, Kus T, Savard P, Fromer M, Page P (1988) Termination of sustained ventricular tachycardia by ultrarapid subthreshold stimulation in humans. Circulation 78:1135–1143
86. Camm J, Ward D, Washington HG, Spurrell RAJ (1979) Intravenous disopyramide phosphate and ventricular overdrive pacing in the termination of paroxysmal ventricular tachycardia. PACE 2:395–402
87. Naccarelli GV, Zipes DP, Rahilly GT, Heger JJ, Prystowsky EN (1983) Influence of tachycardia cycle length and antiarrhythmic drugs on pacing termination and acceleration of ventricular tachycardia. Am Heart J 105:1–5
88. Keren G, Miura DS, Somberg JC (1984) Pacing termination of ventricular tachycardia: influence of antiarrhythmic-slowed ectopic rate. Am Heart J 107:638–643
89. Escher DJW, Furman S (1970) Emergency treatment of cardiac arrhythmias: emphasis on use of electrical pacing. JAMA 214:2028–2034
90. Fisher JD (1990) Electrical therapy in the acute control of tachycardias. A. Antitachycardia pacing in the acute care setting. In: Saksena S, Goldschlager N (eds) Electrical therapy for cardiac arrhythmias. Saunders, Philadelphia, pp 411–423
91. Benson DW (1987) Transesophageal electrocardiography and cardiac pacing: state of the art. Circulation 75:88–90
92. Guarnerio M, Furlanello F, DelGreco M, Vergara G, Inama G, Disertori M (1989) Transesophageal atrial pacing: a first-choice technique in atrial flutter therapy. Am Heart J 117:1241–1252
93. Luck JC, Grubb BP, Artman SE, Steckbeck RT, Markel ML (1988) Termination of sustained ventricular tachycardia by external noninvasive pacing. Am J Cardiol 61:574–577
94. Luck JC, Davis D (1987) Termination of sustained tachycardia by external noninvasive pacing. PACE 10:1125–1129
95. Estes NAM, Deering TF, Manolis AS, Salem D, Zoll PM (1989) External cardiac programmed stimulation for noninvasive termination of sustained supraventricular and ventricular tachycardia. Am J Cardiol 63:177–183
96. Waldo AL, MacLean W, Cooper TB, Kouchoukos NT (1978) Use of temporarily placed epicardial atrial wire electrodes for the diagnosis and treatment of cardiac arrhythmias following open-heart surgery. J Thorac Cardiovasc Surg 76:500–505
97. Neumann G, Funke H, Simon H, Aulepp H, Grube E, Schaede A (1978) Successful treatment of supraventricular reentry tachycardia by implantation of demand overdrive pacemakers. Societe de la Nouvelle Imprimerie Fournie, Toulouse, pp 193–196
98. Griffin JC, Mason JW, Calfee RV (1980) Clinical use of an implantable automatic tachycardia-terminating pacemaker. Am Heart J 100:1093–1096
99. den Dulk K, Brugada P, Waldecker B, Bergemann M, van der Schatte Olivier T, Wellens HJJ (1985) Automatic pacemaker termination of two different types of supraventricular tachycardia. J Am Coll Cardiol 6:201–205

100. Sowton E (1984) Clinical results with the tachylog antitachycardia pacemaker. PACE 7:1313–1317
101. Pless BD, Sweeney MB (1984) Discrimination of supraventricular tachycardia from sinus tachycardia of overlapping cycle length. PACE 7:1318–1324
102. Fisher JD, Goldstein M, Ostrow E, Matos JA, Kim SG (1983) Maximal rate of tachycardia development: sinus tachycardia with sudden exercise vs. spontaneous ventricular tachycardia. PACE 3:221–228
103. Furman S, Brodman R, Pannizzo F, Fisher JD (1984) Implantation techniques of antitachycardia devices. PACE 7:572–579
104. Furman S, Pannizzo F (1985) The role of implantable pacemakers in the therapy of tachycardias. Arch Mal Coeur 78:29–34
105. Furman S, Fisher JD, Pannizzo F (1982) Necessity of signal processing in tachycardia detection. In: Barold SS, Mugica J (eds) The third decade of cardiac pacing. Futura, Mount Kisco, pp 265–274
106. Klementowitz PT, Furman S (1986) Selective atrial sensing in dual chamber pacemakers eliminates endless loop tachycardia. J Am Coll Cardiol 7:590–594
107. Davies DW, Wainwright RJ, Tooley MA, Lloyd D, Nathan AW, Spurrell RAJ, Camm AJ (1986) Detection of pathological tachycardia by analysis of electrogram morphology. PACE 9:200–208
108. Merando AD, Furman S (1986) Measurement of differences in timing and sequence between two ventricular electrodes as a means of tachycardia differentiation. PACE 9:1069–1088
109. Aubert AE, Denys GB, Ector H, DeGeest H (1986) Detection of ventricular tachycardia and fibrillation using ECG processing and intramyocardial pressure gradients. PACE 9:1084–1088
110. Mirowski M (1985) The automatic implantable cardioverter-defibrillator: an overview. J Am Coll Cardiol 6:461–466
111. Arzbaecher R, Bump T, Jenkins J, Glick K, Munkenbeck F, Brown J, Nandhakumar N (1984) Automatic tachycardia recognition. PACE 7:541–547
112. Jenkins J, Bump T, Munkenbeck F, Brown J, Arzbaecher R (1984) Tachycardia detection in implantable antitachycardia devices. PACE 7:1273–1277
113. den Dulk K, Brugada P, Wellens HJJ (1984) A case report demonstrating spontaneous change in tachycardia terminating window. PACE 7:867–870
114. Fahraeus T, Lassvik C, Sonnhag C (1984) Tachycardias initiated by automatic antitachycardia pacemakers. PACE 7:1049–1054
115. Tanabe A, Ikeda H, Fujiyama M, Furuta YI, Matsumura J, Ohbayashi J, Utsu F, Toshima H (1985) Termination of ventricular tachycardia by an implantable atrial pacemaker and external pacemaker activator. PACE 8:532–538
116. Medina-Ravell V, Castellanos A, Portillo-Acosta B, Maduro-Maytin C, Rodriquez-Salas S, Hernandez-Arenas M, LaSalle-Toro R, Mendoza-Mujica I, Ortega-Maldonado M, Berkovitz BV (1984) Management of tachyarrhythmias with dual-chamber pacemakers. PACE 7:173–178
117. Fisher JD, Furman S, Kim SG, Matos JA, Waspe LE (1984) DDD/DDT pacemakers in the treatment of ventricular tachycardia. PACE 7:173–178

118. Bertholet M, Demoulin JC, Waleffe A, Kulbertus H (1985) Programmable extrastimulus pacing for long-term management of supraventricular and ventricular tachycardias: clinical experience in 16 patients. Am Heart J 110:582–589
119. Zipes DP, Prystowsky EN, Miles WM, Heger JJ (1984) Initial experience with Symbios model 7008 pacemaker. PACE 7:1301–1305
120. Goyal SL, Lichstein E, Gupta PK, Chadda KD (1975) Refractory reentrant atrial tachycardia: successful treatment with a permanent radio frequency triggered atrial pacemaker. Am J Med 58:586–590
121. Wyndham CR, Wu D, Denes P, Sugarman D, Levitsky S, Rosen KM (1978) Self-initiated conversion of paroxysmal atrial flutter utilizing a radiofrequency pacemaker. Am J Cardiol 41:1119–1122
122. Solti F, Szabo Z, Bodor A, Renyivamos F Jr (1982) Refractory supraventricular reentry tachycardia treated by radiofrequency atrial pacemaker. PACE 5:275–277
123. Peters RW, Scheinman MM, Morday F, Jacobson L (1985) Long-term management of recurrent paroxysmal tachycardia by cardiac burst pacing. PACE 8:35–44
124. O'Keefe DB, Curry PVL, Sowton E (1981) Treatment of paroxysmal nodal tachycardia by dual demand pacemaker in the coronary sinus. Br Heart J 45:105–108
125. den Dulk K, Bertholet M, Brugada P, Bar FW, Demulin JC, Waleffe A, Bakels N, Lindeman F, Bourgeois I, Kulbertus HE, Wellens HJJ (1984) Clinical experience with implantable devices for control of tachyarrhythmias. PACE 7:548–556
126. Portillo B, Medina-Ravell V, Portillo-Leon N, Castor M, Mejias J, Berkovits BV, Castellanos A (1982) Treatment of drug resistant A-V reciprocating tachycardias with multiprogrammable dual demand A-V sequential (DVI, MN) pacemakers. PACE 5:814–825
127. Abinader EG (1976) Recurrent supraventricular tachycardia: success and subsequent failure of termination by implanted endocardial pacemaker. JAMA 236:2203–2205
128. Arbel ER, Cohen CH, Langendorf R, Glick G (1978) Successful treatment of drug-resistant atrial tachycardia and intractable congestive heart failure with permanent coupled atrial pacing. Am J Cardiol 41:336–340
129. Lüderitz B, d'Alnoncourt CN, Steinbeck G, Beyer J (1982) Therapeutic pacing in tachyarrhythmias by implanted pacemakers. PACE 5:366–371
130. Nilsson G, Ringqvist I (1982) Long-term control of reciprocating paroxysmal tachycardia by ventricular pacing in a case of Wolff-Parkinson-White syndrome. Br Heart J 47:609–612
131. Mandel WJ, Laks MM, Yamaguchi I, Fields J, Berkovits B (1976) Recurrent reciprocating tachycardias in the Wolff-Parkinson-White syndrome: control by the use of a scanning pacemaker. Chest 69:769–774
132. Saksena S, Pantopoulos D, Parsonnet V, Rothbart ST, Hussain SM, Gielchinsky I (1986) Usefulness of an implantable antitachycardia pacemaker system for supraventricular or ventricular tachycardia. Am J Cardiol 58:70–74

133. Kahn A, Morris JJ, Citron P (1976) Patient-initiated rapid atrial pacing to manage supraventricular tachycardia. Am J Cardiol 38:200–204
134. Griffin JC, Sweeney M (1987) The management of paroxysmal tachycardias using the Cybertach-60. PACE 7:1291–1295
135. Rothman MT, Keefe JM (1984) Clinical results with Omni-Orthocor[r], an implantable antitachycardia pacing system. PACE 7:1306–1312
136. Palakurthy PR, Slater D (1988) Automatic implantable scanning burst pacemakers for recurrent tachyarrhythmias. PACE 11:185–192
137. Kappenberger L, Valin H, Sowton E (1989) Multicenter long-term results of antitachycardia pacing for supraventricular tachycardias. Am J Cardiol 64:191–193
138. Occhetta E, Bolognese L, Magnani A, Francalacci G, Rognoni G, Rossi P (1989) Clinical experience with orthocor II antitachycardia pacing system for recurrent tachyarrhythmia termination. J Electrophysiol 3:289–300
139. Moller M, Simonsen E, Arnsbo PI, Oxho H (1989) Long-term follow-up of patients treated with automatic scanning antitachycardia pacemaker. PACE 12:425–430
140. Moreira DA, Shepard RB, Waldo AL (1989) Chronic rapid atrial pacing to maintain atrial fibrillation: use to permit control of ventricular rate in order to treat tachycardia induced cardiomyopathy. PACE 12:761–775
141. Schnittger I, Lee JT, Hargis J, Wyndham CRC, Echt DS, Swerdlow CD, Griffin JC (1989) Long-term results of antitachycardia pacing in patients with supraventricular tachycardia. PACE 12:936–941
142. Nürnberg M, Biber B, Frohner K, Rabitsch C, Steinbach K (1989) Problems of sensing tachyarrhythmias by an antitachycardia pacemaker (Symbios 7008). PACE 12:537–541
143. Van Hemel NM, Bakema H (1979) Treatment of supraventricular tachycardia by chronic demand atrial rapid burst pacing. In: Meere C (ed) Proceedings of the 6th World Symposium on Cardiac Pacing. Pacesymp, Montreal, chap 9-8, pp 1–4
144. Waxman RW, Bonet JF, Sharma AD, MacGregor DC, Goldman BS (1979) Patient initiated rapid atrial stimulation for treatment of paroxysmal supraventricular tachycardia. In: Meere C (ed) Proceedings of the 6th World Symposium on Cardiac Pacing. Pacesymp, Montreal, chap 9-9, pp 1–5
145. Todo K, Kaneko S, Fjuiwara T, Sugiki K, Tanaka N, Komatsu S (1979) Patient-controlled rapid atrial pacing in the long-term management of recurrent supraventricular tachycardias. In: Meere C (ed) Proceedings of the 6th World Symposium on Cardiac Pacing. Pacesymp, Montreal, chap 9-6, pp 1–5
146. Pistolese M, Boccadamo R, Altamura G (1979) Permanent right ventricular pacing in the treatment of refractory supraventricular tachycardia. In: Meere C (ed) Proceedings of the 6th World Symposium on Cardiac Pacing. Pacesymp, Montreal, chap 9-12, pp 1–5
147. Simonsen E, Fabricius J (1985) Frequent attacks of supraventricular tachycardia in a patient treated with an automatic scanning pacemaker (PASAR): Holter documentation of 554 episodes. PACE 8:740–745

148. Critelli G, Grassi G, Chiariello M, Perticone F, Adinolfi L, Condorelli M (1979) Automatic "Scanning" by radiofrequency in the long-term electrical treatment of arrhythmias. PACE 2:289–296
149. Krikler D, Curry P, Buffet J (1976) Dual-demand paçing for reciprocating atrioventricular tachycardia. Br Med J 1:1114–1116
150. Case CL, Gillette PC, Zeigler VL, Oslizlok PC (1990) Successful treatment of congenital atrial flutter with antitachycardia pacing. PACE 13:571–573
151. Li CK, Shandling AH, Nolasco M, Thomas LA, Messenger JC, Warren J (1990) Atrial automatic tachycardia-reversion pacemakers: their economic viability and impact on quality-of-life. PACE 13:639–645
152. Den Dulk K, Brugada P, Smeets JL, Wellens HJ (1990) Long-term antitachycardia pacing experience for supraventricular tachycardia. PACE 13:1020–1030
153. Reddy CP, Todd EP, Kuo SC, DeMaria AN (1984) Treatment of ventricular tachycardia using an automatic scanning extrastimulus pacemaker. J Am Coll Cardiol 3:225–230
154. Hartzler GO (1979) Treatment of recurrent ventricular tachycardias by patient-activated radiofrequency ventricular stimulation. Mayo Clin Proc 54:75–82
155. Ruskin JN, Garan H, Poulin F, Harthorne JW (1980) Permanent radiofrequency ventricular pacing for management of drug-resistant ventricular tachycardia. Am J Cardiol 46:317–321
156. Herre JM, Griffin JC, Nielsen AP, Mann DE, Luck JC, Magro SA, Scheunemeyer T, Wyndham CRC (1985) Permanent triggered antitachycardia pacemakers in the management of recurrent sustained ventricular tachycardia. J Am Coll Cardiol 6:206–212
157. Higgins JR, Swartz JF, Dehmer GH, Beddingfield GW (1985) Automatic scanning extrastimulus pacemaker to treat ventricular tachycardia. PACE 8:101–109
158. Newman DM, Lee MA, Herre JM, Langberg JJ, Scheinman MM, Griffin JC (1989) Permanent antitachycardia pacemaker therapy for ventricular tachycardia. PACE 12:1387–1395
159. Fromer M, Shensa M, Kus T, Page P (1987) Management of a patient with recurrent sustained ventricular tachycardia with a new software-based antitachycardia pacemaker. J Electrophysiol 1:133–139
160. Manz M, Gerckens U, Funke HD, Kirchhoff PG, Lüderitz B (1986) Combination of antitachycardia pacemaker and automatic implantable cardioverter/defibrillator for ventricular tachycardia. PACE 9:676–684
161. Falkoff MD, Barold S, Goodfriend MA, Ong LS, Heinle RL (1986) Long-term management of ventricular tachycardia by implantable automatic burst tachycardia-terminating pacemakers. PACE 9:885–895
162. Greene HL, Gross BW, Preston TA, Werner JA, Kime GM, Hessel EA, Weaver WD, Duncan JL (1982) Termination of ventricular tachycardia by programmed extrastimuli from an externally-activated permanent pacemaker. PACE 5:434–439
163. Lown B, Axelrod P (1972) Implanted standby defribrillators. Circulation 46:637–639

164. Mirowski M, Mower MM, Staewen WS, Tabatznik B, Mendeloff AI (1970) Standby automatic defibrillator. Arch Intern Med 126:158–161
165. Mirowski M, Mower MM, Staewen WS, Denniston RH, Mendeloff AI (1972) The development of the transvenous automatic defibrillator. Arch Intern Med 129:773–779
166. Mirowski M, Mower MM, Gott VL, Brawley RK (1973) Feasibility and effectiveness of low-energy catheter defibrillation in man. Circulation 47:79–85
167. Pycha C, Gulledge AD, Hutzler J, Kadri N, Maloney J (1986) Psychological responses to the implantable defibrillator: preliminary observations. Psychosomatics 27:841–845
168. Pycha C, Calabrese JR, Gulledge AD, Maloney J (1990) Patient and spouse acceptance and adaptation to implantable cardioverter defibrillators. Cleve Clin J Med 57:441–444
169. Fricchione GL, Olson LC, Vlay SC (1989) Psychiatric syndromes in patients with the automatic internal cardioverter defibrillator: anxiety, psychological dependence, abuse, and withdrawal. Am Heart J 117:1411–1414
170. Deeb GM, Gardesty RL, Griffith BP, Thompson ME, Heilman MS, Myerowitz RL (1983) The effects of cardiovascular drugs on the defibrillation threshold and the pathological effects on the heart using an automatic implantable defibrillator. Ann Thorac Surg 4:361–366
171. Singer I, Guarnieri T, Kupersmith J (1988) Implanted Automatic Defibrillators: effects of drugs and pacemakers. PACE 11:2250–2262
172. Marinchak RA, Friehling TD, Kline RA, Stohler J, Kowey PR (1988) Effect of antiarrhythmic drugs on defibrillation threshold: case report of an adverse effect of mexiletine and review of the literature. PACE 11:7–12
173. Guarnieri T, Datorre SD, Bondke H, Brinker J, Myers S, Levine JH (1988) Increased pacing threshold after an automatic defibrillator shock in dogs: effects of class I and class II antiarrhythmic drugs. PACE 11:1324–1330
174. Haberman RJ, Veltri P, Mower MM (1988) The effect of amiodarone on defibrillation threshold. J Electrophysiol 2:415–423
175. Manz M, Gerckens U, Luderitz B (1986) Erroneous discharge from an implanted automatic defribrillator during supraventricular tachycardia induced ventricular fibrillation. Am J Cardiol 57:343–344
176. Kim SG, Furman S, Waspe LE, Brodman R, Fisher JD (1986) Unipolar pacer artifacts induced failure of an automatic implantable cardioverter/defibrillator to detect ventricular fibrillation. Am J Cardiol 57:880–881
177. Bardy GH, Ivey TD, Stewart R, Graham EL, Greene HL (1986) Failure of the automatic implantable defibrillator to detect ventricular fibrillation. Am J Cardiol 58:1107–1108
178. Roth JA, Fisher JD, Furman S, Kim SG (1987) Termination of slower ventricular tachycardias using an automatic implantable cardioverter-defibrillator triggered by chest wall stimulation. Am J Cardiol 59: 1209–1210
179. Kelly PA, Wallace S, Tucker B, Hurvitz RJ, Ilvento J, Mirabel GS, Cannom DS (1988) Postoperative infection with the automatic implantable car-

dioverter defibrillator: clinical presentation and use of the gallium scan in diagnosis. PACE 11:1220–1225
180. Almassi GH, Chapman PD, Troup PJ, Wetherbee JN, Olinger GN (1987) Constrictive pericarditis associated with patch electrodes of the automatic implantable cardioverter-defibrillator. Chest 92:369–372
181. Walls JT, Schuder JC, Curtis JJ, Stephenson HE, McDaniel WC, Flaker GC (1989) Adverse effects of permanent cardiac internal defibrillator patches on external defibrillator. Am J Cardiol 64:1144–1147
182. Jackman WM, Zipes DP (1982) Low-energy synchronous cardioversion of ventricular tachycardia using a catheter electrode in a canine model of subacute myocardial infarction. Circulation 66:187–195
183. Zipes DP, Jackman WM, Heger JJ, Chilson DA, Browne KF, Naccarelli GV, Rahilly GT, Prystowsky EN (1982) Clinical transvenous cardioversion of recurrent life-threatening ventricular tachyarrhythmias: low energy synchronized cardioversion of ventricular tachycardia and termination of ventricular fibrillation in patients using a catheter electrode. Am Heart J 103:789–794
184. Waspe LE, Kim SG, Matos JA, Fisher JD (1983) Role of a catheter lead system for transvenous countershock and pacing during electro-physiologic tests: an assessment of the usefulness of catheter shocks for terminating ventricular tachyarrhythmias. Am J Cardiol 52:477–484
185. Saksena S, Chandran P, Shah Y, Boccadamo R, Pantopoulos D, Rothbart S (1985) Comparative efficacy of transvenous cardioversion and pacing in patients with sustained ventricular tachycardia: a prospective, randomized, crossover study. Circulation 72:153–160
186. Nathan AW, Bexton RS, Spurrell RAJ, Camm AJ (1984) Internal transvenous low energy cardioversion for the treatment of cardiac arrhythmias. Br Heart J 52:377–384
187. McComb JM, McGovern B, Garan H, Ruskin JN (1986) Management of refractory supraventricular tachyarrhythmias using low-energy transcatheter shocks. Am J Cardiol 58:959–963
188. Dunbar DN, Tobler G, Petter J, Gornick CG, Benson DW, Benditt DG (1986) Intracavitary electrode catheter cardioversion of atrial tachyarrhythmias in the dog. J Am Coll Cardiol 7:1015–1027
189. Chang M, Inoue H, Kallok MJ, Zipes DP (1986) Double and triple sequential shocks reduce ventricular defibrillation threshold in dogs with and without myocardial infarction. J Am Coll Cardiol 8:1393–1405
190. Fontaine G, Cansell A, Lechat PH, Pavie A, Grosgogeat Y (1984) Unipolar electrode system for an implantable defibrillator: new experimental approaches. PACE 7:1351–1356
191. Lindsay BD, Saksena S, Rothbart ST, Wasty N, Pantopoulos D (1987) Prospective evaluation of a sequential pacing and high-energy bidirectional shock algorithm for transvenous cardioversion in patients with ventricular tachycardia. Circulation 76:601–609
192. Bardy GH, Stewart RB, Ivey TD, Graham EL, Adhar GC, Greene HL (1987) Intraoperative comparison of sequential-pulse and single-pulse

defibrillation in candidates for automatic implantable defibrillators. Am J Cardiol 60:618–624

193. Wetherbee JN, Chapman PD, Bach SM, Troup PJ (1988) Sequential shocks are comparable to single shocks employing two current pathways for internal defibrillation in dogs. PACE 11:696–703
194. Saksena S, Tullo NG, Krol RB, Mauro AM (1989) Initial clinical experience with endocardial defibrillation using an implantable cardioverter/defibrillator with a triple-electrode system. Arch Intern Med 149:2333–2339
195. Yee R, Jones DL, Klein GJ, Sharma AD, Kallok MJ (1989) Sequential pulse countershock between two transvenous catheters: feasibility, safety, and efficacy. PACE 12:1869–1877
196. Jones DL, Klein GJ, Rattes MF, Sohla A, Sharma AD (1988) Internal cardiac defibrillation: single and sequential pulses and a variety of lead orientations. PACE 11:583–591
197. Jones DL, Klein GJ, Guiraudon GM, Sharma AD (1988) Sequential pulse defibrillation in humans: orthogonal sequential pulse defibrillation with epicardial electrodes. J Am Coll Cardiol 11:590–596
198. Jones DL, Klein GJ, Guiraudon GM, Sharma AD, Kallok M, Bourland JD, Tacker WA (1986) Internal cardiac defibrillation in man: pronounced improvement with sequential pulse delivery for two different lead orientations. Circulation 73:484–491
199. Fain ES, Sweeney MB, Franz MR (1989) Improved internal defibrillation efficacy with a biphasic waveform. Am Heart J 117:358–364
200. Winkle RA, Mead RH, Ruder MA, Gaudiani V, Buch WS, Pless B, Sweeney M, Schmidt P (1989) Improved low energy defibrillation efficacy inman with the use of a biphasic truncated exponential waveform. Am Heart J 117:122–127
201. Tang ASL, Seitaro YA, Wharton M, Dolker M, Smith WM, Ideker RE (1989) Ventricular defibrillation using biphasic waveforms: the importance of phasic duration. J Am Coll Cardiol 13:207–214
202. Bardy GH, Ivey TD, Allen MD, Johnson G, Mehra R, Greene L (1989) A prospective randomized evaluation of biphasic versus monophasic waveform pulses on defibrillation efficacy in humans. J Am Coll Cardiol 14:728–733
203. Flaker GC, Schuder JC, McDaniel WC, Stoeckle H, Dbeis M (1989) Superiority of biphasic shocks in the defibrillation of dogs by epicardial patches and catheter electrodes. Am Heart J 118:288–291
204. Kavanagh KM, Tang AS, Rollins DL, Smith WM, Ideker RE (1989) Comparison of the internal defibrillation thresholds for monophasic and double and single capacitor biphasic waveforms. J Am Coll Cardiol 14:1343–1349
205. Kadish AH, Childs K, Levine B (1989) An experimental study of transvenous defibrillation using a coronary sinus catheter. J Electrophysiol 3:253–260
206. Watkins L Jr, Mower MM, Reid PR, Platia EV, Griffith SC, Mirowski M (1984) Surgical techniques for implanting the automatic implantable defibrillator. PACE 7:1357–1362

207. Brodman R, Fisher JD, Furman S, Johnston DR, Kim SG, Matos JA, Waspe LE (1984) Implantation of automatic cardioverter-defibrillators via medical sternotomy. PACE 7:1363–1369
208. Winkle RA, Stinson EB, Echt DS, Mead RH, Schmidt P (1984) Practical aspects of automatic cardioverter/defibrillator implantation. Am Heart J 108:1335–1346
209. Lawrie GM, Griffin JC, Wyndham CRC (1984) Epicardial implantation of the automatic implantable defibrillator by left subcostal thoracotomy. PACE 7:1370–1374
210. Santel DJ, Kallok MJ, Tacker WA Jr (1985) Implantable defibrillator electrode systems: a brief review. PACE 8:123–131
211. Troup PJ, Chapman PD, Olinger GN, Kleinman LH (1985) The implanted defibrillator: relation of defibrillating lead configuration and clinical variables to defibrillation threshold. J Am Coll Cardiol 6:1315–1321
212. DeBelder MA, Camm AJ (1989) Implantable cardioverter-defibrillators (ICDs) 1989: how close are we to the ideal device? Clin Cardiol 12:339–345
213. Zipes D, Heger JJ, Miles WM, Mahomed Y, Brown JW, Spielman SR, Prystowsky EN (1984) Early experience with an implantable cardioverter. N Engl J Med 311:485–490
214. Mirowski M, Reid PR, Mower MM, Watkins L, Gott VL, Schauble JF, Langer A, Heilman MS, Kolenik SA, Fischell RE, Weisfeldt ML (1980) Termination of malignant ventricular arrhythmias with an implanted automatic defibrillator in human beings. N Engl J Med 303:322–324
215. Mirowski M (1985) The automatic implantable cardioverter-defibrillator: an overview. J Am Coll Cardiol 6:461–466
216. Echt DS, Armstrong K, Schmidt P, Oyer PE, Stinson EB, Winkle RA (1985) Clinical experience, complication, and survival in 70 patients with the automatic implantable cardioverter defibrillator. Circulation 71: 289–296
217. Gabry MD, Brodman R, Johnston D, Frame R, Kim SG, Waspe LE, Fisher JD, Furman S (1987) Automatic implantable cardioverter defibrillator: patient survival, battery longevity and shock delivery analysis. J Am Coll Cardiol 9:1349–1356
218. Winkle RA, Mead RH, Rucer MA, Gaudiani VA, Smith NA, Buch WS, Schmidt P, Shipman T (1989) Long-term Outcome with the Automatic Implantable cardioverter-defibrillator. J Am Coll Cardiol 13:1353–1361
219. Kelly PA, Cannom DS, Garan H, Mirabal GS, Harthorne WJ, Hurvitz RJ, Vlahakes GJ, Jacobs ML, Ilvento JP, Buckley MJ, Ruskin JN (1988) The automatic implantable cardioverter-defibrillator: efficacy, complications and survical in patients with malignant ventricular arrhythmias. J Am Coll Cardiol 11:1278–1286
220. Myerburg RJ, Luceri RM, Thurer R, Cooper DK, Zaman L, Interian A, Fernandez P, Cox M, Glicksman F, Castellanos A (1989) Time to first shock and clinical outcome in patients receiving an automatic implantable cardioverter-defibrillator. J Am Coll Cardiol 14:508–514
221. Tchou PJ, Kadri N, Anderson J, Caceres JA, Jazayeri M, Akhtar M (1988) Automatic implantable cardioverter defibrillators and survival of patients

with left ventricular dysfunction and malignant ventricular arrhythmias. Ann Intern Med 109:529–534

222. Fisher JD, Fink D, Matos JA, Kim SG, Waspe LE (1982) Programmed stimulation and ventricular tachycardia therapy: benefits of partial as well as complete "cures". PACE 6:A139 (abstr)
223. Swerdlow C, Winkle RA, Mason JW (1983) Determinants of survival in patients with ventricular tachyarrhythmias. N Engl J Med 308:1436–1442
224. Graboys TB, Lown B, Podrid PJ, DeSilva R (1982) Long-term survival of patients with malignant ventricular arrhythmia treated with antiarrhythmic drugs. Am J Cardiol 50:437–443
225. Dicarlo LA, Morday F, Sauve MJ, Malone P, David JC, Evans-Bell T, Winston S, Scheinman MM (1985) Cardiac arrest and sudden death in patients treated with amiodarone for sustained ventricular tachycardia or ventricular fibrillation: risk stratification based on clinical variables. Am J Cardiol 55:372–374
226. Horowitz LN, Greenspan AM, Spielman SR, Webb CR, Morganroth J, Rotmensch H, Sokoloff NM, Rae AP, Segal BL, Kay HR (1985) Usefulness of electrophysiology testing in evaluation of amiodarone therapy of sustained ventricular tachyarrhythmias associated with coronary heart disease. AM J Cardiol 55:367–371
227. Cobb LA, Baum RS, Alvarez H, Schaffer WA (1975) Resuscitation from out-of-hospital ventricular fibrillation: 4 year follow-up. Circulation 51:111–117
228. Weaver WD, Cobb LA, Hallstrom AP (1982) Ambulatory arrhythmias in resuscitated victims of cardiac arrest. Circulation 66:212–218
229. Brodman R, Fisher JD, Johnston DR, Kim SG, Matos JA, Waspe LE, Scavin GM, Furman S (1984) Results of electrophysiologically guided operations for drug-resistant recurrent ventricular tachycardia and ventricular fibrillation due to coronary artery disease. J Thorac Cardiovasc Surg 87:431–438
230. Borggrefe M, Podzek A, Ostermeyer J, Breithardt G, and the Surgical Ablation Registry (1987) Long-term results of electrophysiologically guided antitachycardia surgery in ventricular tachyarrhythmias: a collaborative report on 665 patients. In: Breithardt GM, Borggrefe DP, Nonpharmacological therapy of tachyarrhythmias. Futura, Mount Kisco, pp 109–132
231. Josephson ME, Harken AH, Horowitz LN (1982) Long-term results of endocardial resection for sustained ventricular tachycardia in coronary disease patients. Am Heart J 104:51–57
232. Luceri RM, Habal SM, Castellanos A, Thurer RJ, Waters RS, Brownstein SL (1988) Mechanism of death in patients with the automatic implantable cardioverter defibrillator. PACE 11:2015–2022
233. Gross J, Zilo P, Ferrick KJ, Fisher JD, Furman S (1990) Sudden death mortality in AICD patients. RBM, Cardiostim 90, Nice, 20–23 June 1990, vol 12:114

234. Zilo P, Gross J, Benedek M, Fisher JD, Furman S (1990) Occurrence of AICD shocks and patient survival. PACE 13:510 [North American Society of Pacing and Electrophysiology (NASPE) abstr]
235. Fisher JD, Brodman RF, Kim SG, Ferrick KJ, Roth JA (1990) VT/VF: 60/60 protection. PACE 13:218–222 (editorial)
236. Veltri EP (1989) Re: AICD benefit. PACE 12:1964–1967 (letter)
237. Kay GN, Vance JP, Dailey SM, Epstein AE (1990) Current role of the automatic implantable cardioverter-defibrillator in the treatment of life-threatening ventricular arrhythmias. Am J Med 88:1–25N–1–34N
238. Fisher JD, Kim SG, Roth JA, Ferrick KJ, Brodman RF, Gross JN, Furman S (1990) Ventricular tachycardia/fibrillation: therapeutic alternatives. In: Mugica J (ed) Cardiostim proceedings (in press)
239. Nisam S, Thomas A, Moser S, Winkle R, Fisher JD (1988) AICD: standardized reporting and appropriate categorization of complications. PACE 11:2045–2052
240. Kim SG, Fisher JD, Furman S, Brodman R, Gross J, Zilo P, Roth JA, Ferrick KJ, Brodman R (1991) Benefits of implantable defibrillators: sudden death rates and better represented by the total arrhythmic death rate. J Am Coll Cardiol 17:1587–1592
241. Reid PR, Griffith SC, Mower MM, Platia EV, Watkins L Jr, Juanteguy J, Mirowski M (1984) Implantable cardioverter-defibrillator: patient selection and implantation protocol. PACE 7:1338–1344
242. Echt DS, Winkle RA (1985) Management of patients with the automatic implantable cardioverter defibrillator. Clin Prog 3:4–16
243. Fisher JD, Mercando AD, Kim SG (1986) Antitachycardia strategies. PACE 9:1309
244. Platia EV, Griffith LSC, Watkins L Rk, Mower MM, Guarnieri T, Mirowski M, Reid PR (1986) Treatment of malignant ventricular arrhythmias with endocardial resection and implantation of the automatic cardioverter-defibrillator. N Engl Med 314:213–216
245. Manolis AS, Rastegar H, Estes NAM (1989) Prophylactic automatic implantable cardioverter-defibrillator patches in patients at high risk for postoperative ventricular tachyarrhythmias. J Am Coll Cardiol 13:1367–1373
246. Pekarsky V, Astrakhantsev Y, Belenkov Y, Gimrikh E, Oferkin A, Maslov M, Popov S, Pekarskmaya M, Markov V, Vasiltsev Y (1986) Use of electrical pacing and automatic cardioversion fibrillation for normal cardiac function recovery. PACE 9:1349–1355
247. Den Dulk K, Brugada P, Smeets JL, Wellens HJ (1990) Long-term antitachycardia pacing experience for supraventricular tachycardia. PACE 13:1020–1030
248. Song SL (1991) Performance of implantable cardiac rhythm management devices (Bilitch Report). PACE 14:1198–1200
249. Fisher JD, Furman S, Kim SG, Ferrick KJ, Roth JA, Gross J, Brodman RF, Barold S (ed) (1991) Tachycardia management by devices. Futura, Mount Kisco (in press)

Treatment Algorithm for Patients with Life-Threatening Ventricular Tachyarrhythmia

H. Klein, J. Trappe

Various therapeutic modalities are now available for the treatment of patients with ventricular tachyarrhythmias. This can be achieved by either removing or modulating the arrhythmogenic substrate, suppression of trigger mechanism, or delivery of electric current that terminates the tachycardia or ventricular fibrillation. Increasing attention is being given to the role of the autonomic nervous system that may either enhance or suppress the onset of ventricular arrhythmias, and there can be no doubt that factors such as ischemia, electrolyte imbalance or metabolic disturbances have to be restored before a potential life-threatening situation can be abolished. Approaches currently available include antiarrhythmic drugs and various nonpharmacological methods such as electrophysiologically-guided surgery, catheter ablation, and the implantable cardioverter-defibrillator (ICD) with or without antitachycardia pacing modalities [1, 2]. As a last resort even heart transplantation can be considered an approach for life-threatening arrhythmias in patients with severe heart failure.

Prior to the widespread acceptance of defibrillator therapy, the "gold standard" of antiarrhythmic therapy was serial electrophysiologic testing with antiarrhythmic drugs [3–5]. However, despite the introduction of new antiarrhythmic compounds, suppression of arrhythmia is achieved in no more than about 50% of cases [6, 7]. Apart from the high failure rate there is increasing concern about serious pro-arrhythmic effects, especially with Class I drugs, and up to now no specific drug has yielded a significant reduction in mortality [8–10].

Suppression of ventricular tachycardia during serial testing is regarded as "drug response," and various reports have shown that drug responders have a relatively good prognosis with a low incidence of sudden cardiac death. However, patients with arrhythmias that remain inducible – and these are often those with poor ventricular function – have shown a poor outcome and are considered non-responders, with the arrhythmia being refractory to drug therapy [5, 6].

So far nonpharmacological treatment is indicated only in cases of refractoriness to drug therapy. The problem with drug refractoriness is, however, that there is no generally accepted definition of such refractoriness.

Theoretically, drug efficacy can be evaluated by noninvasive or invasive approaches [11–13]. The noninvasive approach includes ambulatory monitoring and exercise testing and is based on the concept of trial and error [14]. Although the criteria for drug efficacy or refractoriness are well-defined when Holter monitoring is used, there are major limitations associated with this technique [15]. Complex ventricular arrhythmias frequently fail to be documented during baseline examination; in addition, there is an enormous spontaneous variability in arrhythmia occurrence [16], and, most important, it has recently been demonstrated that suppression of extrasystoles alone does not necessarily imply freedom from recurrence of ventricular tachycardia or fibrillation. Therefore, there can be no doubt that noninvasive testing for establishing drug efficacy is unreliable.

Today, drug refractoriness is acceptable if sustained ventricular tachycardia remains inducible after a series of electropharmacological trials. The number of drugs to be tested is yet unclear, and there are reports indicating that only the first trial yields the highest probability of identifying the drug with long-term efficacy, whereas subsequent trials have a low probability of finding the appropriate drug [17, 18].

How a partial response to a specific antiarrhythmic drug should be interpreted, is still a matter of debate [19]. Reduction in tachycardia rate, the use of a more aggressive stimulation protocol or induction of unsustained ventricular tachycardia may be acceptable and advantageous for the patient; however, it remains an uncertain situation. The role of amiodarone and beta-blocking agents as drugs requiring to be tested prior to drug refractoriness being established is not yet clear.

Patients in whom a previously documented ventricular tachycardia is not inducible at baseline electrophysiologic study, are not candidates for serial electrophysiologic testing, and the meaning of an induced "nonclinical" tachycardia whether at baseline study or during drug testing requires definition.

Drug refractoriness also depends on the clinical condition of the patient. Coronary artery disease is more suitable for serial electrophysiologic testing than cardiomyopathy or cases summarized as primary electrical disease of the heart. The degree of ventricular dysfunction has a nonnegligible influence on the reproducibility and hemodynamic tolerance of an induced tachycardia, and it is of great importance that personal experience and electrophysiologic training of the physician guide the repeated testing procedure, considering the potential risk of morbidity and even mortality, the age and psychological situation of the patient as well as possible side effects of an antiarrhythmic drug even if noninducibility can be achieved.

Therefore, both the infrequently achieved noninducibility of ventricular tachycardia and the uncertainty of the end-point of electrophysiologic testing have reduced the percentage of patients treated with antiarrhythmic drugs alone, and have, on the other hand, given support to the application of various nonpharmacological approaches.

With several therapeutic options on hand, the selection of the most appropriate approach for the individual patient becomes difficult. It appears to be necessary that a treatment algorithm is designed that helps in choosing the appropriate therapy and may favor one therapeutic option over another in order to optimize the risk-benefit ratio for the patient [20–22].

Pivoting Points of a Treatment Algorithm

Each therapeutic approach has its advantages as well as disadvantages and drawbacks. In setting up a treatment algorithm for ventricular tachycardia or ventricular fibrillation, both the positive and the negative experience gathered so far with various treatment modalities must necessarily be considered. Such an algorithm has its pivoting points where questions have to be answered which then, step by step, lead to the most suitable therapeutic approach for the individual patient.

Factors guiding the treatment algorithm are:

- Arrhythmia event
- Ventricular function
- Underlying disease
- Coronary anatomy
- Baseline electrophysiologic study
- Patient's age, life expectancy
- Quality of life
- Experience of physician and equipment in the treating center.

The Arrhythmia Event

It may be assumed that 80–90% of all events of sudden death are caused by tachyarrhythmia, most often ventricular tachycardia degenerating into ventricular fibrillation. Therefore it is of great importance to know whether the initial event was ventricular tachycardia or primarily ventricular fibrillation [23]. Unfortunately, the arrhythmic event often is not documented or the tachycardia is terminated by the emergency squad before an electrocardiographic (ECG) strip can be taken. Therefore the clinical arrhythmic even often remains pure speculation, and we are bound to believe that in such cases the type and morphology of induced ventricular tachycardia corresponds to the actual situation.

We need to know if the patient became unconscious at the time of tachycardia, how long the syncope lasted, and if angina pectoris preceded the onset of tachycardia. Tachycardia provoked during exercise or effort requires different treatment than tachycardia occurring at rest. Frequent tachycardia episodes do not permit the implantation of a defibrillating device because of many disabling and unpleasant discharges. Antiarrhythmic drugs may be necessary to either suppress frequent tachycardia episodes, or to reduce the tachycardia rate in order to prevent unconsciousness or to render ventricular tachycardia terminable by antitachycardia pacing [24].

Ventricular Function

It has been shown that the long-term outcome of patients with ventricular tachyarrhythmias for the most part depends on the degree of left ventricular (LV) dysfunction [25]. Therefore, evaluation of LV ejection fraction is the most important diagnostic procedure prior to selecting the approach. An LV ejection fraction below 20% indicates a very poor prognosis, and in most cases heart transplantation will be the only treatment modality available. Patients with an ejection fraction between 20% and 30% most often are candidates for defibrillator therapy, whereas an ejection fraction of more than 40% generally indicates a better prognosis; and we have learned that many patients with almost normal LV function often need no antiarrhythmic treatment at all. The largest variety of treatment modalities can be found in the group of patients with left ventricular ejection fractions ranging from 30 to 40%.

Measurement of LV ejection fraction, however, has its drawbacks, too. Apart from the fact that echocardiographic or radionuclide measurements may yield results different from angiographical findings, a well-circumscribed akinetic or dyskinetic wall-motion abnormality must lead to a different approach than a globally hypokinetic ventricle, even with a higher ventricular ejection fraction value.

Scar tissue resulting from myocardial infarction has a different meaning than the finding of fibrolipomatosis in patients with so-called right or left ventricular dysplasia. Thrombus material attached to a myocardial scar after infarction may lead to ineffective catheter ablation or bear the risk of embolic complications during catheter mapping or electrophysiologically-guided surgery. An inferior scar not rarely includes the mitral valve apparatus, which may lead to undesirable mitral regurgitation after endocardial resection – a risk that has to be considered with electrophysiologically-guided surgery. Our own experience comprises three cases in which mitral valve replacement was necessary after cryoablation or endocardial resection of the inferior LV wall.

Ventricular ejection fraction may be without bearing if the clinical status of the circulatory system is neglected. Functional class – expressed by the New York Heart Association (NYHA) classification – of patients with ventricular tachyarrhythmias probably is the most important pivoting point of a treatment algorithm. It has been demonstrated that patients with NYHA class III or IV at the time of the arrhythmic event have a very poor outcome of whatever therapeutic approach is chosen [26–28].

Age and Life Expectancy

The age of the individual patient requiring antiarrhythmic treatment must be duly considered. Can we agree to life-long antiarrhythmic drug therapy in young patients who are given compounds which significantly reduce the quality of life or possibly cause irreversible adverse reactions? What is the bearing of an implanted defibrillator in young individuals, if it is obvious that such a device will require several replacements in the years to come?

Today, patients older than 65 years with poor ventricular function are not candidates for heart transplantation, and therefore drug therapy may be the only approach to their life-threatening arrhythmias, even if suppression of ventricular tachycardia is not achieved by serial testing and if device therapy may not be indicated for various reasons. We believe that an expected survival of less than 2 years should not lead to defibrillator implantation if there is no future possibility of heart transplantation. It is, however, not only the limit of 2 years of expected survival that counts, but the quality of life awaiting the patient for the remaining period of his life.

Underlying Disease

The underlying disease that caused the development of the arrhythmogenic substrate has an important impact on the decision-making process. The largest group of patients with ventricular tachycardia or ventricular fibrillation suffer from coronary artery disease with a history of myocardial infarctions. The additional role of ischemia causing ventricular tachycardia or ventricular fibrillation, and its prevention by bypass grafting has intensely been discussed. Whenever possible, ischemia should be avoided in the setting of ventricular arrhythmias, regardless of the therapeutic approach chosen, a goal that will hardly be achieved in most cases of severe three-vessel coronary artery disease [29, 30]. On the other hand, it must be kept in mind that additional coronary artery bypass grafting prolongs the endocardial resection procedure or defibrillator implantation and may increase the incidence of perioperative mortality. We have been able to demonstrate that concomitant coronary bypass grafting with defibrillator implantation increased the perioperative mortality from 1% to almost 5%. The incidence of defibrillator discharges, however, was not significantly lower in patients with concomitant bypass grafting.

Although endocardial resection guided by electrophysiologic mapping is an accepted approach for patients with fairly good ventricular function, long-term follow-up in our series of patients indicates that not a small percentage of patients undergoing this procedure experience severe heart failure a few years after open heart surgery.

Cardiomyopathy, either dilative or hypertrophic, is more unpredictable in respect of survival than are patients with coronary artery disease. The incidence of inducibility of ventricular tachycardia at baseline examination is significantly lower, and serial drug testing is most unreliable. Electrophysiologic testing itself bears a risk of morbidity and even mortality, especially if patients at the time of testing are still under antiarrhythmic therapy with drugs like amiodarone [31]. Antiarrhythmic drugs may increase the defibrillation threshold and tend to produce a higher rate of ventricular acceleration with antitachycardia pacing [32]. In general, cardiomyopathy patients are not candidates for electrophysiologically guided surgery, and detection of a circumscribed arrhythmogenic focus is most difficult if not impossible. It has thus been our experience that patients with cardiomyopathy are not appropriate candidates for catheter ablation either.

Patients with so-called right or left ventricular dysplasia angiographically show in the classical setting well-circumscribed large areas of bulging fibrolipomatosis. In the early days of our experience in electrophysiologically-guided surgery we thought that resection or isolation of these areas using cryoablation could cure the patients and permanently abolish arrhythmias. However, in most of the patients operated upon it we noticed that the fibrolipomatosis was more extensive than had been assumed from angiography. The intraventricular septum was often shown to be involved as well. The recurrence of ventricular tachycardia episodes after cryoablation in ventricular dysplasia patients is rather high, and therefore the surgical approach has almost been abandoned.

The inducibility of ventricular tachycardia in patients with ventricular dysplasia is most reliable; due to the fact that the morphologic changes involve large parts of both ventricles, we often find more than one ventricular tachycardia morphology, however, and various tachycardia rates. In general, ventricular tachycardia is also amenable to pace termination; however, in the setting of various tachycardia rates and morphologies, the antitachycardia stimulation mode has to be most flexible in order to terminate all clinical tachycardias. On the whole, the prognosis of patients with ventricular dysplasia and episodes of ventricular tachycardia is more favorable than that of those patients suffering from coronary artery disease [33].

The problem of patients with so-called idiopathic ventricular tachycardia is due to the fact that our diagnostic procedures are unable to detect morphologic or hemodynamic abnormalities. The definition of a patient with "idiopathic tachycardia" is not unanimously accepted, and the same holds true for the assessment of prognosis. Selecting the proper approach for patients with idiopathic ventricular tachycardia is thus rather difficult and most debatable. It has been shown, however, that patients with idiopathic ventricular tachycardia and compromised ventricular function must be considered to bear the same high risk of sudden death as patients with coronary artery disease or cardiomyopathy in whom ventricular tachycardia cannot be suppressed by serial drug testing [6].

Ventricular tachycardia due to long QT syndrome must also in some way be classified as idiopathic. The prognosis is highly questionable in the case of frequent tachycardia episodes or syncopal attacks; however, the proper therapeutic approach for these patients has not been defined yet. We believe that patients with long QT syndrome and ventricular tachycardia are not amenable to nonpharmacological therapy, except for the interruption of the left ganglion stellatum. There have only been very few cases reported on the use of defibrillator therapy in such patients.

Electrophysiologic Parameters

It has been mentioned already that the tachycardia induced in the electrophysiologic laboratory has to be identical or at least comparable to the clinically documented arrhythmia. Slightly different tachycardia rates may be acceptable. The meaning of a completely different morphology or rate of a tachycardia induced in the laboratory is unclear.

Endocardial mapping during induced ventricular tachycardia – a prerequisite for successful ablation either by catheter-mediated electric current or endocardial resection – requires hemodynamic stability and a sustained reproducibily inducible tachycardia. Various tachycardia morphologies do not necessarily imply a different origin or arrhythmogenic substrate. The spread of activation may vary significantly; however, the reentrant circuit can still use the same area of slow conduction that has to be removed or ablated in order to suppress the tachycardia.

A ventricular tachycardia rate of more than 200 bpm is unlikely to be suitable for reliable antitachycardia pacing. Faster rates, in general, require more aggressive stimulation modes, and the likelihood of tachycardia acceleration is higher with faster stimulation rates. Although the most appropriate stimulation mode for tachycardia termination has to be assessed yet, there is general agreement that adaptive pacing with or without an autodecremental mode is superior to fixed burst pacing [34]. The necessary number of stimuli and pacing attempts per tachycardia episode is most variable. The currently available antitachycardia pacing devices offer sufficient flexibility for tachycardia recognition and termination; however, the 2 years of experience with antitachycardia pacing have shown clearly that there will always be a need for cardioversion or defibrillation back-up even if pace termination has been tested successfully in the laboratory many times.

The second or third generation devices for tachycardia pacing enable antibradycardia pacing to be performed as well. It may be important to consider rate support in patients with depressed sinus node function in cases of bradycardia-dependent tachycardias or especially after shock delivery by the implanted defibrillator. In general, however, we have learned that permanent antibradycardia pacing is rarely necessary in patients with ventricular tachycardia.

Although the significance of antiarrhythmic drug therapy alone keeps decreasing, there will always be a need for antiarrhythmic drugs in addition to nonpharmacological approaches. The influence of an antiarrhythmic agent, however, must be studied very carefully since it may cause hemodynamic impairment of already compromised ventricular function, and it can cause an increase in the defibrillation threshold or even enhance the tendency towards tachycardia acceleration or degeneration into fibrillation [35].

Specific Treatment Algorithms

Since a variety of clinical settings is met in patients referred for treatment of ventricular tachyarrhythmias, an attempt is made to design an algorithm for each specific tachycardia event (see Figs. 1–4).

Ventricular Tachycardia with Sufficient Ventricular Function

It is assumed that the patient has recurrent episodes of sustained ventricular tachycardia refractory to antiarrhythmic drugs. The underlying disease is either coronary artery disease, cardiomyopathy or so-called arrhythmogenic right or left ventricular disease (dysplasia), and the hemodynamic evaluation has shown a LV ejection fraction of more than 25%, i.e., LV function is considered "sufficient", and there is NYHA class I or II.

During baseline electrophysiologic study the clinical ventricular tachycardia is reproducibly inducible, using a generally accepted stimulation protocol [36]. In the case of a monomorphic sustained ventricular tachycardia, the rate is either below or faster than 200 bpm. The important question to be answered, then, is that of the hemodynamic tolerance of the ventricular tachycardia. With a rate below 200 bpm, the hemodynamic situation may be stable or unstable. With a stable hemodynamic situation we perform endocardial catheter mapping in order to identify the arrhythmogenic substrate, i.e., either the earliest endocardial activation or the area of slow conduction, considered as the critical isthmus of the reentrant circuit.

An unstable hemodynamic situation, even with tachycardia rates of less than 200 bpm, will not permit the thorough catheter mapping required for eventual surgical approach or catheter ablation. Therefore, the use of an ICD, using a device yielding additional tired antitachycardia pacing modalities is considered the most appropriate approach. For the selection of the most effective pacing mode, pre-implant testing with the device-specific pacing algorithm must be performed.

With a tachycardia rate faster than 200 bpm, the hemodynamic tolerance is even more important to be assessed. In very few cases antitachycardia pacing modes will be found for reliable pace termination of ventricular tachycardia. This will also be limited by the device characteristics, since in many devices the upper rate limit for pace termination is set to 220 bpm. Faster rates will be terminated automatically by either low or high energy cardioversion or defibrillation. The efficacy of an antiarrhythmic drug in slowing ventricular tachycardia with a view to rendering tachycardia terminable by antitachy pacing, may be checked. Hemodynamic intolerance in cases with tachycardias faster than 200 bpm does not permit many pace termination attempts to the effect that an ICD without antitachycardia pacing modality is most appropriate.

If a polymorphic – most often fast – ventricular tachycardia is induced, sometimes requiring a very aggressive stimulation protocol or even catecholamine help for induction, that may even have a nonclinical

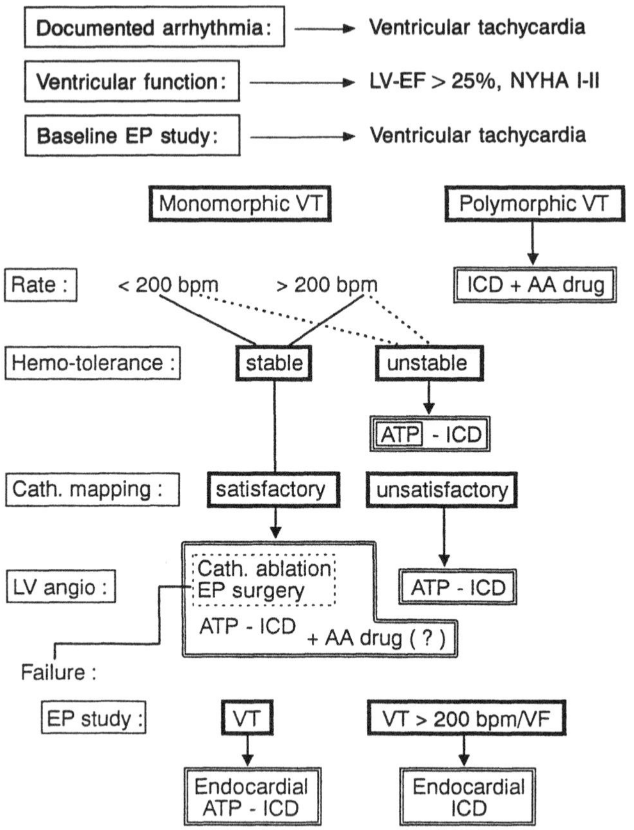

Fig. 1. Flow chart of treatment algorithm for patients with recurrent episodes of sustained ventricular tachycardia refractory to antiarrhythmic drugs, and in whom the underlying disease is coronary artery disease, cardiomyopathy, or arrhythmogenic right or left ventricular disease (dysplasia). *LV-EF*, left ventricular ejection fraction; *VT*, ventricular tachycardia; *ICD*, implantable cardioverter-defibrillator; *ATP*, antitachycardia pacing; *AA* antiarrhythmic; *EP*, electrophysiologic; *VF*, ventricular fibrillation

morphology, for safety reasons our treatment algorithm leads to immediate ICD implantation with or without antiarrhythmic drug support (Fig. 1).

Ventricular Tachycardia Tolerating Catheter Mapping

Either endocardial catheter mapping may yield a satisfactory result or we may fail to localize the critical area for further interventions. If the area to be removed or ablated is identified, the LV angiogram and the underlying disease decide on whether electrophysiologically-guided surgery (endocardial resection or cryoablation) can be performed. Only well-circumscribed LV scars or aneurysms of the anterior or lateral wall favor the surgical approach. Today, some centers prefer catheter ablation attempts with either direct current or radio frequency energy prior to surgery. However, as will be discussed in another chapter, the results of catheter ablation for sustained ventricular tachycardia are not very promising.

Since third-generation ICDs with antitachycardia pacing capabilities are available, implantation of this device will be considered more appropriate in future than catheter ablation attempts or even endocardial resection since it will go along with a lower perioperative mortality and probably less impairment of ventricular function, especially if the endocardial lead technique is used.

In the case of an unsatisfactory catheter mapping result, there is no doubt that ICD device implantation is favorable to "blind" endocardial resection or antiarrhythmic drug therapy alone. Antitachycardia pacing most likely is applicable in patients with coronary artery disease or arrhythmogenic dysplasia, whereas patients with cardiomyopathies may be better off with "simple" ICD devices alone, since pace termination appears to be less reliable in cardiomyopathy patients (Fig. 1).

Ventricular Tachycardia after Surgery or Catheter Ablation

Recurrence of ventricular tachycardia after electrophysiologically-guided surgery has been reported to be 10–15%, the percentage of tachycardia relapse after catheter ablation attempts being 25–30% or more. Drug therapy may be attempted then, remaining most unreliable, however. Most often, a second surgical intervention is not advisable. This then calls for ICD therapy after performance of another re-evaluating electrophysiologic study.

Ventricular tachycardia rates of less than 200 bpm are most likely to permit antitachycardia pacing, whereas rates of induced tachycardia of more than 200 bpm will require an ICD only. The same approach is indicated if programmed stimulation leads to ventricular fibrillation. The patient who has undergone unsuccessful ventricular tachycardia surgery will be a candidate for the endocardial lead system since re-opening of the chest most often is undesirable.

As our experience has shown, electrophysiologically-guided surgery may lead to chronic heart failure with or without recurrence of ventricular tachycardia. Although the endocardial lead system with defibrillator therapy will be appropriate for some patients, not rarely heart transplantation will be the only treatment option that remains. In elderly patients amiodarone therapy – even without serial testing – may be indicated if heart transplantation is not feasible for whatever reason (Fig. 1).

Ventricular Tachycardia with Sufficient Ventricular Function Not Inducible at Baseline Study

This group of patients most often includes cases of so-called primary electrical disease or cardiomyopathies of unknown origin. The main question for this group of patients is whether ventricular tachycardia leads to syncope or whether resuscitation was required. Years ago defibrillator therapy was indicated only if ventricular tachycardia or fibrillation had been inducible during baseline study. Nowadays, this is being handled less strictly and we have learned that noninducible ventricular tachycardia patients have a poor prognosis if syncopal attacks go along with organic heart disease and poor left ventricular function. These patients need defibrillator therapy without antitachycardia pacing modalities [37, 38].

If there are patients who have clinically documented tachycardias which remain noninducible during baseline study and who experience no syncopal attack during the tachycardia event, empiric drug therapy is rather questionable. Perhaps beta-blocking agents are as good in these cases as amiodarone treatment. It is hard to follow the concept of giving no treatment at all in those cases of documented ventricular tachycardia; however, it has been shown that Class I antiarrhythmic drug therapy alone is unable to significantly reduce sudden arrhythmic events or to improve survival. It may thus be justified to refrain from drug therapy altogether (Fig. 2).

Ventricular Tachycardia with Inducible Ventricular Fibrillation

It may occur that only ventricular fibrillation is inducible at baseline electrophysiologic study, although sustained ventricular tachycardia has been documented with the arrhythmia event. The electrophysiologic study should be repeated under oral antiarrhythmic drug therapy. If ventricular fibrillation is inducible again with a beta-blocking agent or amiodarone treatment, we propose defibrillator implant and discontinuation of drug therapy.

In case of sustained ventricular tachycardia being induced under drug therapy, we believe that ICD treatment – most likely in combination with antitachycardia pacing – will be the treatment of choice. The effective antiarrhythmic drug should not be discontinued in order to keep the arrhythmia pace-terminable.

If neither ventricular tachycardia nor ventricular fibrillation will be inducible with one of the drugs referred to above, we tend to leave the patient on this drug regimen. However, patients with cardiomyopathy and poor ventricular function will be given better protection by defibrillator back-up even if arrhythmia is not inducible (Fig. 2).

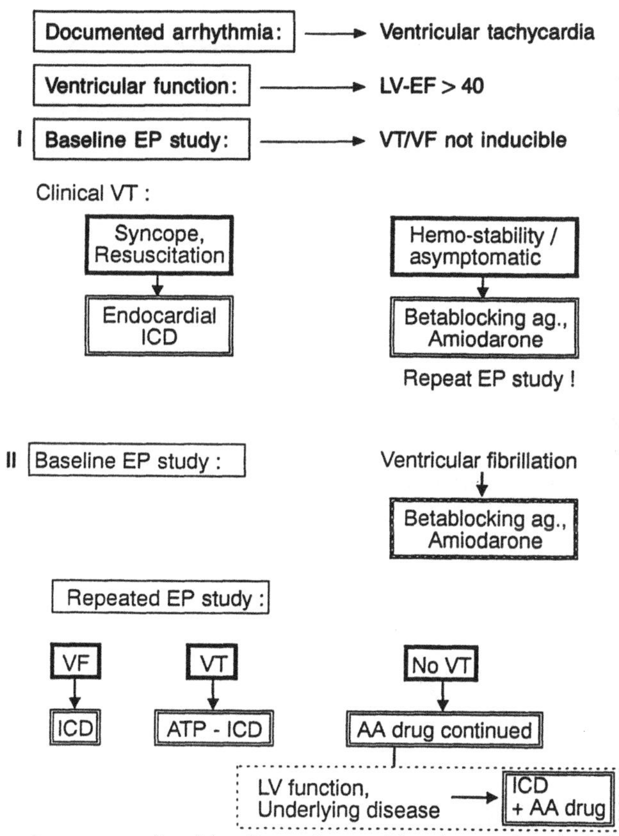

Fig. 2. Flow chart of treatment algorithm for patients with primary electrical disease or cardiomyopathies of unknown origin (abbreviations as in Fig. 1)

Ventricular Tachycardia with Poor Ventricular Function

Patients with poor ventricular function assessed by an ejection fraction of 20% or less, particularly those of NYHA functional class III or even IV, are not appropriate candidates for surgery, catheter ablation, or device treatment. Heart transplantation will be the only choice in patients not older than 65 years. Amiodarone – given even without serial testing – will be the treatment in patients beyond the age of 65 years.

Left ventricular ejection fraction ranging from 20% to 25% clearly indicates defibrillator implantation. With the endocardial lead system being available, we propose to attempt the endocardial lead system first, combined with left-lateral subcutaneous patch placement. In case of a defibrillation energy of more than 20 J being required, epicardial or extrapericardial placement of two patches will be unavoidable. It is strongly recommended, however, that the cardiopulmonary bypass be kept in stand-by position since our experience has shown that heart defibrillation may be impossible using the endocardial lead system, especially if the patient is still under amiodarone.

With the ICD systems currently available, we feel that in 20 to 25% of cases the endocardial lead system with or without combined subcutaneous patch placement will fail to yield an energy low enough for safe defibrillation. The likelihood of cardiopulmonary bypass becoming necessary during endocardial ICD implant underlines the problem of ICD implantation in centers without open-heart surgery (Fig. 3).

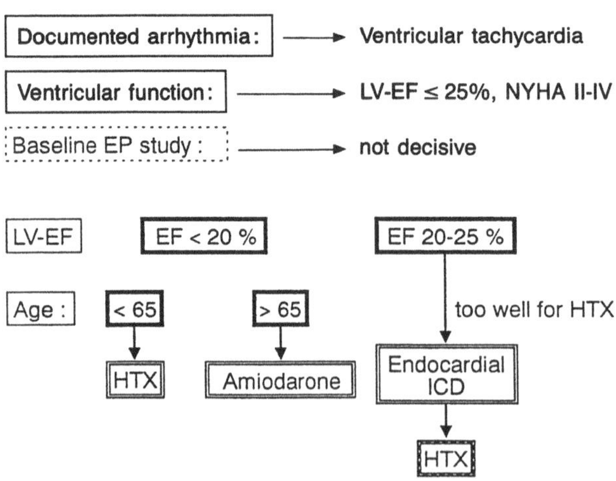

Fig. 3. Flow chart of treatment algorithm for patients with poor ventricular function (*HTX*, heart transplantation; other abbreviations as in Fig. 1)

Primary Ventricular Fibrillation

Patients experiencing cardiac arrest with documented primary ventricular fibrillation should undergo electrophysiologic testing. However, even more important than the result of electrophysiologic testing is the degree of ventricular dysfunction. Ventricular tachycardia induced in patients with good ventricular function or no detectable organic heart disease, showing primary ventricular fibrillation, represents an indication for ICD treatment. The use of a combination with antitachycardia pacing mode will depend on the rate of the ventricular tachycardia induced. There is no doubt that repeatedly induced ventricular fibrillation calls for ICD implantation.

A problem yet unsolved is the patient who survived an episode of ventricular fibrillation unrelated to acute myocardial infarction, ischemia, or remediable causes, who shows good ventricular function, and in whom ventricular arrhythmia is not inducible. Despite the fact of aborted sudden cardiac death, antiarrhythmic treatment is not generally accepted for this type of patients. Should these patients receive beta-blocking agents or even amiodarone? If they do without protection by an implantable defibrillator being provided, we have to repeat the electrophysiologic study on drugs in order to unmask possible proarrhythmic drug effects. It is our personal recommendation, however, that this group of patients should be given a defibrillator since drug therapy alone or no treatment at all appears to be unreliable.

Answering the question of whether patients with primary ventricular fibrillation and reduced ventricular function require defibrillator therapy is less difficult. Irrespective of the type of arrhythmia induced or even without inducible arrhythmia, ICD implantation is strongly recommended. Depending upon the degree of LV ejection fraction, in patients with an ejection fraction of 20–25% defibrillator therapy serves as a bridging therapy prior to future heart transplantation, whereas an LV ejection fraction of less than 20% calls for immediate heart transplantation without preceding defibrillator therapy (Fig. 4).

Discussion

We attempted to set up a treatment algorithm for patients with recurrent episodes of ventricular tachycardia or those who survived cardiac arrest episodes. This algorithm has been based on personal experience with all therapeutic approaches currently available, trying to incorporate decision trees developed by other authors as well [21, 39]. Mention must be made of the fact that personal experience gained in the course of the last

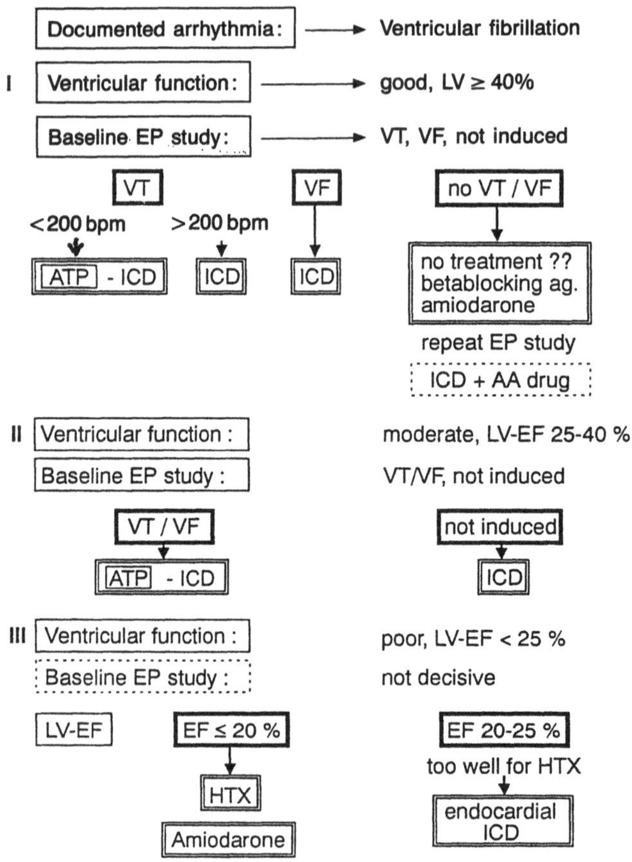

Fig. 4. Flow chart of treatment algorithm for patients with documented primary ventricular fibrillation (*HTX*, heart transplantation; other abbreviations as in Fig. 1)

few years has certainly been based on the patient population referred, and the algorithm outlined will be applicable only to those centers fitted with the whole set of therapeutic modalities.

Our algorithm is subdivided according to the initial arrhythmia event, i.e., either ventricular tachycardia, ventricular fibrillation or cardiac arrest, respectively, with "initial" summarizing reported and/or documented arrhythmia events. However, the majority of patients have been through several drug therapy trials prior to referral to our center or prior to guidance through our treatment algorithm. We are aware of the fact that many arrhythmia patients will be managed with drug therapy outside a treatment center, and drug refractoriness is determined mainly by the behavior of the medical community.

The most important parameters determining the direction of the decision tree are ventricular function and the result of baseline electrophysiologic study. It has previously been discussed that a left ventricular ejection fraction of 25% or less represents an arbitrary value that may be misleading in assessing ventricular function occasionally. However, the application of NYHA functional classes is not precise either, particularly if treatment of heart failure along with antiarrhythmic therapy succeeded in improving the clinical state.

It is obvious that many of the end-points of our decision tree represent ICD therapy. There seems to be no indication reserved for antiarrhythmic drug therapy [40, 41]. In this we differ from the opinion of Brugada [39] who believes that, to date, 77% of patients with infarction-related ventricular tachycardia may be medically managed, with no more than 23% requiring ICD therapy. We agree with Brugada in that in future electrophysiologically guided surgery will be performed in about 15% of ventricular tachycardia patients.

We do not rely on antiarrhythmic drug therapy alone, especially with Class I drugs, after one electropharmacological test has failed. Amiodarone and beta-blocking agents may not be more successful in suppressing inducibility [41]; we have learned, however, that these are potent drugs in slowing the rate of tachycardia or in suppressing undesirable runs or salvos of ventricular tachycardia. Antiarrhythmic drug therapy today is thus an adjuvant rather than a primary therapy for various nonpharmacological approaches in the selected patient population discussed herein. Their role in patients with normally contracting ventricles and noninducible ventricular tachyarrhythmias as an exclusive treatment modality is still pending assessment.

The treatment algorithm outlined here does not include the time of the arrhythmia event after myocardial infarction, which has been assumed to be important in the decision tree proposed by Brugada [39]. Prevention of ischemia, the need for coronary artery bypass grafting, eventual valve replacement, removal of thrombus, or medical therapy for heart failure may significantly affect the decision-making process. However, for the sake of simplicity, we did not include these variables in our algorithm. Treatment of arrhythmia, however, can only be successful or improve the prognosis if considerable attention is paid to the treatment of the underlying disease.

The goal of therapy in patients with recurrent episodes of ventricular arrhythmias is improvement of the poor prognosis. The way of expressing this is still a matter of debate. Consideration of sudden death, cardiac death and noncardiac death with defibrillator therapy may lead only to ICD therapy being overestimated, as some cases of cardiac death may be due to arrhythmic events [42, 43]. Prevention of an arrhythmic event may, on the other hand, also have an impact on improvement in cardiac mortality. Assessing the effectiveness of defibrillator therapy merely after delivery of appropriate discharges represents an approach which is not generally accepted [44–47].

Reduction of sudden death is the main objective of all antiarrhythmic interventions, despite the so-called 60/60 protection, i.e., 60% of all patients treated will stay alive for 60 months of follow-up [48]. However, prevention of sudden death today is not enough. Immediate termination of recurrent episodes of ventricular tachycardia by defibrillator discharge or antitachycardia pacing saves the patient frequent admissions to hospital and may avoid long-term stays in hospital. This can, no doubt, be considered as an improvement in quality of life, achieved by ICD therapy, although the "arrhythmia disease" will not be cured as it may be achieved by electrophysiologically guided surgery or catheter ablation.

The algorithm must be directed by the quality of life to be expected for the individual patient. Although certainly involving some difficulty, a careful life expectancy analysis will be necessary in order to avoid tortuous modes of therapy. For some patients, sudden death may be more desirable than prolongation of a life with chronic heart failure that cannot be improved and leaves no hope for future heart transplantation.

Various treatment modalities cannot be statistically compared in one center as soon as patients are treated according to a specific treatment algorithm. We believe that today random assignment of patients to a certain approach with the object of assessing therapeutic efficacy is not ethical and should not be done since there has been sufficient proof of both advantages and shortcomings for any therapeutic approach already. However, this is true only in respect of patients with documented tachycardia episodes or a history of aborted sudden cardiac death; it does not apply to patients considered to be at high risk, but who have not experienced arrhythmia events. Current studies will show if this group of patients may also be subjected to our treatment algorithm in the near future.

Guidelines have been designed for defibrillator therapy [49, 50], but not for other therapeutic approaches such as surgical intervention or catheter ablation. It is yet unclear if such guidelines are helpful in setting up a treatment algorithm or if such algorithms affect the definition of guidelines. Technical progress in defibrillator devices and the introduction of antibradycardia pacing, antitachycardia pacing, and improved battery longevity and event memory function in particular have changed and extended the indication for defibrillator therapy [51]. Therefore, guidelines as well as the treatment algorithm must constantly be adjusted to the rapidly changing defibrillator technology.

Today, ICD therapy actually represents the "gold standard" of antiarrhythmic treatment for life-threatening ventricular tachyarrhythmias, which other approaches such as drug therapy, surgery, or catheter ablation must compete with [52, 53].

Acknowledgment: We express our appreciation to Mrs. Inge Habel for her assistance in preparing the manuscript.

References

1. Zipes DP, Klein LS, Miles WM (1991) Nonpharmacologic therapy: can it replace antiarrhythmic drug therapy? J Cardiovasc Electrophysiol [Suppl] 2:255–272
2. Dimarco JP (1990) Nonpharmacological therapy of ventricular arrhythmias. PACE 13/II:1527–1532
3. Swerdlow CD, Winkle RA, Mason JW (1983) Determinants of survival in patients with ventricular tachyarrhythmias. N Engl J Med 308:1436–1442
4. Eldar M, Suave MJ, Scheinman HM (1987) Electrophysiologic testing and follow-up of patients with aborted sudden death. J Am Coll Cardiol 10:291–298
5. Waller TJ, Kay HR, Spielman SR, Kutalek SP et al. (1987) Reduction in sudden death and total mortality by antiarrhythmic therapy evaluated by electrophysiologic drug testing: criteria of efficacy in patients with sustained ventricular tachyarrhythmias. J Am Coll Cardiol 10:83–89
6. Wilber DJ, Garan H, Finkelstein D et al. (1988) Out-of-hospital cardiac arrest. Use of electrophysiologic testing in the prediction of long-term outcome. N Engl J Med 318:19–24
7. Rae AP, Spielman SR, Kutalek SP et al. (1987) Electrophysiologic assessment of antiarrhythmic drug efficacy for ventricular tachyarrhythmias associated with dilated cardiomyopathy. Am J Cardiol 59:291–295
8. The Cardiac Arrhythmia Suppression Trial (CAST) Investigators Preliminary Report (1989) Effect of encainide and flecainide on mortality in a randomized trial of arrhythmia suppression after myocardial infarction. N Engl J Med 321:406–412
9. Ruskin JN, McGovern B, Garan H, Kelly E et al. (1983) Antiarrhythmic drugs: A possible cause of out-of-hospital cardiac arrest. N Engl J Med 309:1302–1306
10. Yusuf S, Joon KT (1991) Approaches to prevention of sudden death; Need for fundamental reevaluation. J Cardiovasc Electrophysiol [Suppl] 2:233–239
11. Kim SG (1987) The management of patients with life-threatening ventricular tachyarrhythmias: programmed stimulation or Holter monitoring either or both? Circulation 76:1–5

12. Mitchell LB, Duff HJ, Manyari DE, Wyse DG et al. (1987) A randomized clinical trial of the non-invasive and invasive approaches to drug therapy of ventricular tachycardia. N Engl J Med 317:1681–1687
13. Shale BT, Miles WM, Heger JJ, Zipes DP et al. (1986) Survivors of cardiac arrest. Results of management guided by electrophysiologic testing or electrocardiographic monitoring. Am J Cardiol 57:113–119
14. Moosvi AR, Goldstein S, Medendorp SVB et al. (1990) Effect of empiric antiarrhythmic therapy in resuscitated out-of-hospital cardiac arrest victims with coronary artery disease. Am J Cardiol 65:1192–1197
15. Morganroth J (1988) Evaluation of antiarrhythmic therapy using Holter monitoring. Am J Cardiol 62:18–23
16. Michelson EL, Morganroth J (1980) Spontaneous variability of complex ventricular arrhythmias detected by long-term electrocardiographic recording. Circulation 61:690–695
17. Kavanagh KM, Wyse G, Duff HJ, Gillis AM et al. (1991) Drug therapy for ventricular tachyarrhythmias: How many electropharmacologic trials are appropriate? J Am Coll Cardiol 17:391–396
18. Kuchar DL, Roffman J, Berger E, Freeman CS et al. (1988) Prediction of successful suppression of sustained ventricular tachyarrhythmias by serial drug testing from data derived at the initial electrophysiologic study. J Am Coll Cardiol 12:982–988
19. Borggrefe M, Tampisch HJ, Breithardt G et al. (1988) Reappraisal of criteria for assessing drug efficacy in patients with ventricular tachyarrhythmias: complete versus partial suppression of inducible arrhythmia. J Am Coll Cardiol 12:140–149
20. Wyndham CRC (1991) A clinician's approach to therapy of ventricular arrhythmias. J Cardiovasc Electrophysiol [Suppl] 2:273–283
21. Fisher JD, Kim SG, Roth JA, Ferrick KJ et al. (1991) Ventricular tachycardia/fibrillation: therapeutic alternatives. PACE 14:370–375
22. Hargrove WC, Miller JM (1989) Risk stratification and management of patients with recurrent ventricular tachycardia and other malignant ventricular arrhythmias. Circulation [Suppl I] 79:I178–I181
23. Adhar GC, Larson LW, Bardy GH, Green HL (1988) Sustained ventricular arrhythmias: differences between survivors of cardiac arrest and patients with recurrent sustained ventricular tachycardia. J Am Coll Cardiol 12:159–165
24. Singer J, Guarnieri T, Kupersmith J (1988) Implanted automatic defibrillators: effects of drugs and pacemakers. PACE 11:2250–2262
25. Pratt CM, Eaton T, Frances M, Woolbert S et al. (1989) The inverse relationship between baseline left ventricular ejection fraction and outcome of antiarrhythmic therapy: a dangerous imbalance in risk-benefit ratio. Am Heart J 118:433–441
26. Brugada P, Talajic M, Smeets J et al. (1989) Risk stratification of patients with ventricular tachycardia or ventricular fibrillation after myocardial infarction. The value of clinical history. Eur Heart J 10:747–752
27. Fogoros RN, Elson JJ, Bonnet CA, Fiedler SB, Burkholder JA (1990) Efficacy of the automatic implantable cardioverter-defibrillator in prolonging

survival in patients with severe underlying cardiac disease. J Am Coll Cardiol 16:381–386
28. Marchena ED, Chakko S, Fernandez P, Villa A et al. (1991) Usefulness of the automatic implantable cardioverter defibrillator in improving survival of patients with severely depressed left ventricular function associated with coronary artery disease. Am J Cardiol 67:812–816
29. Kelly P, Ruskin JN, Vlahakes GJ, Buckley MJ et al. (1990) Surgical coronary revascularization in survivors of prehospital cardiac arrest: its effect on inducible ventricular arrhythmias and long-term survival. J Am Coll Cardiol 15:267–273
30. Pinski SL, Mick MJ, Arnold AZ, Golding L et al. (1991) Retrospective analysis of patients undergoing one- or two-stage strategies for myocardial revascularization and implantable cardioverter defibrillator implantation. PACE 14:1138–1147
31. Krafchek J, Lin H, Beckman K, Nielsen A et al. (1988) Cumulative effects of amiodarone on inducibility of ventricular tachycardia: Implications for electrophysiologic testing. PACE 111:434–444
32. Guarnieri T, Levine JH, Veltri EP, Griffith LSC et al. (1987) Success of chronic defibrillation and the role of antiarrhythmic drugs with the automatic implantable cardioverter defibrillator. Am J Cardiol 60:1061–1064
33. Lemery R, Brugada P, Janssen J, Cherieux E et al. (1989) Nonischemic sustained ventricular tachycardia: clinical outcome in 12 patients with arrhythmogenic right ventricular dysplasia. J Am Coll Cardiol 14:96–105
34. Charos GS, Haffajee CI, Gold RJ, Bishop RL et al. (1986) A theoretically and practically more effective method for interruption of ventricular tachycardia: self-adapting autodecremental overdrive pacing. Circulation 73:309–315
35. Haberman RJ, Veltri EP, Mower MM (1988) The effect of amiodarone on defibrillation threshold. J Electrophysiol 2:415–423
36. Freedman RA, Swerdlow CD, Soderholm-Difatte V et al. (1988) Prognostic significance of arrhythmia inducibility or non-inducibility at initial electrophysiologic study in survivors of cardiac arrest. Am J Cardiol 61:578–582
37. Kron J, Kudenchuk PJ, Murphy FS et al. (1987) Ventricular fibrillation survivors in whom tachyarrhythmia cannot be induced. Outcome related to selected therapy. PACE 10:1291–1300
38. Zeutlin TA, Steinman RT, Mattioni TA, Kehoe RF (1988) Long-term arrhythmic outcome in survivors of ventricular fibrillation with absence of inducible ventricular tachycardia. Am J Cardiol 62:1213–1217
39. Brugada P, Andries E (1991) The patient with ventricular arrhythmias can be offered optimal treatment on the basis of simple clinical variables. PACE 14:1201–1204
40. Kim SG (1990) Management of survivors of cardiac arrest: is electrophysiologic testing obsolete in the area of implantable defibrillators? J Am Coll Cardiol 16:756–762
41. Herre JM, Sauve MJ, Malone P et al. (1989) Long-term results of amiodarone therapy in patients with recurrent sustained ventricular tachycardia or ventricular fibrillation. J Am Coll Cardiol 13:442–449

42. Kim SG, Fisher JD, Furman S, Gross J et al. (1991) Benefits of implantable defibrillators are overestimated by sudden death rates and better represented by the total arrhythmic death rate. J Am Coll Cardiol 17:1587–1592
43. Henthorn RW, Waller TJ, Hiratzka LF (1991) Are the benefits of the automatic implantable cardioverter-defibrillator (AICD) overestimated by sudden death rate? J Am Coll Cardiol 17:1593–1594
44. Furman S (1989) AICD benefit. PACE 12:399–400
45. Furman S (1990) Implantable cardioverter defibrillator statistics. PACE 13:1–2
46. Gross J, Zilo P, Ferrick K, Fisher JD, Furman S (1991) Sudden death mortality in implantable cardioverter defibrillator patients. PACE [Suppl II] 14:250–254
47. Guarnieri T, Levine JH, Griffith LSC, Veltri EP (1988) When "sudden cardiac death" is not so sudden: lessons learned from the automatic implantable defibrillator. Am Heart J 115:205–207
48. Fisher JD, Brochman RF, Kim SG et al (1990) VT/VF: 60/60 protection. PACE 13:218–222
49. Dreifus LS, Fish C, Griffin JC, Gilette PC et al (1991) Guidelines for implantation of cardiac pacemakers and antiarrhythmia devices. J Am Coll Cardiol 18:1–13
50. Lehmann MH, Saksena S (1991) Implantable defibrillators in cardiovascular practice: Report of the policy conference of the North American Society of Pacing and Electrophysiology. PACE 14:969–979
51. Leitch JW, Gillis AM, Wyse G, Yee R et al (1991) Reduction in defibrillator shocks with an implantable device combining antitachycardia pacing and shock therapy. J Am Coll Cardiol 18:145–151
52. Winkle RA, Mead RH, Ruder MA, Gaudiani VA et al (1989) Long-term outcome with the automatic implantable cardioverter-defibrillator. J Am Coll Cardiol 13:1353–1361
53. Lehmann MH, Steinman RT, Schuger CD, Jackson K et al (1988) The automatic implantable cardioverter defibrillator as antiarrhythmic modality of choice for survivors of cardiac arrest unrelated to myocardial infarction. J Am Coll Cardiol 12:803–805

PART V

Surgical Aspects of Defibrillation Treatment

Defibrillator Leads: Optimizing of Configuration, Placement, and Energy Delivery

S. Saksena

Introduction

Development of a lead system was an integral part of the development of the implantable defibrillator over the past two decades. The earliest lead systems evaluated included the single right ventricular multielectrode catheter for defibrillation and sensing as well as the combination of an intravascular spring and an epicardial patch electrode [1]. Further research and development has resulted in the development of successive generations of endocardial and epicardial lead systems. These have been designed to deliver a variety of shock patterns, in different intracardiac and extracardiac locations. While the majority of clinically evaluated lead systems have used an epicardial electrode alone or in combination with an intravascular electrode, the trend towards endocardial defibrillation lead systems is now gaining momentum. In general, the latter approach is preferred for a variety of reasons.

The requirements for an ideal lead system for implantable cardioverter defibrillators can now be delineated with the following considerations predominating, but not necessarily in the order listed below:

1) Safety of lead insertion
2) ease of lead insertion
3) reliability of defibrillation
4) reliability of sensing for ventricular tachycardia and ventricular fibrillation
5) reliability of demand pacing for bradyarrhythmias
6) ability to provide low defibrillation thresholds
7) long-term performance characteristics
8) flexibility for use with multiple pulse generators
9) flexibility for delivery of different shock patterns and waveforms
10) ease of lead replacement
11) provide an even electric field during defibrillation including both ventricles and interventricular septum.

These objectives serve as general guidelines for assessment of the lead system and its objectives. However, specific issues relative to each individual lead system arise from time to time and need to be assessed individually.

It is generally convenient to classify currently available defibrillation lead systems into: (a) epicardial lead systems and (b) endocardial lead systems. It needs to be recognized, however, that in individual patients combinations of epicardial and endocardial electrodes have been employed and more recently other more distant electrode locations such as a variety of thoracic electrodes are being considered [2–5]. These lead systems can be monoelectrode or multielectrode and may or may not include pacing electrodes on the same lead body. Individual electrodes may be suitable for epicardial or endocardial placement. It is generally unusual for a single electrode to be suitable for both sites although placement of a catheter defibrillation electrode in both endocardial and subcutaneous locations has been suggested. While the majority of clinically utilized shocks have been monophasic in nature, other approaches such as biphasic or subthreshold endocardial shocks are now being considered [6, 7].

Defibrillation Electrode Systems for Implantable Cardioverter Defibrillators

The defibrillation electrode systems for implantable cardioverter defibrillators can be classified into the following categories, (a) epicardial lead systems: (b) endocardial lead systems, and (c) mixed electrode systems, including both combined endocardial/epicardial and endocardial and subcutaneous electrodes.

Epicardial electrode systems typically utilize two or three electrodes. Electrodes that have been clinically employed include rectangular titanium mesh patch electrodes (CPI model 0041 or 0040 or Telectronics model 040), helical coil patch electrodes (Medtronic model 6897), or contoured titanium mesh patches (Intermedics). While in most clinical situations two epicardial electrodes have been employed, triple electrode configurations are being increasingly utilized. This is most frequently used with the Medtronic epicardial lead system for delivery of simultaneous or sequential shocks with dual current pathways (Fig. 1). This may reduce epicardial defibrillation threshold. Epicardial electrodes are usually available in a variety of surface areas that usually range from 13.5 to 50 cm^2 in different series. These epicardial electrodes vary in degree of stiffness with the rectangular patch electrodes having the highest degree of rigidity and the helical coil electrodes having the

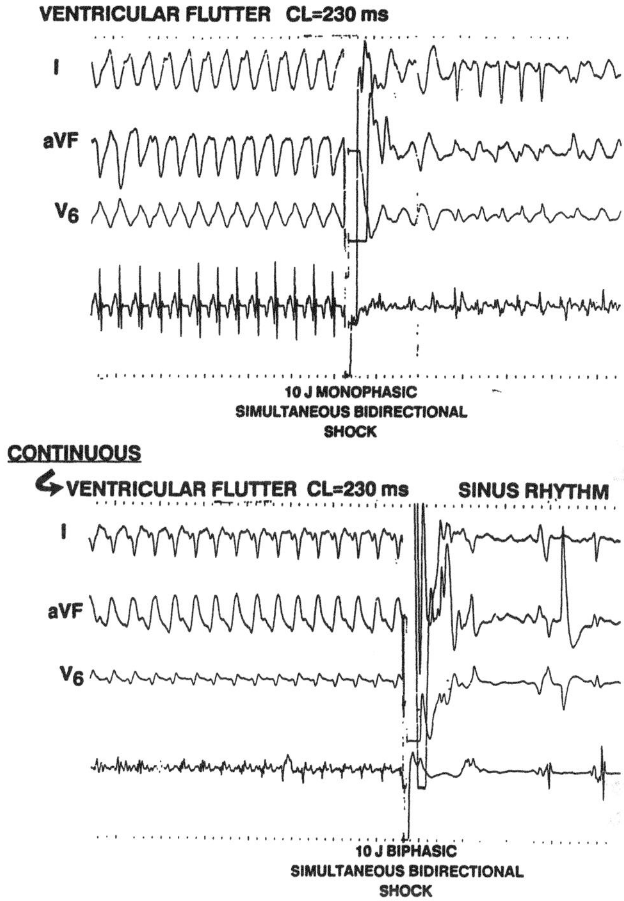

Fig. 1. Defibrillation threshold testing in a patient with sustained VT. Ventricular flutter is induced at implantation of the ICD using alternating current (*top*). A 10 J monophasic simultaneous bidirectional shock is delivered (*arrow*). Tachycardia is accelerated into VF which reorganizes into ventricular flutter (*bottom*). A 10 J biphasic shock using simultaneous bidirectional pathways now converts the ventricular flutter to sinus rhythm. *CL*, cycle length. (Reproduced with permission from Saksena [28])

greatest degree of flexibility in our experience. The electrodes are typically constructed of titanium whereas the lead conductors are usually drawn-brazed-stranded lead conductors (DBS), stainless steel and silver with the back of the electrode and the conductor insulated with silastic or polyurethane [8]. The advantages of biocompatible materials such as titanium include its low cost and inert properties.

Endocardial defibrillation lead systems are under clinical investigation for several third generation implantable cardioverter defibrillators. One lead system used with prototype implantable cardioverter defibrillator consists of a single electrode defibrillation catheter (CPI model 0020 spring electrode). This was largely utilized in mixed lead systems. Other first generation endocardial lead systems used a single multielectrode catheter electrode (Intec Systems ICDC catheter, CPI Endotak, and Medtronic model 6880) [4, 9, 10]. These catheter electrodes utilized stainless steel or titanium spring electrode with surface areas varying from 1.25 to 8 cm^2. The Medtronic 6880 and Endotak catheters include a tip-sensing electrode with a distal right ventricular defibrillating electrode and a more proximal right atrial/superior venacaval defibrillating electrode. These tripolar catheter systems were inserted transvenously for placement in the right ventricular apex. The interelectrode distance between the defibrillation electrodes was adjusted to obtain optimal electrode location and typically ranged from 11 to 15 cm for different heart sizes. Second generation endocardial lead systems utilized individual catheter electrodes at different intracardiac sites (Fig. 2). These systems utilized the concept of a generic pacing and defibrillation catheter (Telectronics Accufix DF and Medtronic models 2100, 2091, 10285 or 6881) [11]. In these electrode catheters, multicatheter (dual or triple) systems are employed for endocardial defibrillation alone or in combination in mixed endocardial lead systems. The Medtronic electrodes are manufactured from platinum/iridium wire and are coil wound electrodes on a polyurethane lead body. The Telectronics Accufix DF lead uses a titanium braid for the endocardial defibrillation electrode. Pacing and sensing are accomplished either in the ambipolar or integrated bipolar mode using a screw-in tip electrode being the cathode and the defibrillation electrode being the indifferent electrode or alternatively with a true bipolar sensing and pacing configuration using a tipped bipolar ring electrode. Active fixation in both lead systems is accomplished by a retractible active fixation screw mechanism.

Mixed lead systems utilize a combination of an endocardial catheter electrode with either an epicardial or subcutaneous extrathoracic patch electrode (Fig. 3). The construction of the endocardial or epicardial electrodes has already been described. The earliest mixed configuration utilized an apical epicardial electrode in conjunction with an intravascular spring (CPI model 0020) [12]. This configuration was largely discarded in favor of a dual epicardial electrode configuration due to higher defibrillation thresholds and the continuing need for both transvenous lead placement and tunnelling and a thoracotomy for epicardial lead placement [13]. This often resulted in a two-stage procedure or an interrupted procedure using two access sites raising concern regarding infec-

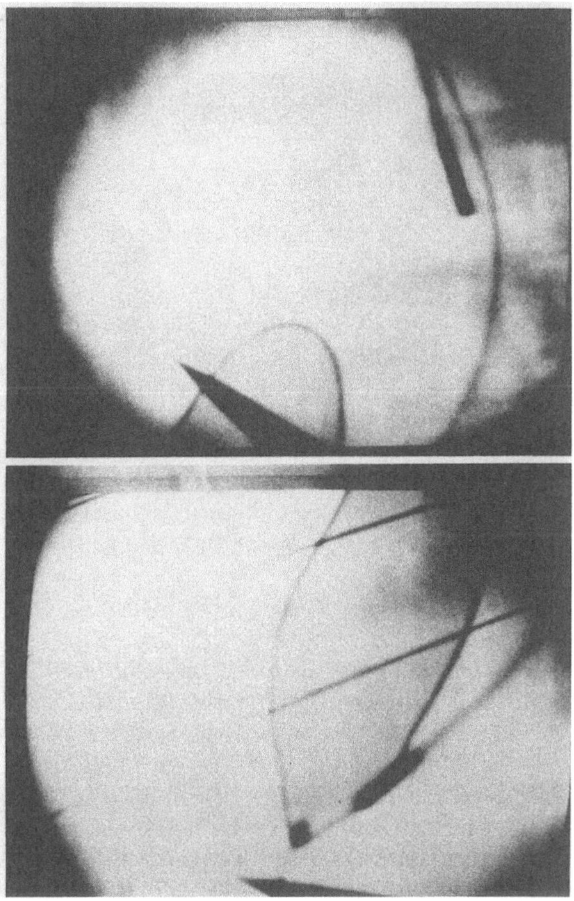

Fig. 2. *Top panel* fluoroscopic image (right lateral projection) of endocardial defibrillation catheters. At the *top* of the figure is the distal end of the right atrial catheter electrode at the superior vena cava/right atrial junction. Traversing the figure is the right ventricular pacing and defibrillation catheter whose strip is seen in the *lower panel* at the ventricular pacing and defibrillation catheter electrode with the lateral thoracic patch electrode. Notice the elliptical shape of the patch electrode. Triple electrode configuration permits unidirectional and bidirectional shocks

tion of two incisions. Early complications included migration of the spring electrode. More recently, mixed electrode systems using two endocardial electrodes in conjunction with a subcutaneous left extrathoracic patch have been used for a nonthoracotomy lead implantation [4]. This electrode configuration utilizes a right ventricular common

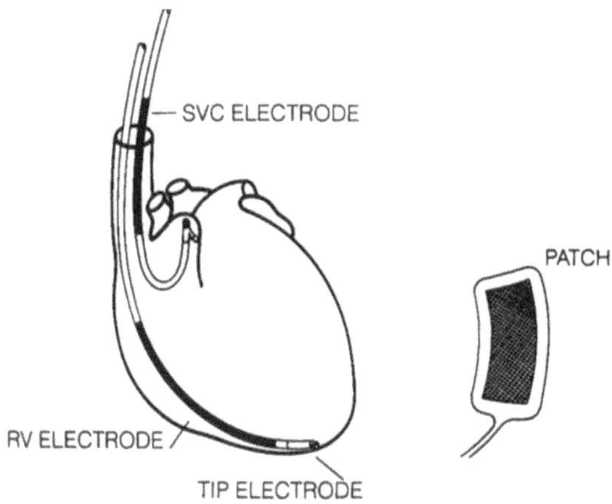

Fig. 3. Electrode placement. Second generation endocardial pacing and defibrillation lead system. One lead is fixed in the atrium while the other is fixed in the right ventricular apex, akin to conventional dual chamber pacing leads. This can be used in conjunction with a subcutaneous patch electrode system to achieve a bidirectional shock

cathode and dual anodes in the right atrium/superior vena cava and left thoracic patch [3]. The subcutaneous patch is similar in construction to the epicardial patch with increased reinforcement of the back surface with insulation and use of more supple materials to withstand chest wall stress [10]. The defibrillation electrode utilizes either a titanium wire or mesh. The lead conductor used in the CPI subcutaneous patch model is DBS wire in a double helical coil configuration. Early clinical experience shows evidence of stress fracture and insulation breakdown in the conductor coil with the patch electrode as well as the catheter electrode (CPI Endotak). Second generation lead systems utilize similar conductors to currently available pacing leads using a multifilar conductor of MP35N or Elgiloy. Connector pins on epicardial and endocardial leads have varied in design. These have depended on the individual device header. The endocardial lead systems also utilize a bifurcated Y-connector.

Lead Location

Epicardial electrode location has varied at different centers due to the use of different surgical access techniques, electrode dimensions, and results of defibrillation threshold testing. It is generally recommended for dual epicardial electrode systems that one electrode be placed on the left ventricle and another as diametrically opposite as possible on the right ventricle. The left ventricular electrode is most often placed on the lateral or posterior aspect and the right ventricular electrode on the inferior or lateral aspect. It is generally desirable to avoid extension of the electrode margin above the atrioventricular groove. However, exact electrode positioning has depended on the results of defibrillation threshold testing in most instances. While inclusion of the bulk of the right and left ventricular myocardium and the intraventricular septum in the shock vector has been deemed desirable, individual instances of specific positions providing lower defibrillation thresholds and greater safety margins which do not incorporate these principles are well documented. In some instances, positioning of the right ventricular patch electrode to include the right atrial lateral margin has been suggested as a method for reducing high defibrillation thresholds [14]. Crossing the atrioventricular groove causes concern when the sensing circuit of the device includes a patch electrode which may be crossing the groove. This would result in sensing of atrial and ventricular potentials and inaccurate VT detection.

Triple epicardial electrode systems have been used in an effort to provide lower defibrillation thresholds with dual current pathways. In addition, newer shock waveforms such as simultaneous biphasic, sequential monophasic or biphasic shocks can be utilized in addition to single simultaneous monophasic shocks (Figs. 4 and 5) [6, 15]. The advantages of alternative shock pulsing techniques in the monophasic shock waveform remain uncertain. It has been suggested that at the very least sequential shocks have equivalent efficacy to simultaneous shocks in dual current pathways. Comparison with single unidirectional shocks has suggested that sequential bidirectional shocks may be superior with respect to reducing defibrillation thresholds. However, this advantage, which has been disputed in large surface area epicardial electrode systems [16], may be related to the bidirectional nature of the shock rather than its sequential nature. Epicardial electrode location could be intra- or extrapericardial depending on the access route, the need for concomitant cardiac surgery or the existence of prior cardiac surgery. In general, extrapericardial electrodes have provided satisfactory defibrillation thresholds although patch location has been limited by the reflections of the pericardium. Typically, extrapericardial electrodes can be placed on the anterior and lateral margins of both ventricles. Inferior and posterior locations require pericardial incision and intrapericardial placement. Access to all epicardial locations is best achieved with a median sternotomy or a left lateral thoracotomy. Subxiphoid and subcostal incisions provide access to most extrapericardial sites except the extreme right lateral locations and a lesser degree of access to superior locations.

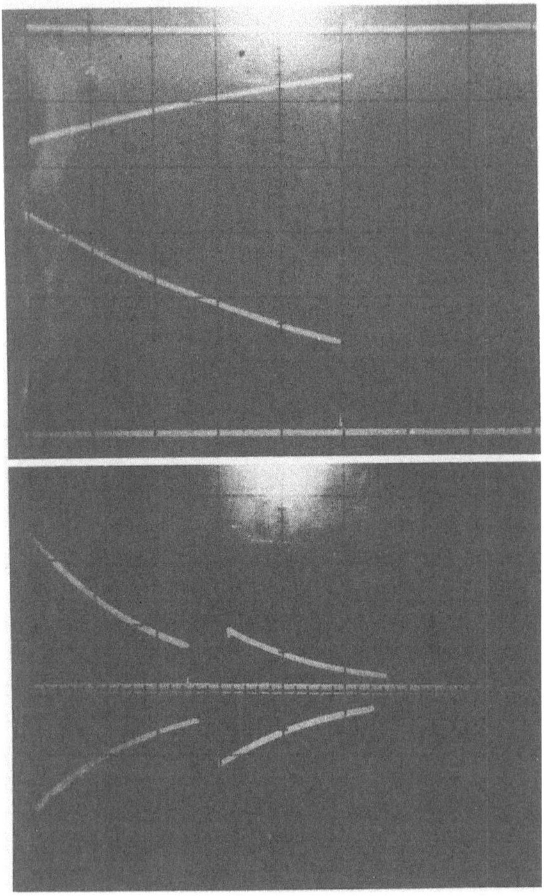

Fig. 4. *Top*, monophasic and biphasic truncated exponential shock waveforms utilized with unidirectional pulses. Vertical divisions are 200 V/cm and the horizontal divisions represent 2 m time intervals. The monophasic waveform is 5 m in duration and the biphasic waveform consists of a positive truncated exponential pulse duration of 5 ms followed by a 1 ms delay and a subsequent negative truncated voltage pulse of 5 ms duration whose leading voltage magnitude is 50% of the positive pulse

Sensing electrode placement for epicardial sensing is also determined to some extent by the access incision, the existence of prior cardiac surgery, and cardiac pacemaker leads. Older generation ICDs, in whom demand pacing was not present, considerations of endocardial pacing lead location with reference to epicardial defibrillator sensing lead loca-

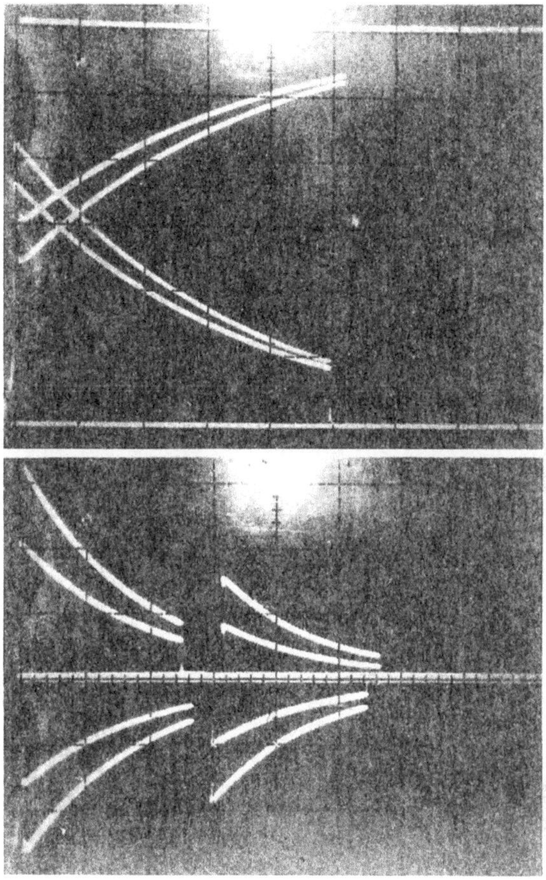

Fig. 5. Monophasic and asymmetric biphasic shock waveforms utilized with bidirectional shocks

tion also were important. In more recent systems, e.g., Medtronic 7216A/7217, Telectronics Guardian, Venitrex Cadence, the existence of sensing and pacing circuits utilizing the same epicardial lead system has obviated this concern. With median sternotomy and lateral thoracotomy incisions, anterior right ventricular or left ventricular sensing electrode placement along the basal aspects of either ventricle is common. With subxiphoid and subcostal incisions, inferior or apical placement may be more frequent. However, the final location of such electrodes is determined by the sensing electrogram amplitude and duration during sinus rhythm, ventricular tachycardia and ventricular fibrillation. It has been recently recognized, particularly for endocardial lead systems, that sensing electrogram amplitude in monomorphic sustained ventricular tachycardia, polymorphic ventricular tachycardia and ventricular fibrillation may not be equivalent [17]. Furthermore, electrogram characteristics in sinus rhythm are not predictive of its characteristics during ventricular fibrillation. Thus, it is incumbent at the time of lead placement and lead testing, to determine adequate sensing and electrogram characteristics during sinus rhythm for purpose of demand pacing and sensing as well as during ventricular tachycardia and ventricular fibrillation for tachycardia detection and therapy.

In contrast, to epicardial lead location, endocardial lead location has been limited by catheter access and safety issues. Left heart locations for chronic in-dwelling catheters have not been considered due to safety considerations. Right-sided cardiac locations have included the right ventricle (apex and outflow tract), right atrium (appendage and lateral margin), superior venacava, pulmonary artery, or coronary sinus [18–20].

Safety issues at all these sites must be considered. In-dwelling spring electrodes in the superior vena cava/right atrium have been chronically employed as part of mixed endocardial/epicardial lead systems for several years. Clinical evidence for increased thrombosis or embolism in these patients has not been presented. A higher incidence of lead complications has been reported. While migration of such electrodes into the inferior venacava and even pelvis has been documented, careful lead fixation at the venous entry site or the use of active fixation second generation endocardial electrodes similar to pacing leads may eliminate this problem. Atrial sensing and pacing would also be feasible with this configuration. This is available in the Telectronics Accufix DF braid endocardial defibrillation lead system. Right ventricular locations for defibrillation electrodes have typically employed an apical site [18]. Active fixation using tined electrodes (Endotak C) or screw-in electrodes (Medtronic model 2100/10285 or Telectronics Accufix DF) is feasible [11, 21–23]. The alternative locations include the right ventricular outflow tract which has been used only for acute testing (Medtronic model 2091). Pulmonary arterial locations have been used during experimental studies but have thus far not been investigated in a significant measure in the clinical situation. Sensing for endocardial lead systems has been typically accomplished using an electrogram obtained through an integrated bipolar set of electrodes or a true bipolar set of electrodes. The former employ one of the defibrillation electrodes as an indifferent sensing electrode with the tip electrode in the right ventricle. An alternative intravascular site that is currently being considered is the coronary sinus [20]. Defibrillation electrodes have been placed in the distal coronary sinus or the main body of the coronary sinus. In the former location, the defibrillation electrode has been wedged to achieve a location along the left cardiac border with the tip in the lesser cardiac vein. Sensing is accomplished in a similar manner to the right ventricular electrodes. Endocardial pacing is typically accomplished using the right ventricular sensing electrodes.

A variety of patch electrode locations have been evaluated. While animal studies suggested an apical location could be utilized, human studies did not support this approach [24, 25]. Our clinical studies over the past six years have evaluated a number of anterior, lateral and posterior thoracic locations. Early evidence suggests that anterior and lateral sites along the left cardiac border provide clinical locations with acceptable efficacy [18, 26, 27].

Energy Delivery Modes

Energy delivery modes to endocardial and epicardial lead systems employ similar concepts. Inclusion of the majority of the ventricular mass in the shock pathway is generally desired. This may be accomplished with unidirectional or bidirectional shock vectors using single or dual current pathways respectively. In single current pathways, this objective is frequently achieved by appropriate positioning of the electrodes as well as increasing surface area of the defibrillation electrodes. Thus, a large patch/large patch configuration is frequently employed for epicardial electrode systems with single current pathways and monophasic shocks. This may lower defibrillation thresholds. Particular electrode positions may also achieve this. Finally, this may be achieved by inscription of dual current pathways with triple electrode systems. In this situation, a single shock achieves simultaneous dual current pathways and two shock vectors (Fig. 4). This achieves the same objective of inclusion of a larger mass of ventricular myocardium in the shock vectors. Alternatively, pulsing in the two pathways may be temporarily separated using sequential shocks. This separation may be a fraction of or a few milliseconds. Finally, pulsing in the two pathways may involve reversal of shock polarity in a biphasic shock (Fig. 5). This may be accomplished with no temporal separation resulting in a simultaneous biphasic shock. Alternatively, there may be temporal separation resulting in a sequential biphasic shock. Finally, biphasic shocks can also be delivered with single current pathways thus resulting in a unidirectional biphasic shock. The duration of each of the components of sequential and biphasic shocks can often be independently controlled with the external or internal cardioverter defibrillator programming. The individual current flow in dual pathways in simultaneous shocks, however, cannot be similarly controlled. This is dependent on tissue impedance in the two pathways at the time of shock delivery.

Clinical Application

The majority of present day clinical experience has been derived from epicardial and mixed endocardial/epicardial lead systems. The latter were employed in the early experience with the automatic implantable defibrillator (Intec Systems, Pittsburgh, PA) and have been largely supplanted by the former. Comparison of lead efficacy, safety and performance has not been feasible in most series. Defibrillation thresholds vary widely in individual patients with one lead system due to lead position. In the absence of standardized positions, particularly for epicardial electrodes, truly accurate comparative data are absent. However, it is widely accepted in clinical practice and documented in several studies that lower defibrillation thresholds are achieved in the majority of patients with larger epicardial lead systems as compared to the spring/patch mixed lead system. Individual exceptions to this have also been observed. Lead performance of patch electrodes has also been superior. Lead-related complications occurred in 10% of patients with spring leads and 2% of patients with patch leads in one series [2]. Data on endocardial lead systems are very limited. One first generation lead (CPI Endotak C) in a small series had a 30% incidence of catheter conductor core fracture and a similar incidence of subcutaneous patch conductor fracture [10]. The most widely used endocardial electrode configuration reported used a triple electrode configuration (right ventricular common cathode with dual right atrial and subcutaneous patch anodes) permitting bidirectional shocks (Fig. 6) [8]. In individual and multicenter experience the configuration proved superior to other electrode configurations with the same electrode sites [18, 19]. More recently the addition of a coronary sinus site has provided an option for defibrillation in selected patients [20]. The use of endocardial dual electrode systems has been clinically disappointing [25]. The use of the right ventricular outflow tract or increasing endocardial right ventricular cathode surface area greater than 4 cm^2 has not provided improvement in the efficacy of dual endocardial electrode systems [22, 23]. This area remains a field for active investigation and considerable progress remains to be made. Currently available information suggests that 50% – 70% of patients can be reliably defibrillated with first and second generation endocardial lead systems using bidirectional monophasic truncated exponential waveform shocks using a right ventricular common cathode and dual anodes in the right atrium/superior vena cava and left thoracic patch. Our preliminary

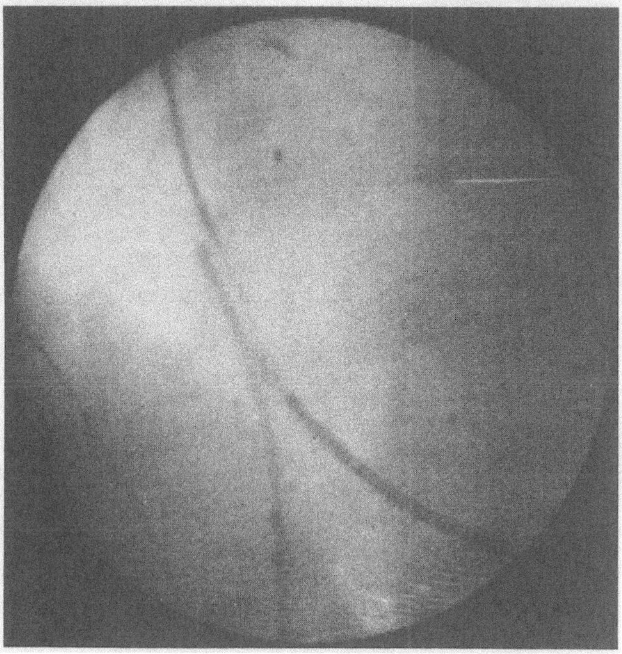

Fig. 6. Fluoroscopic image (posteroanterior view) of a second generation endocardial defibrillation lead system (Medtronic models 2100 and 10285 leads) used alone or in conjunction with a thoracic patch electrode. The model 2100 lead is placed in the right ventricular apex and consists of a spring electrode with an active fixation screw-in pacing electrode. This permits endocardial pacing and delivery of defibrillation shocks. The right atrial electrode can be used for atrial sensing above and in conjunction with the defibrillation electrode. (Reproduced with permission from Saksena [28])

data indicate that simultaneous bidirectional shocks have higher efficacy. Higher efficacy may be obtained by optimizing patch anode position by "patch mapping" using a temporary cutaneous patch electrode or biphasic simultaneous shocks [29]. Larger clinical trials will be needed to validate these early observations.

References

1. Mirowski M, Mower MM, Gott VL et al. (1973) Feasibility and effectiveness of low energy catheter defibrillation in man. Circulation 47:79
2. Winkle RA, Mead RH, Ruder MA et al. (1989) Long-term outcome with the automatic implantable cardioverter-defibrillator. J Am Coll Cardiol 13:1353

3. Saksena S, Calvo RA, Pantopoulos D et al. (1988) A prospective evaluation of single and dual current pathways for transvenous cardioversion in rapid ventricular tachycardia. PACE 10:1130
4. Saksena S, Parsonnet V (1988) Implantation of a cardioverter/defibrillator without thoracotomy using a triple electrode system. JAMA 25:69
5. Obel IWP, Poluta M, Jardine R et al. (1987) Electrode system for closed chest ventricular defibrillation: In: Belhassen B, Feldman S, Copperman Y (eds) Cardiac pacing and electrophysiology. R & L Creative Communications, Tel Aviv, p 465
6. Schuder JC, McDaniel WC, Steckle H (1982) Defibrillation of 100 kg calves with asymmetrical, bidirectional rectangular pulses. Cardiovasc Res 18:419–426
7. Dixon EG, Tang ASL, Wolf PD et al. (1987) Improved defibrillation thresholds with large contoured epicardial electrodes and biphasic waveforms. Circulation 76:1176
8. Bach SM Jr, Shapland JE (1990) Engineering aspects of implantable defibrillators. In: Saksena S, Goldschlager N (eds) Electrical therapy for cardiac arrhythmias. Saunders, Philadelphia, p 371
9. Saksena S, Lindsay BD, Parsonnet V (1987) Development of future implantable cardioverters and defibrillators. PACE 10:1342
10. Tullo NG, Krol RB, Mauro AM et al. (1990) Management of complications associated with a first-generation endocardial defibrillation lead system for implantable cardioverter-defibrillators. Am J Cardiol 66:411
11. Saksena S, Scott SE, Accorti PR et al. (1990) Efficacy and safety of monophasic and biphasic waveform shocks using a braided endocardial defibrillation lead system. Am Heart J 120:1342
12. Winkle RA, Stinson EB, Bach SM et al. (1984) Measurement of cardioversion/defibrillation threshold in man by a truncated exponential waveform and an apical patch-superior venacaval spring electrode configuration. Circulation 69:766
13. Troup PJ, Chapman PD, Olinger GN et al. (1985) The implanted defibrillator: relation of defibrillating lead configuration and clinical variables to defibrillation threshold. J Am Coll Cardiol 6:1315
14. Kaushik RR, Lawrie GM, Havill LF, Pacifico A (1989) Left ventricular-right atrial patch orientation for optimal theshold in AICD implants. PACE 12:6898
15. Jones DL, Klein GJ, Kallok MJ (1985) Improved internal defibrillation with train pulse sequential energy delivery to different lead evaluations in pigs. Am J Cardiol 55:821
16. Wetherbee JN, Chapman PD, Bach SB Jr et al. (1986) "Split" single versus sequential pulse defibrillation: are two pulses better than one? Circulation 74:111
17. Tullo NG, Saksena S, Krol R et al. (1990) Sensing characteristics of endocardial lead systems for implantable defibrillators. PACE 13:546 (abstr)
18. Saksena S, Tullo NG, Krol RB et al. (1989) Initial clinical experience with endocardial defibrillation using an implantable cardioverter/defibrillator with a triple electrode system. Arch Intern Med 149:2333

19. Bach SM Jr, Barstad J, Harper N et al. (1989) Initial clinical experience: Endotak-implantable transvenous defibrillator system. J Am Coll Cardiol 13:65 A (abstr)
20. Bardy GH, Allen MD, Mehra R et al. (1990) Transvenous defibrillation in humans via the coronary sinus. Circulation 81:1252
21. Saksena S (1990) Initial experience with second generation. Rev Eur Tec Bio 12:112 (abstr)
22. Saksena S, Krol RB, Tullo NG et al. (1990) Implantable cardioverter-defibrillators for the 1990s: pulse generators, lead systems and patient selection. In: Furlanello F (ed) New trends in arrhythmias. Libbey, Rome, p 81
23. An H, Saksena S, Mehra R et al. (1990) Effect of right ventricular cathode configuration on endocardial cardioversion and defibrillation with dual electrode systems and monophasic shocks. PACE 13:511
24. An HL, Saksena S, Pantopoulos D (1988) Prospective comparison of combined transvenous catheter and cutaneous electrodes with catheter electrodes alone for ventricular tachycardia cardioversion. PACE 11:492 (abstr)
25. Saksena S, An H (1990) Clinical efficacy of dual electrode systems for endocardial cardioversion of ventricular tachycardia: a prospective randomized crossover trial. Am Heart J 119:15
26. An H, Saksena S (1989) Optimal location of patch electrode for non-thoracotomy cardioversion/defibrillation lead systems. PACE 12(I):681 (abstr)
27. Krol RB, Saksena S, Tullo NG et al. (1989) Electrode configuration for optimal defibrillation with nonepicardial lead systems for cardioverter/defibrillators. PACE 12(I):646 (abstr)
28. Saksena S (1990) Current application of implantable cardioverter – defibrillators in the management of malignant ventricular tachyarrhythmias. Cardiology 77:181
29. Saksena S, An H, Krol RB, Burkhardt E (1991) Simultaneous biphasic shocks entrance efficacy endocardial defibrillation in man. PACE 14:1935

Surgical Techniques of Defibrillator Implantation

F. Siclari, H. Klein, J. Trappe

Introduction

The automatic implantable cardioverter defibrillator (AICD) was developed by Mirowski in order to treat patients surviving sudden cardiac death [1]. After early studies had confirmed that the device was able to reliably sense malignant tachycardias and could terminate them, this therapeutic modality rapidly gained in popularity [2].

After the successful experience with the first device, new features and refined algorithms were successively introduced. In addition to the antitachycardia function, the latest generation of devices also includes an antibradycardia one. At present five devices are under investigation for clinical use (Table 1).

In general, the AICD weighs 250 g and measures approximately 10.8×7.6×2.0 cm. It can be connected to various electrode systems which are inserted transvenously or applied directly to the heart surface (Table 2). The superior vena cava electrode was often used in the beginning, but durability problems forced most investigators to switch to the epicardial patch-patch configuration, which at present is the perferred combination. Sensing electrodes are usually placed epicardially.

Median Sternotomy

The classical approach was chosen initially when concomitant open heart surgery had to be performed. Due to the familiarity of the surgeon with this approach, it has also been proposed for primary implantation of the device alone [3]. Following sternotomy the pericardium is opened longitudinally and suspended at the skin edges. Two screw-in electrodes are then usually placed on the anterior aspect of the right ventricle, trying to keep the interelectrode distance at a minimum (the skirts of the electrodes should overlap). Two patch electrodes are then gently applied to the heart surface, generally in inferior and anterolateral positions. We

Table 1. New defibrillator devices

CPI	Ventak PRX I
CPI	Ventak PRX II
Medtronic	PCD 7216/7217
Intermedics	Res Q
Ventritex	Cadence
Siemens	Thor
Telectronics	Guardian 4210

Table 2. Possible electrode configurations

Electrodes	1	2	3	4
Bipolar transvenous			×	×
Sutureless myocardial	×	×		
Large patch	×	××		
			×	×
Standard patch	×		×	
Vena cava lead				×

use the large patch lead (28 cm^2) anterolaterally and the standard-sized patch lead (14 cm^2) inferiorly (Fig. 1). Only in case of cardiomegaly do we prefer to use two large patch leads. After connecting the four electrodes to the external cardioverter defibrillator unit (ECD) via extension cables, defibrillation threshold tests are preformed. Once the test protocol has been satisfied, the patch electrodes are sutured in place to the epicardium or pericardium using 5-O polypropylene sutures. We prefer epicardial fixation since we believe it minimizes rubbing of the coarse surface on the patch against the epicardium which might cause injury to the coronary arteries. Through the second set of cables the AICD generator is then connected to the ECD-electrode system and the AICD conversion tests performed. The AICD device is then connected with the electrodes and introduced into a pocket within the abdominal wall. There are two possible locations for the pocket, subcutaneous or subfascial. The subcutaneous pocket is easily performed, usually through a separate horizontal incision in the left epigastrium. The electrodes are then tunnelled into the pocket. In fashioning the pocket, one should try to stay on the fascial plane and leave a generous subcutaneous fat layer in order to avoid pressure necrosis from the generator. A pocket too small will run the same risk, whereas a too large one may fill with

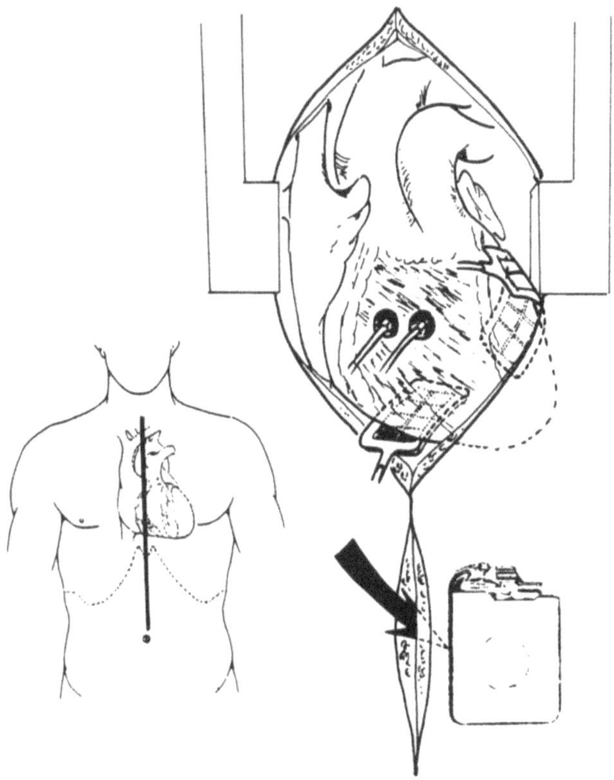

Fig. 1. The median sternotomy approach

serous fluid. The subfascial location of the generator may be above or below the left rectus muscle. Good access to this region is achieved by prolonging the sternotomy incision for about 10 cm below the xiphoid and then preparing the subcutaneous tissue to identify the linea alba. A vertical incision of the left rectus fascia is then performed 2 cm lateral of the linea alba. The rectus muscle is easily mobilized from the posterior fascia to achieve enough room for the placement of the device. Sometimes, in thin patients, it is necessary to incise the lateral reflection of the fascia to accommodate the AICD. This is particularly important since a tight pocket may provoke localized muscle necrosis. We prefer the subfascial location of the device below the muscle because it gives a superior cosmetic result and does not bulge; in addition, the overlying skin is not at risk for pressure necrosis. A small redon drain is then inserted into the pocket and the fascia closed with interrupted silk stitches.

Pericardium is left open and routine closure of the sternotomy follows after insertion of a retrosternal drain.

Anterolateral Thoracotomy

Through a left anterolateral thoracotomy there is a good exposure of the heart and the placement of both patches and the sensing electrodes is easily performed [4]. This approach is particularly useful in cases of previous open heart surgery when resternotomy may pose an increased risk. The chest is usually entered in the fifth intercostal space. After preparation of the pericardium a small incision is performed parallel and anterior to the phrenic nerve. The screw-in electrodes are placed at the base of the left ventricle. The two patch electrodes are then applied to the heart surface, usually in the anteroposterior position. Some surgeons

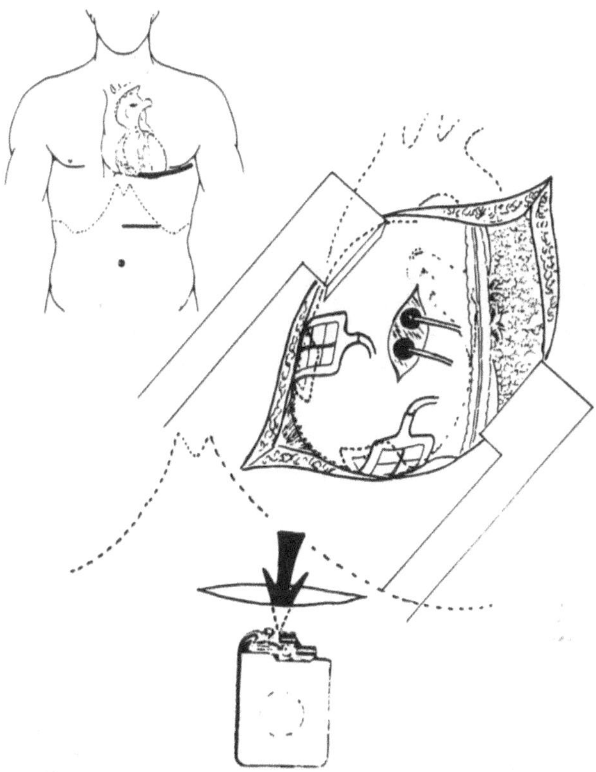

Fig. 2. The anterolateral thoracotomy approach

prefer to apply the patches directly to the pericardium which would be opened only for the insertion of the sensing electrodes (Fig. 2). Although no prospective study has been performed comparing the two approaches it seems that equally good results can be obtained with either method without a significant increase in threshold [5]. Significant postoperative pericardial effusion may lead to threshold elevation in routine predischarge testing [6]. The pocket is usually prepared subcutaneously through a separate incision in the left epigastrium. The electrodes are then tunnelled from the left hemithorax into the pocket. After testing, the patches are then secured to the pericardium with 5-O polypropylene stitches at the corner of the patch. Routine closure of the thoracotomy follows after insertion of one large chest drain.

Subxiphoidal Approach

First described by Watkins [7] with insertion of the single epicardial patch in the spring-coil/patch configuration, this approach has also been used to insert all four electrodes. By avoiding thoracotomy it is well tolerated by the patient, but, since the access is limited, it is rather difficult to change patch position or perform open heart massage. Moreover, it cannot be used in case of concomitant open heart surgery. The incision is performed from the xiphoid for a length of 15 cm and a self-retaining retractor inserted. To allow better exposure the xiphoid is often resected. After preparation of the prefascial fat tissue the space between pericardium and diaphragm is dissected free. The pericardium is incised vertically and suspended at the skin edges. Sensing electrodes are usually placed on the inferior aspect of the right ventricle. The two patches in anteroposterior position are secured as usual (Fig. 3). Alternatively, one can proceed with the pericardial dissection and apply the patches to the pericardium. The latter will only be opened for the insertion of the sensing screw-in electrodes. Establishment of the pocket is then performed (subcutaneous or subfascial).

Subcostal Approach

In order to obviate the limited access provided by the subxiphoidal approach and at the same time maintain the advantages of avoiding thoracotomy, Lawrie [8] introduced the left subcostal approach. The skin incision begins at the xiphoid and runs parallel to the left costal margin. The left rectus muscle is divided along with the anterior and posterior sheath. Through dissection beneath the costal margin, the

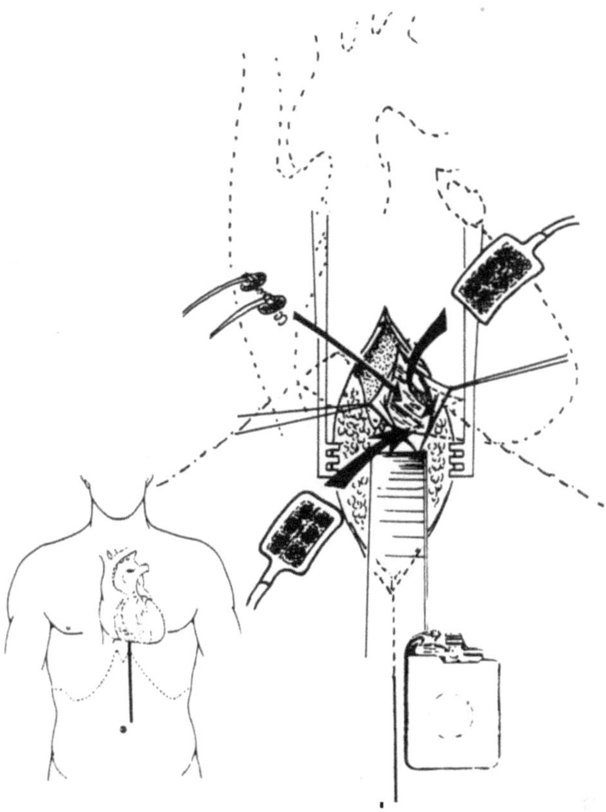

Fig. 3. The subxiphoidal approach

costal attachment of the diaphragm is incised and the pericardium exposed extrapleurally. After this incision, sensing electrodes are applied to the apex of the right ventricle and patch leads are then inserted as usual mainly in an anteroposterior position and secured in the usual fashion (Fig. 4). In case high defibrillation thresholds are encountered, one of the patches may be positioned at the apex of the heart and the second one on the pericardium overlying the right atrium through a right lateral minithoracotomy [9]. The AICD generator is placed beneath the left rectus muscle.

Transdiaphragmal Approach

As with the subcostal approach, the intent was to gain good access to the heart without thoracotomy. This is achieved through the same inci-

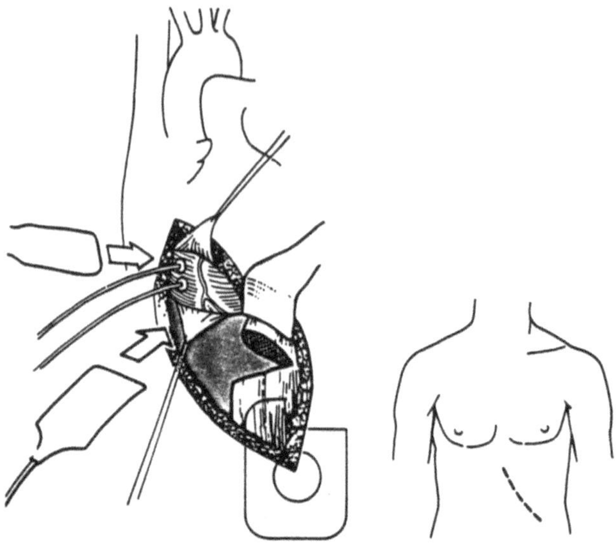

Fig. 4. The subcostal approach

sion as for the subxiphoidal approach, with partial resection of the xiphoid [10] (Fig. 5). The linea alba is incised, the preperitoneal fat dissected and the central tendon of the diaphragm exposed. Through a horizontal "T" incision, diaphragm and pericardium are then exposed. Placement of the leads is similar to the subcostal approach. The generator is usually placed prefascially in the left upper abdomen.

Combined Approach

In case of previous open heart surgery, resternotomy for AICD implantation may be dangerous. Therefore left lateral thoracotomy has been considered to be the approach of choice in these cases. Not rarely, thoracotomy may lead to splinting, pleural effusion and lasting postoperative pain. In such cases a limited subcostal or subxiphoidal approach will safely provide sufficient exposure for the epicardial placement of the sensing leads and the standard-sized patch. Left anterior minithoracotomy (12 cm) in the fifth or sixth intercostal space will enable easy placement of the large sized patch on the pericardium overlying the anterolateral aspect of the ventricle [11]. The patches are secured as usual, and the generator lies in a subfascial pocket in the left upper abdomen (Fig. 6).

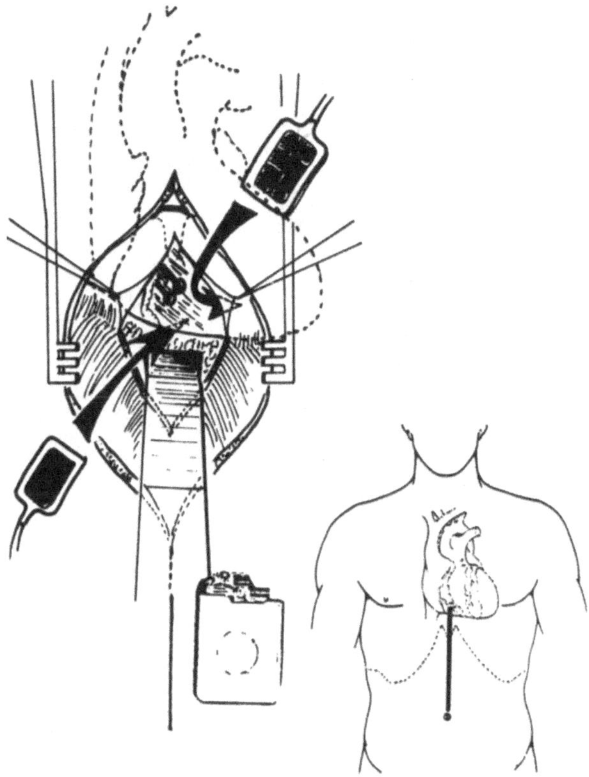

Fig. 5. The transdiaphragmal approach

Alternative Pocket for the Generator

The standard location of the AICD generator is in the left upper abdomen. If for some reason this is not feasible the generator can be incorporated into the thorax wall as described recently by Hartz [12]. After placing the leads through lateral thoracotomy, part of the sixth and seventh rib are removed subperiostially and the intercostal musculature approximated. The AICD can be accommodated in the newly formed extrapleural pouch. Fixation of the device will be achieved by pericostal mersilene sutures around the fifth and the eighth ribs. At the same time, the thoracotomy closure serves to secure the AICD.

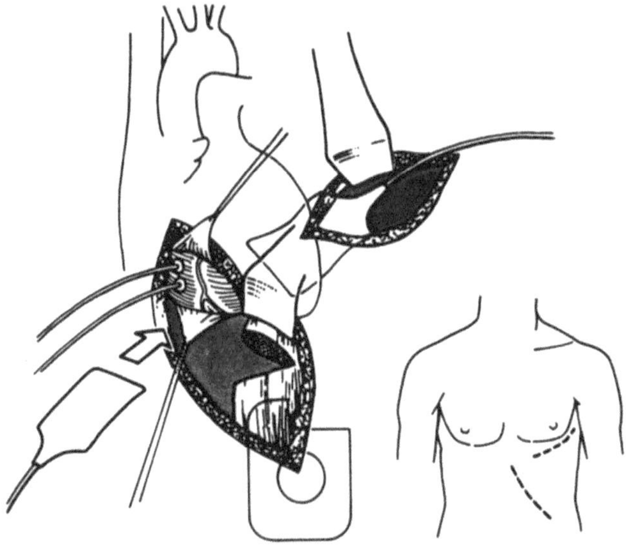

Fig. 6. The combined approach

General Considerations

The choice of the surgical technique for AICD implantation is strongly influenced by the surgeon's preference. Nevertheless, the preoperative evaluation of the patient will be of great value in the decision process. Most of the patients eligible for AICD implantation have coronary heart disease and not rarely have associated chronic obstructive pulmonary heart disease. These patients would probably be better off by avoiding lateral thoracotomy and using rather a subxiphoidal or subcostal approach. Patients with extremely reduced ventricular function may rapidly deteriorate into cardiogenic shock during the testing protocol if prompt defibrillation does not occur. Therefore one would rather be prepared for cardiopulmonary bypass by choosing median sternotomy. In patients who had previous open heart surgery, lateral thoracotomy would offer a good exposure but, as a better tolerated alternative, a combined subcostal approach plus right minithoracotomy may be used.

Infection Prophylaxis

The most common complication of AICD implantation is infection of the system. It seems now that the incidence is about 5% [13]. Perioperative systemic antibiotic prophylaxis is therefore particularly important. There is growing evidence that *Staphylococcus epidermidis* is the bacterium most commonly involved in contaminating the system at the site of implantation [14]. In order to avoid adhesion of bacteria to the polyurethane surface of the devices, we rinse all the electrodes in antibiotic solution (e.g., neomycin) prior to implantation. Using this technique in the last 50 patients the incidence of infection has dropped to zero. We perform routinely a high dose prophylaxis with cephalosporin for 48 h, starting 10 min before skin incision. In order to reduce the risk of contamination from the patient's skin, adhesive plastic sheets are used and the incision edges covered with towels soaked in dilute Betadine solution.

Hannover Experience

From January 1984 to June 1990, 205 AICD devices were implanted in 146 patients. There were 134 men and 12 women with a mean age of 56 years (31–76). Coronary artery disease was present in 116 patients, cardiomyopathy in 19 and an arrhythmogenic ventricular dysplasia in 11. Open heart surgery had previously been performed in 29 patients, coronary artery bypass grafts in 19, valve replacement in 4 and aneurysmectomy with or without endocardial resection in 7. Median sternotomy was the standard approach. In the last seven patients presenting with previous sternotomy, a subxiphoidal approach combined with a small left thoracotomy was chosen. Left lateral thoracotomy was performed in two patients undergoing reimplantation of the entire system following explantation because of infection of the first one. The main complication was infection of the system (8/146 = 5.4%). No infection was observed in the last 50 patients following rinsing of the device with neomycin solution. Early mortality was 6% (9/146), mainly due to low output syndrome (6/9) especially with concomitant open heart surgery (4/6).

Conclusions

We believe there is no "gold standard" as far as the surgical approach is concerned. This must be individualized according to the patient's characteristics. Patients with intermediate ventricular function (cardiomyopathy, arrhythmogenic ventricle) not requiring concomitant surgery are probably good candidates for a nonthoracotomy approach. Patients requiring concomitant open heart surgery and/or having limited ventricular reserves are better off with a median sternotomy. For patients with previous open heart surgery, lateral sternotomy or a combined approach would be the procedure of choice.

References

1. Mirowski M, Reid PR, Mower MM et al. (1980) Termination of malignant ventricular arrhythmias with an implanted automatic defibrillator in human beings. N Engl J Med 303:322
2. Reid PR, Mirowski M, Mower MM et al. (1983) Clinical evaluation of the internal automatic cardioverter-defibrillator in survivors of sudden cardiac death. Am J Cardiol 51:1608
3. Brodman R, Fisher JD, Furman S, Johnston DR, Kim SG, Matos JA, Waspe LE (1984) Impantation of automatic cardioverter-defibrillators via median sternotomy. PACE 7:1363
4. Watkins L Jr, Mower MM, Reid PR, Platia EV, Griffith LSC, Mirowski M (1984) Surgical techniques for implanting the automatic implantable defibrillator. PACE 7:1357
5. Lemmer JH Jr, Faber LA, Mariano DJ, Drews TA, Kienzle MG (1990) Pericardial influence on internal defibrillation energy requirements. Presented at the Annual Meeting of the American Association for Thoracic Surgery 4:1990
6. Schamp DJ, Langberg JJ, Lesh MD, Witherell CL, Scheinman MM, Griffin JC (1990) Post-implant/pre-discharge automatic implantable defibrillator testing: is it mandatory? PACE 13:510, A62
7. Watkins L Jr, Mirowski M, Mower MM, Reid PR, Freund P, Thomas A, Weisfeldt ML, Gott VL (1982) Implantation of the automatic defibrillator: the subxiphoid approach. Ann Thorac Surg 34 (5):515
8. Lawrie GM, Griffin JC, Wyndham CRC (1984) Epicardial implantation of the automatic implantable defibrillator by left subcostal thoracotomy. PACE 7:1370
9. Lawrie GM, Kaushik RR, Pacifico A (1989) Right mini-thoracotomy: an adjunct to left subcostal automatic implantable cardioverter defibrillator implantation. Ann Thorac Surg 47:780
10. Shapira N, Cohen AI, Wish M, Weston LJ, Fletcher RD (1989) Transdiaphragmatic implantation of the automatic implantable cardioverter defibrillator. Ann Thorac Surg 48:371
11. Siclari F, Klein H (1990) Automatic implantable cardioverter defibrillator implantation after previous open heart surgery. Subcostal incision and small left anterior thoracotomy. PACE 13:715–718
12. Hartz RS, Kehoe R, Frederiksen JW, Zheutlin T, Shields TW (1989) New approach to defibrillator insertion. J Thorac Cardiovasc Surg 97:920
13. Olinger GN, Chapman PD, Troup PJ, Almassi GH (1988) Stratified application of the automatic implantable cardioverter defibrillator. J Thorac Cardiovasc Surg 96:141

Complications Associated with the Automatic Implantable Cardioverter Defibrillator

P. J. Troup, S. Nisam

Introduction

Complications associated with automatic implantable cardioverter defibrillator implantation have been reported in isolated case reports, in clinical series, and by the device manufacturer. It is difficult to assess the prevalence of specific complications because data reporting methods vary in the literature and complications involving devices not implanted under the aegis of FDA clinical trials may not be reliably reported to the device manufacturer. There is no uniform agreement regarding what should be defined as a complication and the manufacturer's perspective as the custodian of the largest data base regarding these devices has been the subject of editorial comment [1].

We reviewed the literature to attempt to group complications reported in association with implantable cardioverter defibrillators. Table 1 summarizes a review of ten published series [2–11] involving a total of 913 patients, published between 1987 and 1990 which forms the index group for this analysis. These series include populations ranging in size from 22 to 270 patients with a mean follow-up of 18 months. Most pool data from implants dating to the early 1980s with more recent ones, which may obscure any "learning curve" effect. When multiple reports were published from the same institution, we included the more recent one in our analysis and assumed it contained previously reported cases. However, as indicated in Table 1, early reports sometimes alluded to complications not mentioned in later reports.

Prevalence of complications was determined by inclusion of patients for whom a particular complication was reported and the population for which the risk of that complication was evaluated.

When data integrity was not compromised, we categorically grouped complications according to our definitions, which sometimes were not used by authors in the original series. When effects of our categorization were unclear, definitions and grouping of the original study authors were maintained.

Table 1. Complications (%) reported in ten series of patients with automatic implantable defibrillators

	Winkle et al. [2]	Reid et al. [3]	Kelly et al. [6]	Hargrove et al. [9]	Manolis et al. [8]	Tchou et al. [5]	Fogoros et al. [4]	Myerburg et al. [7]	Borbola et al. [11]	Gabry et al. [10]
Total shocks	58	58	66	NA[a]	54	57	57	64	39	64
Problematic	21	NA	NA	NA	NA	NA	NA	NA	NA	NA
Inappropriate	NA	12	9	31	20	NA	17	NA	9	41
Unknown	NA	NA	10	14	NA	23	31	NA	NA	NA
Pulmonary NS	NA	NA	29	NA[a]	NA	NA	NA	NA	NA	NA
Pleural effusion	0	0	NA	10	5	100	NA	NA	4	0
Hemothorax	0	0	0	NA	0	1	NA	NA	0	0
Pneumothorax	0	0	NA	NA[a]	0	1	NA	NA	0	0
Pneumonia	0	5	NA	NA[a]	0	0	NA	NA	4	0
Pulmonary edema	NA	1	2	NA	0	0	NA	NA	0	0
Amiodarone toxicity	0.7	0	NA	NA	0	4	NA	7	0	0
Device infections	2.2	7.2	2.2	3	2.6	2.9	NA	NA	0	9.1
Other infections	1.9	0	0	NA[a]	0	0	NA	NA	16	0
Perioperative death	1.5	3.3	3.2	3	2.6	1.4	NA	1.7	8	0
Elevated DFTs	3.3	?	5.3	NA[a]	0	0	0	NA	0	NA
Defibrillating lead	6.6	23	2.2	NA[a]	0	0	NA	NA[a]	0	4.5
Rate counting lead	2.2	23	6.7	NA[a]	0	0	NA	NA[a]	0	4.5
Pacer interactions	3.5	0	15.4	NA[a]	NA	NA	NA	NA[a]	0	0
MI	0	1.3	1.1	NA	0	2.9	NA	1.7	4.4	0
Tamponade	0	1.3	0	NA	2.6	0	NA	NA	0	0
DVT	0	0	2.2	NA	1.3	0	NA	NA	0	4.6
Bleeding	0.7	2.6	0	1.3	0	0	NA	NA	0	0
CVA	1.5	0	1.1	NA[a]	0	0	NA	NA	0	0
Follow-up (months)	NA	17	17	14	15	18	25	25	12	20

These 10 series comprise the index group for complications.
NA, category was not addressed or insufficient information was provided to compute percentage.
[a] A previously published series from the same institution that reported complications in that category. All are perioperative except shocks, infections, lead complications, and pacemaker interactions.

Since many complications may be time-dependent, we emphasized complications surrounding the implant procedure because they are unaffected by follow-up duration. The perioperative period began at operation to implant the defibrillating electrodes and ended 30 days after implantation of the pulse generator.

To compare previously reported complications with present implant techniques and device function, we included patients from CPI's clinical data base [clinical evaluation of the Ventak P Model 1600, Cardiac Pacemakers Incorporated (CPI), St. Paul, MN 1990] on patients receiving the Model 1600 Ventak P device (currently undergoing clinical investigation in the US) in Table 2. Implant procedures and many functional aspects of Model 1600 device are similar to the approved devices reported in the index group and these data are subject to scrutiny by the FDA and are unlikely to be biased.

Table 2. Summary of complications (%) from the series reported in Table 1 and those from the US clinical trials of the Ventak P model 1600 series of devices

	Index Series ($n = 913$)	CPI Ventak P Series ($n = 295$)
Total shocks	58	47
Inappropriate	18	3
Unknown	19	7
Pulmonary		
Pleural effusion	20	0.7
Hemothorax	0.2	0
Pneumothorax	0.3	0
Pneumonia	2.3	0.3
Pulmonary edema	1	1
Amiodarone toxicity	1.4	–
Device infections	3.4	2.7
Other infections	1.3	–
Perioperative death	2.6	2.4
Elevated DFTs	2.1	0.7
Defibrillating lead	4.8	–
Rate counting lead	1.9	1
Pacer interactions	5	0.7
MI	0.9	0.3
Tamponade	0.5	0
DVT	0.8	0
Bleeding	0.8	0
CVA	0.7	0
Follow-up (months)	18	6.8

Since many other studies have emphasized the long-term efficacy of implantable defibrillators and their impact on patient mortality, we did not address this area.

Any analysis of this sort is limited. Cognizance of the facts that complications are subjective phenomena, that investigators included complications which they considered to be of clinical significance, possibly excluding others, and that patients with multiple complications may have been multiply counted is implicit in this presentation.

Shocks

Other than patient survival, no other aspect of implantable defibrillators has been the subject of more analysis than shock delivery. Some authors have found it unproductive to attempt to classify all shocks [2], grouping them as "problematic" while others have employed various criteria to attempt to categorize them, sometimes including "false positive discharges" as complications [6].

Analysis of the index group revealed that 58% of patients experienced defibrillator shocks with a range of 39% [11] –66% [6]. Analysis of shocks is a function of time, patient selection, pharmacologic therapy, and investigator interpretation. The majority of initial defibrillator shocks occur within the first year after implant and most [3–5], but not all [7], studies suggest these continue at reduced frequency well beyond the first year. Since follow-up duration is a major determinant of percentage of patients receiving initial shocks, actuarial analytical methodology is preferred. Fogoros et al. [4] (Fig. 1) found the actuarial incidence of shocks for any reason to be 81% at 4 years and we found it to be 66% at 4 years [12].

Within the index series, shocks not thought to have resulted from sustained VT/VF were classified as "inappropriate," "unknown," or "problematic." On average, about 18% of all patients received shocks in these categories, while 42% received shocks which were considered "appropriate." Classification of implanted defibrillator shocks is difficult in the absence of electrocardiographic documentation or hemodynamic collapse and shock classification was often speculative. Since defibrillators may rapidly correct arrhythmias prior to symptom onset, requiring hemodynamic symptoms for "appropriate" shock classification may underestimate shocks for true ventricular tachyarrhythmias and overestimate the prevalence of "inappropriate" shocks. Conversely, nonspecific symptoms such as palpitations and lightheadedness may be associated with rhythms other than VT/VF so these criteria may overestimate "appropriate" defibrillator discharges.

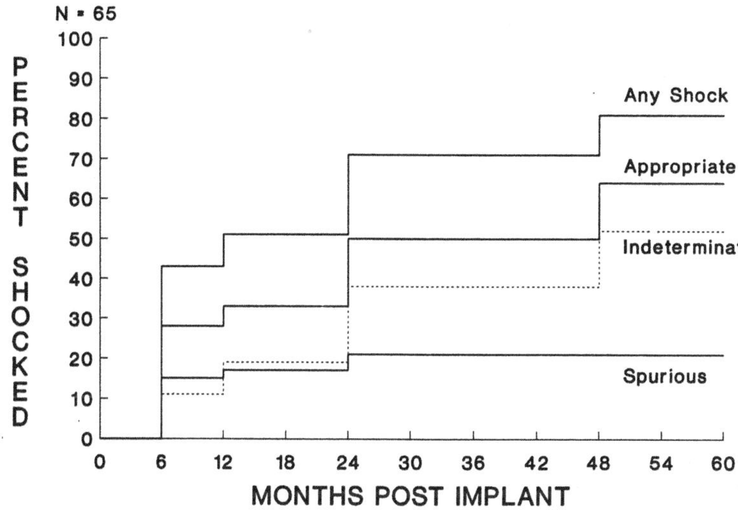

Fig. 1. Actuarial probability of receiving shocks. Data for the graph were taken from the report of Fogoros et al. [4]. Appropriate shocks were defined as those preceded by symptoms of severe lightheadedness, presyncope, or syncope, followed immediately by relief of symptoms or electrocardiographically documented to be associated with sustained ventricular tachycardia or ventricular fibrillation. Spurious shocks were electrocardiographically documented not to be associated with ventricular tachycardia or ventricular fibrillation. Indeterminate shocks were those which could not be classified as appropriate or spurious based upon the criteria above

Causes of shocks in the "inappropriate," "unknown," or "problematic" categories include supraventricular tachycardias (including sinus tachycardia), nonsustained and sustained ventricular tachycardia, rate sensing lead fracture, insulation disruption or migration, loose set screws, interaction with implanted pacemakers, and defibrillator pulse generator malfunction. Supraventricular tachycardia was the most common cause of undesired shocks in the index series.

In the assessment of "problematic shocks," which occurred in 21% of their patients, Winkle et al. [2] found supraventricular tachycardia to be the most common cause, accounting for shocks in 36% of patients in this category. The second most common cause of "problematic" shocks was shocks of undetermined cause (18% of "problematic" shocks). This is similar to another large study [6] which evaluated "false positive discharges," which occurred in 19% of patients. Supraventricular tachycardias (sinus tachycardia and atrial fibrillation) were the most common causative factors, accounting for about half of such shocks and next were shocks of undetermined cause, accounting for about one-third of "false positive discharges." Sensing lead problems (fracture, missing lead capscrews), pacemaker interactions, and device malfunctions rounded out the list of both series of problematic or false positive discharges.

Fogoros et al. [4] found "spurious shocks," all due to supraventricular tachycardia, were responsible in 30% of their patients who were shocked and 17% of their entire population. "Spurious shocks" occurred relatively soon after device implantation and more often consisted of multiple shocks per episode in contrast to "appropriate" shocks, which were typically characterized by one or two shocks per episode.

Some 91% of patients with "problematic shocks" in Winkle's series [2] (i.e., 98.2% of all implantees) and 73% of patients with "spurious shocks" in Fogoros' series [4] were ultimately controlled by changes in drug therapy, AV junctional ablation, restriction of exercise, or correction of a lead or generator problem.

Addition of programmability of rate cutoff, delay of delivery of the initial shock, and the ability to program morphology detection criteria on/off have favorably influenced occurrence of "inappropriate" shocks. Thus far (6.8 months mean follow-up) 47% of patients have received shocks in the Ventak P clinical trials (clinical evaluation of the Ventak P 1600 model, CPI 1990), but "inappropriate shocks" have been reported in only 3% of the population (7% of all patients who received shocks), suggesting that programmability has improved shock specificity.

The groundwork for future troubleshooting device discharges should begin *prior* to implant and is facilitated by knowledge of device function and by antecedent experience, such as the results reported above. A preoperative symptom limited stress test is of value in determining the device rate cutoff and selection of pharmacologic agents. The maximum possible separation of the maximum sinus rate and the slowest VT rate is desirable. The minimum acceptable rate cutoff is 10 beats/min below the slowest monomorphic VT and 30% below the rate of the slowest polymorphous VT according to the manufacturer. Reciprocating tachycardias should be identified at preoperative electrophysiologic testing and appropriately managed to ensure they will not recur at rates above the rate cutoff. Older nonprogrammable devices were inflexible. Drugs and procedures had to be devised to change patients' rhythm and rate characteristics to coexist with the implanted device, often at the expense of side effects. Programmability should obviate the need for many of these interventions since the device can be better tailored to individual patient characteristics after implant. The utility of the morphology detection (PDF) algorithm has been assessed in vivo postoperatively with atrial and ventricular pacing as well as with exercise [13] and, if satisfied by VT, but not supraventricular rhythms, may be useful to enhance specificity of device response. Tomaselli et al. reported morphology detection algorithm had a sensitivity of 91% and specificity of 69% [13].

Atrial flutter and fibrillation have been reported commonly following other cardiac surgical procedures [14–18], but reported in only 9%–19% of patients receiving defibrillators [6, 8]. One study noted such atrial arrhythmias were more commonly observed in patients with two patch electrodes as contrasted to those with spring-patch systems [6]. Lehmann et al. [19], surveying implant centers that practice postoperative device deactivation because of concern over undesired shocks for supraventricular tachycardia, found the average period of deactivation to be 1.7 days (range 0–7 days). However, 14% of those centers observed one or more deaths prior to postoperative device activation [19]. In the index series, VT/VF was primary or, at least, an associated factor in 23% of perioperative deaths. In most instances it is unclear whether defibrillators were active at the times of these deaths or whether active devices would have changed the outcome since most deaths were multifactorial and VT/VF was often described as incessant or nearly so.

Evaluation of shocks following hospital discharge is strongly dependent upon the history of events surrounding the episode and facilitates decision making regarding need for hospital admission. We do not advocate hospitalization for isolated single shocks, but do advocate admission for multiple shocks. We instruct patients who experience multiple shocks to contact paramedics and to go to the nearest hospital. Patients are encouraged to contact us regardless of the time of day and the defibrillator is interrogated as soon thereafter as is feasible. Symptoms such as syncope and presyncope and a history of a single discharge are typical of shocks for ventricular tachyarrhythmias. Repetitive discharges over a short period of time suggest a rhythm disturbance of which the device is incapable of terminating, a recurrent or incessant arrhythmia, or a hardware problem. If the cause for device discharge is obvious, appropriate treatment is initiated. If supraventricular tachycardia is the cause, the defibrillator is deactivated until the arrhythmia is eliminated or the rate is controlled. If the cause of the discharge is not apparent, we initiate monitoring and perform a "beepogram" [20] (Fig. 2) in hopes of documenting a spontaneous discharge and the device is not deactivated. A chest X-ray is obtained to assess the lead system for dislodgement or fracture. Stress testing may be useful to assess the maximum heart rate relative to the defibrillator rate cutoff, whether the PDF criterion is fulfilled (in devices using this criterion) and, perhaps, elicit exercise-related arrhythmias.

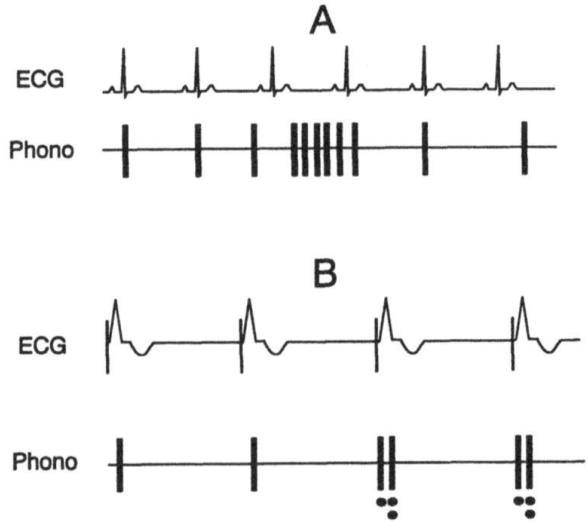

Fig. 2A,B. Example of a "beepogram" obtained by placing the AICD in the electrophysiologic test mode. This mode is accessed by placing a magnet over the AICD, during which it emits audible tones synchronous with each event sensed by the rate counting leads. These tones are recorded through a microphone, amplified, and displayed as a phonogram on an oscillographic recorder producing the trace labeled *Phono*. **A** The first two QRS complexes are appropriately sensed, but the third QRS complex is undersensed, preceded and followed by tones which are not synchronous with any surface ECG event and representing oversensing of true ventricular signals. The combination of undersensing and oversensing suggests dislodgement, conductor fracture, or insulation disruption of the rate counting lead(s). **B** representative of a recording from a patient with a VVI pacemaker; the first two QRS complexes are appropriately sensed while the corresponding pacemaker pulse artifacts are appropriately not sensed. The third and fourth pacemaker pulse artifacts are (inappropriately) sensed (*single dots*) along with their respective depolarization events (*double dots*). The AICD refractory period of 140 ms precludes sensing of the initial portion of the QRS, but the terminal portion is sensed. This situation arises when the pacemaker artifact is relatively large in comparison to the true ventricular depolarization signal and the ventricular signal duration is long

Pulmonary Complications

Pulmonary complications were reported in approximately 44% of cases, but ranged from 0% to 100%, the extremes reflecting individual definitions probably more than any other factor. These were grouped according to the authors' descriptions into subcategories including pleural effusion, pneumothorax, hemothorax, atelectasis, pneumonia, adult respiratory distress syndrome, pulmonary edema, and pulmonary complications which were not otherwise specified. In one series pulmonary complications occurred in 38% of patients with the left anterior thoracotomy approach, 5% of patients with the median sternotomy approach and 25% of patients in whom the subxiphoid approach was used [6]. In another series, pleural effusions were noted in all patients, regardless of the surgical approach, which was a left anterior thoracotomy in 77% of cases [5].

Amiodarone was mentioned as an etiologic factor for pulmonary complications in 1.4% of all patients, although it is possible this drug could have been involved in other cases without being specifically implicated.

Since pulmonary complications relate to the surgical approach more than to any direct effect of the defibrillator device, a more meaningful approach to reporting device-related complications is to report complications beyond those customarily expected with a thoracotomy procedure alone. Using this reporting methodology, total pulmonary complications reported by Ventak P clinical investigators was 1.3% (clinical evaluation of the Ventak P model 1600, CPI 1990).

Infections

The pulse generator pocket and/or lead system was involved in 3.4% of all patients and device hardware was involved in over 50% of all reported infections. The pulse generator, and usually the lead system, was explanted in 74% of patients with infected devices. Infection not directly involving the defibrillator hardware was reported in approximately 2% of cases. The range for any type of perioperative infection ranged from 0% to 16% and infections directly involving implanted device hardware occurred in 0% – 7.2% of patients. The latter series, from the institution which implanted the first defibrillator devices, included a number of infections from the era in which devices were implanted in stages: intravascular electrodes were implanted in the cardiac catheterization lab and the patch lead was implanted later in the operating room.

Infections are time-dependent, as evidenced by infection of the AICD patch electrodes in one of our patients (without a pulse generator or interim instrumentation) 32 months after implant [22].

Concomitant cardiac surgical procedures, in addition to AICD hardware, were performed in 23% of patients. Insufficient information was available to compare infection frequency in patients receiving AICDs alone with those who underwent concomitant cardiac surgical procedures. No significant relationship was found between the percentage of infections and the percentage of concomitant surgical procedures performed in this index group. Our data, independent of the index group, suggests the possibility of a relationship between concomitant cardiac surgery and infection [22].

Diagnostic methods leading to the conclusion of device infection were seldom discussed. In a separate communication, Kelly et al. [6] reported on the utility of gallium scans for the diagnosis of device infections presenting 13 days to 6 months after initial implant. All of their patients with infected devices presented with fever, fluid in the generator pocket, and leukocytosis.

We have found computed tomographic images of the ventricular patch electrodes to be useful for electrodes placed intrapericardially. Fluid between patch electrodes and the epicardium normally resorbs by the fourth postoperative week and is an unusual finding (4.5%) in uncomplicated implants, but fluid collections were found in all patients with infected electrode systems in whom they were sought. Fluid beneath the patch electrodes more than a month after implant in the setting of generator pocket infection should raise concern over intrathoracic electrode involvement.

In the index series, pathogens were described for ten patients with device infections: eight were due to *Staphylococcus aureus*, one due to *Staphylococcus epidermidis*, and one due to *Serratia*. The time of infection discovery was seldom detailed. At least one infection due to *Staphylococcus aureus* was identified 6 months following implant, but may have resulted from a remote cutaneous infection rather than infection dating to implant.

We previously reported 7 infections of 160 patients (4.4%) with defibrillator hardware, five of which involved the patch electrodes. Only two of these seven patients had pulse generators; the remaining five patients had undergone surgical VT ablation with no VT/VF inducible postoperatively. Pathogens identified in the patch electrode infections were *Staphylococcus aureus, Staphylococcus epidermidis, Candida albicans*, mixed infection with *Propionibacterium* and *Peptostreptococcus*, and in one case no organism was grown (although Gram stain revealed Gram-positive cocci). All patients received preoperative antibiotics, for several months in one instance, which may have influenced the culture results. *Staphylococcus aureus* was cultured only from the generator pocket in one patient and from a sternal wound infection in close proximity to the anterior patch electrode in another. Neither had gross infection of the patch electrodes at surgery and the patient with infection confined to the generator pocket had no evidence of fluid beneath the patch electrodes by CT scan [22].

In cases of suspected infection, we found evidence on chest X-ray of "crumpling" (deformation of the radiopaque wire marker around the patch perimeter) of one or both of the patch electrodes in four of five of patients found to have infection involving the patch electrodes. Crumpling of the patch electrodes, however, was a nonspecific finding, present in 21% of patch electrodes implanted in 51 patients with uncomplicated and presumably normal clinical courses. Posterior patches were crumpled more than twice as frequently as anterior ones in this series [22].

Diagnosis of defibrillator hardware infections requires a high index of suspicion. Although evidence is inconclusive, infection may be increased by concomitant cardiac surgical procedures.

Discoloration, fluctuance, and draining sinuses are all signs of possible device infection. Fluctuance of the generator pocket is a nearly universal finding in our experience immediately following implant and the fluid usually spontaneously resorbs 4–6 weeks after surgery. This was been reported as a complication in approximately 1.3% of the index series. Aspiration of these effusions for symptom relief has been described when they are painfully tense. When fluctuance within the pocket fails to resolve or reappears in concert with other signs such as fever, leukocytosis, pocket discoloration, or warmth, aspiration may be justified for diagnostic purposes.

Although it may occasionally be possible to treat infected devices with protracted courses with antibiotics and pulse generator explantation alone, our experience with this approach has been disappointing and we have ultimately explanted the entire system in all patients harboring a device infection. We have employed a polyvidone-iodine pericardial irrigation system in conjunction with systemic antibiotics for approximately 10 days after removal of the patch electrodes and epimyocardial rate counting leads. Irrigation is continued and (non-bacteriostatic) saline infused for 24 h and, when the effluent becomes clear, cultures are obtained. Irrigation is discontinued and the drainage system removed when the saline effluent is sterile [23].

Perioperative Mortality

The average 30 day perioperative mortality for the index series was 2.6% and ranged from 0% to 8%. In the ongoing Ventak P series (clinical evaluation of the Ventak P model 1600, CPI 1990) perioperative mortality is 2.4%. Causes and percentages of total deaths in the index series were: VT/VF (23%), myocardial infarction (15%), congestive failure (9%), sepsis (9%), vascular tears (9%), pulmonary embolism (5%), CVA (5%), adult respiratory distress syndrome (5%), electromechanical dissociation (5%), amiodarone toxicity (5%), and no cause of death was reported in 9%. For the same reasons outlined in the section above, it was impossible to relate perioperative mortality and concomitant cardiac surgical procedures, which were performed at the time of AICD implant in 23% of patients in the index series. Edel et al. [24] found the perioperative mortality to be more than *five times higher* (9.6% vs 1.7%) in patients who underwent *concomitant* cardiac surgical procedures compared with those who underwent implantation of an AICD alone. Hargrove et al. [9] compared operative mortality for patients undergoing subendocardial resection with that for defibrillator implant alone. They found mortality was five times higher with subendocardial resection (15% vs 3%) than for AICD implant alone. These two groups had similar ventricular function and similar long-term survival after the perioperative period, with heart failure (not arrhythmias) the most common cause of death in both groups. It was emphasized that the surgical approach for patients with arrhythmias must be tailored to the disease process, target arrhythmia, and "intangible factors" [9].

Evaluated Defibrillation Energy Requirements

The ideal safety margin for defibrillation remains unknown although 10 J has been suggested [25, 26] and a defibrillation threshold (DFT) of 15 J or less was the goal of most investigators surveyed [19]. While no uniform definition of elevated defibrillation requirement exists, DFTs greather than 25 J compromise the 10 J safety margin for the majority of most implantable devices available during the period covered by this report. When stated, the maximum acceptable DFT was 25 J [2, 5, 6] or 20 J [3, 8]. Using the criteria set forth by the investigators in their own studies, 2.1% of patients (range 0%–8%) exhibited high DFTs during implant or follow-up testing. Winkle et al. [2] found high DFTs in 3.3% of their patients and noted the occurrence of high DFTs was six times higher (6% vs 1%) in their early patients compared to later ones in their series. This may have related to the predominant use of two patch electrode systems later in their series, but also suggests that a learning curve exists. In the Ventak P series (clinical evaluation of the Ventak P model 1600, CPI 1990) 0.7% of patients demonstrated defibrillation energy requirements above 25 J and this was corrected by reversing lead polarity.

Kelly et al. [6] felt that *amiodarone* may have been responsible for high DFTs in at least 75% their patients with unacceptable DFTs at the time of initial implant. They found significant differences between DFTs for patients who had received this drug within 1 month of implant compared to patients not so treated. Others have also reported a similar effect on DFTs induced by amiodarone [27] and we found amiodarone to be an independent predictor of higher DFTs, but we did not observe unacceptably high DFTs (i.e., 25 J) associated with this drug [28]. Winkle et al. did not implicate drugs in any of their patients with high DFTs [2].

When high DFTs are encountered, electrode repositioning, replacement, and/or reversal of defibrillating electrode polarity is often effective in achieving an acceptable DFT. These maneuvers were reportedly necessary in 20% of patients in one study [11]. Electrode repositioning is probably frequently performed, but infrequently reported unless acceptable DFTs cannot be obtained.

Antiarrhythmic drug effects should always be considered in the setting of elevated DFTs. Many antiarrhythmic agents have been shown in dogs and in humans to increase defibrillation energy requirements [29]. Under some circumstances, such as hemodynamic deterioration with protracted testing, it may be appropriate to suspend testing, discontinue potentially deleterious drugs, and repeat testing at a later time. A single operative fatality resulting from inability to terminate an induced arrhythmia has been reported [11].

Fortunately, cardiopulmonary bypass, cardioplegia, and prior hypothermia have not been found to substantially alter defibrillation energy requirements [30, 31] and thresholds remain relatively stable over time [32].

Under extenuating circumstances, 64% of implanting centers surveyed acknowledged they would proceed with pulse generator implantation if the best defibrillation threshold which could be obtained was 25 J, but 96% would strive to achieve a lower energy requirement [19].

Lead Complications

The spring electrode, now rarely used, was implicated in many of the early lead complications prior to the availability of a device to anchor the lead. The reported complications approximated 4.8% considering all complications involving the high voltage electrodes. Migration was the most common complication, with fracture, vascular injury and obstruction less commonly reported. Complications were reported nearly four times more often with spring electrodes than with patch electrodes (approximately 1% of patients in the index series) and inclusion of spring lead complications inflate the complication rate. Patch lead fracture, insulation break, or deformation developed in 2% of implanted patch electrodes in the largest published series [2]. Of these, all fractures and the single insulation break occurred in the abdomen. Sensing lead problems were noted in 3% of patients, of which 58% involved epicardial and 42% involved endocardial leads. Half of these problems were insulation breaks, 25% were related to implant difficulties (lead unintentionally severed, loose set screws, capscrews left off), 17% were lead fractures, and 8% were due to endocardial lead migration. There have been no patch lead complications in the Ventak P series (clinical evaluation of the Ventak P model 1600, CPI 1990) and migration or fracture of the rate counting leads have occurred in 1% of patients.

Patch and rate-counting electrode problems in the index series were most often diagnosed at the time of pulse generator change. Only approximately 25% of sensing lead problems came to attention because of inappropriate device discharges.

We have found "beepograms" to be of value in the diagnosis of sensing lead fracture and insulation breaks [20] (Fig. 2). Another clue to the diagnosis of lead fracture or insulation break is a noisy signal which cannot be corrected at the time of lead system testing. A pacing system analyzer is useful when the lead system is accessed for testing. As with any pacing lead, the rate counting lead impedance will be infinite at least intermittently when an open circuit exists and the impedance may be abnormally low in the case of insulation disruption.

Pacemakers

Approximately 11% of patients in the index series had electronic pacemakers. Several papers have addressed the problem of defibrillator-pacemaker interactions [20, 25, 34–38]. These interactions fall into three categories: defibrillator oversensing of pacemaker mediated rhythms, pacemaker undersensing of tachyarrhythmias, and post-shock pacemaker malfunction. In the index series the prevalence of interaction was in the range of 5% and in the Ventak P series it was 0.7%. Three pacemakers were bipolar devices and pacemaker defibrillator interaction was recognized at implant in three patients. These consisted of defibrillator oversensing of far field pacemaker pulses in one VVI and one DDD pacemaker, with post-shock loss of DDD sensing and capture in one of these. The third patient had "significant interactions" between an AICD and an antitachycardia pacemaker. An additional report of defibrillator discharge during magnet application to a permanent pacemaker occurred in one patient [10]. In an earlier report from this group, the pacemaker was identified as a unipolar VVI device [34].

Unipolar pacemakers have been implicated in all reports of pacemaker-mediated inhibition of AICD tachyarrhythmia recognition [25, 34–37]. Unipolar pacemakers are contraindicated in conjunction with AICDs by the device manufacturer [39].

Pulse Generator Malfunction

Generator failure, misdirected shocks, and detection failure were grouped into the rather broad category of pulse generator malfunction. These complications were reported in approximately 5% of patients. We did not attempt to correlate reports of device malfunction with the manufacturer's analysis of devices returned for verification of such problems.

Phenomena such as premature battery depletion due to glass corrosion of the battery terminal feedthroughs and devices prophylactically replaced because of argon backfill of the generator case, etc., were excluded unless they were associated with failure of resuscitation and/or patient death. These were early problems which are primarily of historical interest, but of little relevance to presently manufactured devices which have much longer life expectancies because of new battery chemistry as well as reduced device current drain.

Malfunction was manifest as lack of output in at least 38% of the cases in which generator malfunction was documented. Three deaths were associated with devices found to be nonfunctional. Some 38% of generator failures were labeled "component malfunction" without description of the circumstances in which the devices failed, 15% of generator failures were manifest as inappropriate shocks for which no other explanation could be found, and 8% of failures were manifest as "sensing difficulties."

Misdirected shocks are those delivered to the patient instead of dumping into the internal load during a magnet test. These occurred in 1.3% of all patients and accounted for 26% of all cases of generator malfunction. Ventricular fibrillation resulted in 60% of the reported cases of misdirected pulses and required external resuscitation in one-third of these instances, but no misdirected shock was implicated in a patient death.

Detection failure was difficult to analyze and the exact cause was frequently unclear. It reportedly occurred in 0.97% of devices and accounted for 19% of all generator failures. Although causes of detection failure were sometimes proffered, these were often speculative and lacking confirmation by manufacturer's device analysis.

Miscellaneous Complications

A number of other complications have been reported, which have not been included above. Our goal has been to emphasize those complications which are likely to be seen with present and future implants, particularly those which may be preventable.

Fever was reported in only approximately 7% of patients and was probably underreported because of its nonspecificity or temperature elevation did not exceed 101 °F orally, or was considered a part of the usual postoperative course.

Pericarditis was reported in only approximately 4% of patients and there appeared to be no diagnostic criteria which were generally accepted. One study reported pericardial friction rubs in all patients postoperatively, but "clinical pericarditis" in only 4% [8] of which half developed cardiac tamponade. Another series reported asymptomatic pericardial friction rubs "frequently," but symptomatic pericarditis in only 3% [6] and no cases of tamponade. Cardiac tamponade was reported in less than 2% of patients and there were no fatalities attributed to this complication.

In the index series myocardial infarction was reported in about 0.9% of implants, deep venous thrombosis in 0.8%, bleeding associated with the implant surgery in 0.8%, cerebrovascular accidents in 0.7%, and gastrointestinal bleeding in less than 1%.

Even less frequent complications, occurring in less than 1% of patients were superior vena caval obstruction, pulmonary embolism, vascular tears (but two had fatal outcomes), and inadvertent pulse generator deactivation presumably due to contact with magnets.

In the Ventak P series (clinical evaluation of the Ventak P model 1600, CPI 1990), perioperative myocardial infarction occurred in 0.3% of patients, and there have been no known cases of deep venous thrombosis, bleeding, or cerebrovascular accidents.

References

1. Furman S (1990) Implantable cardioverter defibrillator statistics. PACE 13:1–2
2. Winkle RA, Mead RH, Ruder MA, Gaudiani VA, Smith NA, Buch WS, Schmidt P, Shipman T (1989) Long-term outcome with the automatic implantable cardioverter-defibrillator. J Am Coll Cardiol 13:1353–1361
3. Reid PR, Griffith LSC, Platia EV, Mower MM, Veltri EP, Mirowski M, Guarnieri T, Singer I, Juanteguy J, Watkins L (1987) The automatic implantable cardioverter-defibrillator: five year clinical results. In: Breithardt G, Borggrefe M (eds) Nonpharmacologic treatment of tachyarrhythmias. Futura, Mount Kisco, pp 477–486
4. Fogoros RN, Elson JJ, Bonnet CA (1989) Actuarial incidence and pattern of occurrence of shocks following implantation of the automatic implantable cardioverter defibrillator. PACE 12:1465–1473
5. Tchou PJ, Kadri N, Anderson J, Caceres JA, Jazayeri M, Akhtar M (1988) Automatic implantable cardioverter defibrillators and survival of patients

with left ventricular dysfunction and malignant ventricular arrhythmias. Ann Intern Med 109:529–534
6. Kelly PA, Cannom DS, Garan H, Mirabal GS, Harthorne JW, Hurvitz RJ, Vlahakes GJ, Jacobs ML, Ilvento JP, Buckley MJ, Ruskin JN (1988) The automatic implantable cardioverter-defibrillator: efficacy, complications and survival in patients with malignant ventricular arrhythmias. J Am Coll Cardiol 11:1278–1286
7. Myerburg RJ, Luceri RM, Thurer R, Cooper DK, Zaman L, Interian A, Fernandez F, Cox M, Glicksman A, Castellanos A (1989) Time to first shock and clinical outcome in patients receiving an automatic implantable cardioverter-defibrillator. J Am Coll Cardiol 14:508–514
8. Manolis AS, Tan-DeGuzman W, Lee MA, Rastegar H, Haffajee C, Huang SKS, Estes NAM (1989) Clinical experience in seventy-seven patients with the automatic implantable cardioverter defibrillator. Am Heart J 118: 445–449
9. Hargrove WC, Josephson ME, Marchlinski FE, Miller JM (1989) Surgical decisions in the management of sudden cardiac death and malignant ventricular arrhythmias. J Thorac Cardiovasc Surg 97:923–928
10. Gabry MD, Brodman R, Johnston D, Frame R, Kim SG, Waspe LE, Fisher JD, Furman S (1987) Automatic implantable cardioverter-defibrillator: patient survival, battery longevity, and shock delivery analysis. J Am Coll Cardiol 9:1349–1356
11. Borbola J, Denes P, Ezri MD, Hauser RG, Serry C, Goldin MD (1988) The automatic implantable cardioverter-defibrillator: clinical experience, complications, and follow-up in 25 patients. Arch Intern Med 148:70–76
12. Wetherbee J, Troup P, Peterson P, Thakur R, Tucker V, Veseth-Rogers J, Chapman P, Almassi GH, Olinger G (1990) Actuarial probability of initial appropriate AICD shocks over long-term follow-up. J Am Coll Cardiol 15:199A
13. Tomaselli GF, DeBorde R, Griffith LSC, Guarnieri T (1990) Does AICD probability density function improve tachycardia discrimination? PACE 13:506
14. Rubin DA, Nieminski KE, Reed GE, Herman MV (1987) Predictors, prevention, and long-term prognosis of atrial fibrillation after coronary bypass graft operations. J Thorac Cardiovasc Surg 94:331–335
15. Williams JB, Stephenson LW, Holford FD, Langer T, Dunkman WB, Josephson ME (1982) Arrhythmia prophylaxis using propranolol after coronary artery surgery. Ann Thorac Surg 34:435–438
16. Stephenson LW, MacVaugh H III, Tomasello DN, Josephson ME (1979) Propranolol for prevention of postoperative cardiac arrhythmias: a randomized trial. Ann Thorac Surg 29:113–116
17. White HD, Antmann EM, Glynn MA, Collins JJ, Cohn LH, Shemin RJ, Friedman PL (1984) Efficacy and safety of timolol for prevention of supraventricular tachyarrhythmias after coronary artery bypass surgery. Circulation 70:479–484
18. Davison R, Hartz R, Kaplan K, Parker M, Feiereisel P, Michaelis L (1985) Prophylaxis of supraventricular tachyarrhythmia after coronary bypass

surgery with oral verapamil: a randomized double blind trial. Ann Thorac Surg 39:336–339
19. Lehmann MH, Steinman RT, Schuger CD, Jackson K (1989) Defibrillation threshold testing and other practices related to AICD implantation: do all roads lead to Rome? PACE 12:1530–1537
20. Chapman PD, Troup P (1986) The automatic implantable cardioverter-defibrillator: evaluating suspected inappropriate shocks. J Am Coll Cardiol 7:1075–1078
21. Kelly PA, Wallace S, Tucker B, Hurvitz RJ, Ilvento J, Mirabel GS, Cannom DS (1988) Postoperative infection with the automatic implantable cardioverter defibrillator: clinical presentation and use of the gallium scan in diagnosis. PACE 11:1220–1225
22. Goodman LR, Almassi GH, Troup PJ, Gurney JW, Veseth-Rogers J, Chapman PD, Wetherbee JN (1989) Complications of automatic implantable cardioverter defibrillators: radiographic, CT, and echocardiographic evaluation. Radiology 170:447–452
23. Almassi GH, Olinger GN, Troup PJ, Chapman PD, Goodman LR (1988) Delayed infection of the automatic implantable cardioverter-defibrillator: current recognition and management. J Thorac Cardiovasc Surg 95:908–911
24. Edel TB, Castle LW, Morant VA, Simmons TW, Wilkoff BL, Trohman R, Maloney JD (1990) Effect of combined cardiac surgery during implantable defibrillator placement on operative mortality and morbidity, late mortality and shock analysis. PACE 13:529A
25. Marchlinski FE, Flores B, Miller JM, Gottlieb CD, Hargrove WC (1988) Relationship of the intraoperative defibrillation threshold to successful postoperative defibrillation with an automatic implantable cardioverter defibrillator. Am J Cardiol 62:393–398
26. Cannom DS, Winkle RA (1986) Implantation of the automatic implantable cardioverter defibrillator (AICD): practical aspects. PACE 9:793–809
27. Guarnieri T, Levine JH, Veltri EP, Griffith LSC, Watkins L, Juanteguy J, Mower MM, Mirowski M (1987) Success of chronic defibrillation and the role of antiarrhythmic drugs with the automatic implantable cardioverter defibrillator. Am J Cardiol 60:1061–1064
28. Troup PJ, Chapman PD, Olinger GN, Kleinman LH (1985) The implanted defibrillator: relation of defibrillating lead configuration and clinical variables to defibrillation threshold. J Am Coll Cardiol 6:1315–1321
29. Troup P (1989) Implantable cardioverters and defibrillators. In: O'Rourke RA, Crawford MH, Beller GA, Rahimtoola SH, Schlant RC, Shah P (eds) Current problems in cardiology. Yearbook, Chicago 14:788–789
30. Blakeman BM, Pifarre R, Scanlon PJ, Wilber DJ (1989) Coronary revascularization and implantation of the automatic cardioverter/defibrillator: reliability of immediate intraoperative testing. PACE 12:86–91
31. Klein GJ, Jones DL, Sharma AD, Kallok MJ, Guiraudon GM (1986) Influence of cardiopulmonary bypass on internal cardiac defibrillation. Am J Cardiol 57:1194–1195

32. Wetherbee JN, Chapman PD, Troup PJ, Veseth-Rogers J, Thakur RK, Almassi GH, Olinger GN (1989) Long-term internal cardiac defibrillation threshold stability. PACE 12:443–449
33. Marchlinski FE, Flores BT, Buxton AE, Hargrove WC III, Addonizio VP, Stephenson LW, Harken AH, Doherty JU, Grogan EW, Josephson ME (1986) Automatic implantable cardioverter-defibrillator: efficacy, complications and device failures. Ann Intern Med 104:481–488
34. Brodman R, Fisher JD, Furman S, Johnston DR, Kim SG, Matos JA (1984) Implantation of automatic cardioverter-defibrillators via median sternotomy. PACE 7:1363–1369
35. Mirowski M (1983) Management of ventricular arrhythmias with implanted cardioverter-defibrillators. Mod Concepts Cardiovasc Dis 52:41–44
36. Kim SG, Furman S, Waspe LE, Brodman R, Fisher JD (1986) Unipolar pacemaker artifacts induce failure of the automatic implantable cardioverter/defibrillator to detect ventricular fibrillation. Am J Cardiol 57:880–881
37. Cohen AI, Wish MH, Fletcher RD, Miller FC, McCormick D, Shuck J, Shapira N, DelNegro AA (1988) The use and interaction of permanent pacemakers and the automatic implantable cardioverter defibrillator. PACE 11:704–711
38. Echt DS (1984) Potential hazards of implanted devices for the electrical control of tachyarrhythmias. PACE 7:580–587
39. Bach SM Jr (1983) Technical communication: AID-B cardioverter-defibrillator: possible interactions with pacemakers. Intec Systems, Pittsburgh, 29 Aug 1983

Safety Margin for Defibrillation

D. J. Lang, D. K. Swanson

There are two goals when performing clinical defibrillation testing protocols. The first is to verify an adequate safety margin for the patient's automatic implantable cardioverter defibrillator (AICD) system. The second is to determine the defibrillation threshold characteristics of that system. In practice, one can accomplish the first goal without addressing the second. However, given the programmable nature of current AICD devices and their longer life, it has become more important to do both: to establish the device safety margin by determining the patient's defibrillation threshold.

We can define the safety margin as the difference in energy between the AICD output and the minimum energy for consistent defibrillation. Since the relationship between percent successful defibrillation and shock energy is a defibrillation success curve (Fig. 1), the lower boundary of the safety margin corresponds to the curve's upper corner (near E_{95}, i.e., the shock energy yielding 95% defibrillation success). Thus, the safety margin is a measure of the width of the plateau between the AICD output and the energies that fail to defibrillate the patient. Obviously, one should have a safety margin large enough such that a shift in the defibrillation success curve to higher energies would not surpass the output of the device. Such shifts in the defibrillation requirements may result from prolonged fibrillation time if the later rescue shocks are needed from the device, further disease progression, or a modification in the patient's drug regimen.

Defibrillation Threshold Testing. In practice, the safety margin is estimated by the measurement of a defibrillation threshold (DFT). A DFT is determined using a test sequence of several fibrillation trials with defibrillation attempted at selected energies using a cardioverter-defibrillator. If the initial shock energy is successful, defibrillation shock energies are decreased in successive fibrillation trials until a failed defibrillation attempt is encountered. If the initial energy fails to defibrillate, shock energies are increased in successive fibrillation trials

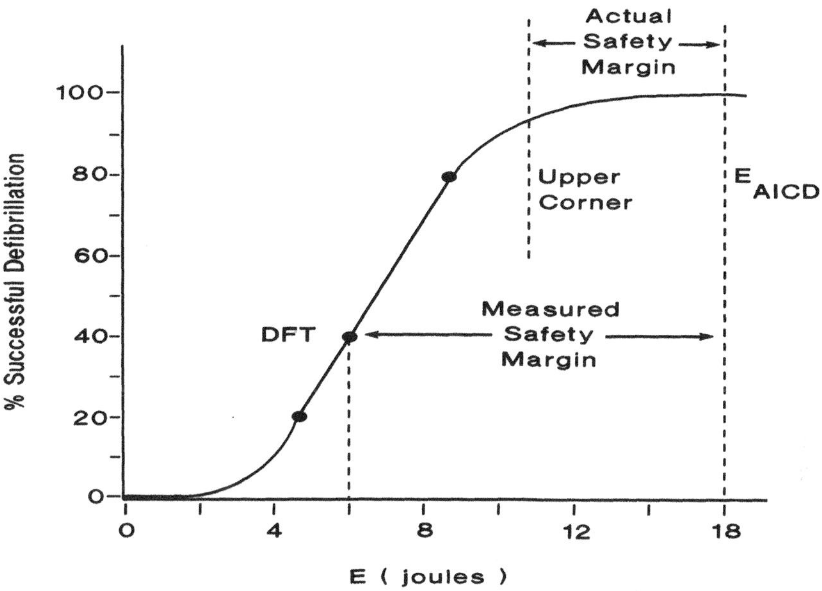

Fig. 1. Percent probability for successful defibrillation vs shock energy. The actual safety margin for the AICD system is the difference in energy between the output of the device and the upper corner of the defibrillation success curve (approximately E_{95}, the energy with 95% defibrillation success). The measured safety margin (DFT$-E_{AICD}$) can often be larger than the actual safety margin due to variability in the location of the DFT along the defibrillation curve

until conversion is obtained. With this protocol, the DFT is defined as the minimum energy producing defibrillation success.

If the DFT always identified the upper corner of the defibrillation success curve, the difference in energy between the AICD output and the DFT would equal the patient's safety margin. However, due to the probabilistic nature of defibrillation, the DFT can be located anywhere along the sloping portion of the curve [1]. This can cause problems with the safety margin assessment.

Numerical Modeling of DFT Protocol. To determine the variability of repeated DFT measurements, we performed numerical DFT simulations similar to that used by Schuder and McDaniel [1, 2]. The hypothetical defibrillation success curve, based on experimental data, is given in Fig. 1 ($E_{20} = 4.8$ J, $E_{40} = 6$ J, $E_{80} = 8.5$ J). The DFT protocol in our simulation began at 18 J with decreasing energy steps of 2 J until a defibrillation attempt failed. The success or failure of each trial was determined

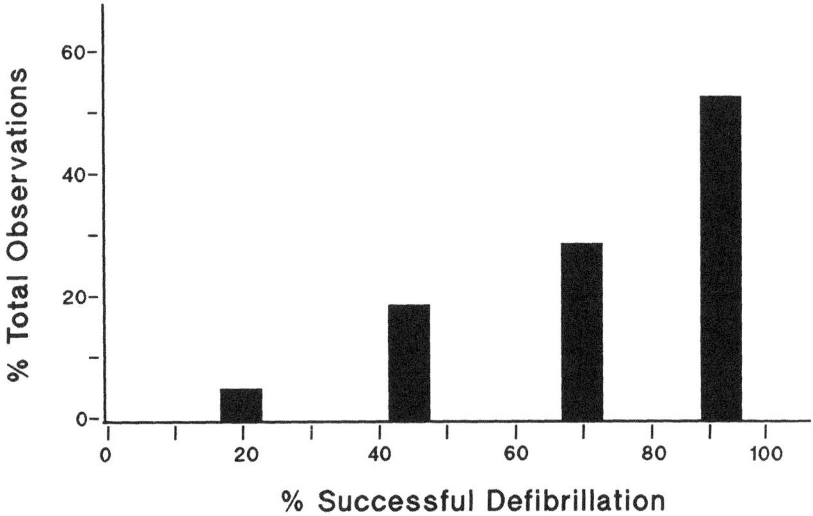

Fig. 2. Distribution of DFTs along the sloping portion of the defibrillation curve (from 0% to 100% probability of successful defibrillation) for 50 numerical simulations of the decreasing-step DFT protocol. The defibrillation curve used in the simulation is shown in Fig. 1. The starting energy for the DFT protocol was 18 J and the step size was 2 J

by the generation of a random number between 0 and 100. Defibrillation was considered to be terminated successfully if the random number was less than or equal to the curve's percent probability for successful defibrillation (% SDF) at the shock energy being tested.

The mean DFT energy after 50 repeated DFT protocols was 10.8 ± 2.2 J (SD). On the average, the DFTs were positioned approximately one-quarter of the way down the defibrillation success curve: the mean % SDF for all 50 DFTs was 75.2% ± 21.6%, with success values ranging from 20% to 98%. The distribution of DFTs along the sloping portion of the curve was skewed to higher energy (Fig. 2). Half of the DFTs were located high, at 80% success and above. However, there was an equal probability that DFTs were located low on the curve, at 70% and below. Most of these lower DFTs lay between 40% and 70% on the curve, with 22% being below 60% SDF and only 4% below 40% SDF. Thus, the DFT protocol yielded only a gross estimate of the curve location. Repeated DFT measures could vary by as much as 40% above or below the expected DFT energy, based on variation due to probability alone.

Experimental DFT Protocols. The estimate of the DFT variability from our simulation is similar to that seen *in vivo* [3–5]. Although the defibrillation energies varied between animals, the range of DFT positions along the sloping part of the defibrillation success curve was similar to our modeling results (canine mean % SDF for the DFTs = 71% ± 27%, range 10% – 100%) [3]. Due to this variability, one can use the DFT to identify the energy range of the sloping part of the curve for a particular lead system, but not to locate particular points on the curve.

Safety Margin Overestimation. The variability of the DFT can cause problems in measuring a patient's safety margin. If the DFT is located low on the defibrillation curve, the measured safety margin ($E_{AICD} - DFT$) will be larger than the actual margin of safety for the device ($E_{AICD} - E_{95}$) (Fig. 1). Thus, one could be fooled into thinking that the buffer of safety is larger than it really is.

Our numerical and experimental models suggest that for a defibrillation protocol with decreasing steps, the probable location of the DFT is approximately one-quarter down the success curve (mean $DFT_{decreasing\ steps} = E_{75}$), with DFTs distributed between 40% and 100% SDF. Thus, the maximum error in overestimating the margin of safety would be approximately 50% of the defibrillation curve width ($E_{95} - E_5$). From canine studies, the partial width of this curve between E_{80} and E_{20} was 48% ± 9% of the DFT energy [5]. This is comparable to the measurements of curve width from a compilation of our canine defibrillation studies (partial width: $E_{80} - E_{20} = 0.48 \times E_{50}$; full width: $E_{95} - E_5 = 1.1 \times E_{50}$). With the caveat that human and dog defibrillation curve widths may differ, one can infer from our numbers that the overestimate of the safety margin could be as large as half the curve width, or $0.5 \times E_{50}$. As a worse case, if a 10 J DFT were at E_{50}, the actual safety margin would be 5 J less than the margin measured from the DFT. With a 25 J AICD output, the measured safety margin would be 15 J and the actual safety margin 10 J. For a 20 J DFT, however, the possible overestimation of the safety margin may be as large as 10 J. If the device output were 30 J in this case, no margin of safety would exist. The AICD energy would be located at the top of the defibrillation success curve, with no room for movement of the curve to higher energies.

These estimates of safety margin errors are consistent with clinical work on prediction of defibrillation success using single DFT measurements [6]. Test shocks had to be elevated more than twice the DFT to assure 100% defibrillation success in all patients (factor tested = 2.6). The defibrillation protocol in this study involved increasing steps until conversion success was obtained. This DFT method tends to place the

DFTs further down on the sloping portion of the success curve than the decreasing step protocol (mean $DFT_{increasing\ steps}$ near E_{30}), with DFTs distributed between 0% and 60% SDF [1]. The error in overestimating the safety margin with an increasing-step DFT could be as large as the full width of the defibrillation curve, $1.1 \times E_{50}$ or $1.4 \times E_{20}$. With the low position of their DFTs (approximately E_{20}), one would expect test shock energies to be at least 2.4×DFT before 100% defibrillation success is obtained for all patients: 100% success energy = DFT+curve width = DFT+1.4 DFT = 2.4 DFT. This agrees directly with their results. While the authors have used the term "safety margin" in referring to this extra energy needed for 100% success, they are only referring to the energy needed to reach the top of the success curve. A device safety margin or buffer should be measured from this 100% success energy to the output of the AICD device.

DFT+Testing. For high thresholds (≥20 J), the variability of the DFT placement along the curve could have a significant impact on device safety margin. However, this could also be true if the AICD energy is aggressively programmed lower near the DFT, such that the safety margin is small. In both cases, uncertainty over the DFT position could lead to an error in the safety margin and an inflated sense of security. If the DFT is located near the upper corner, the estimate of safety will be accurate, but if the DFT is located further down, which is also possible, safety is overestimated.

Lang et al. have proposed an augmented DFT+protocol to help clarify the safety margin in these uncertain situations [3]. They recommend doing one or possibly two additional defibrillation trials at the DFT energy. If the extra test is successful (DFT+), there is greater chance that the safety margin is accurate. If the extra test fails (DFT−), it suggests that the DFT is on the sloping portion of the curve. If one encounters a DFT−, one should revise the lead system if the DFT is high, or increase the AICD output energy to obtain an adequate safety margin.

Clinical practice to this date has sought to obtain a safety margin of 10 J for an AICD implant. If the difference between the DFT and the programmable AICD output is greater than 10 J, possible errors in the safety margin will not be a major issue. In this case, the DFT alone is adequate for clinical assessment of the patient. The extrashock protocols only need to be invoked when the measured safety margin is less than or equal to the minimum accepted value. While it is unknown at this time, it is possible that minimum safety margins may be smaller than 10 J for low-energy AICD systems.

Alternative Safety Margin Protocols. Defibrillation testing with the DFT or DFT+protocols not only permits the selection of an adequate safety margin, but leads to a minimum safe setting for the shock energy. Safety margins could also be assessed with an efficacy protocol which tests defibrillation success at a certain energy one or two times (1 S and 2 S protocols). Success with these single-energy protocols will have varying degrees of accuracy in assessing whether the safety margin tested ($E_{AICD} - E_{test}$) is adequate. They do not locate the defibrillation curve, but only establish an upper boundary. More information about the curve location is needed to select the lowest AICD output with an adequate safety margin, taking full advantage of the programmable shock energies. In addition, more specific information on DFTs is helpful in the clinical management of the patient, e.g., in the reassessment of defibrillation requirements after drug modifications, disease progression, or device replacement.

These single-energy protocols have limited accuracy in evaluating safety margins, since they are subject to the same safety margin overestimation errors encountered with the DFT. The energy tested for a 1 S protocol could lie anywhere above 5% – 10% SDF on the defibrillation success curve. Since the position is not known, one must take the worst case and assume that the 1 S energy lies at the bottom of the curve. Because of this, the safety margin with the 1 S protocol must be increased to include the full width of the defibrillation success curve plus the minimum safety buffer between the upper corner and the AICD output, similar to case of the increasing-step DFT protocol. In humans, the upper corner of the defibrillation curve is more than twice the energies located low on the curve (assume a factor of 2.4 from above) [6]. Adding the 10 J safety margin to this would result in a 1 S safety margin that is twice or more than the margin for standard decreasing-step DFT protocols. For example, a single conversion success at 10 J can be used to justify the use of a 34 J AICD output: the upper corner for a 1 S shock at 10 J could be as high as 24 J [6], and adding a 10 J margin to this yields a minimum device output of 34 J. The measured safety margin required for the 1 S protocol at this 10 J test level is 24 J. The 1 S protocol cannot be used to test energies higher than 10 J, since its poor accuracy could result in large overestimates of the patient's safety margin.

The restriction of large measured safety margins can be relaxed slightly with the 2 S protocol. If one obtained 2 successful conversions, the test energy could lie along the upper two-thirds of the defibrillation success curve, between 30% and 100% SDF. This protocol is more precise than the 1 S, so the safety margin will be slightly smaller. The maximum error in overestimating the safety margin for the 2 S protocol is two-thirds the curve width, or $0.7 \times E_{50}$. For a 2 S result at 10 J, the AICD output could be set to 27 J or above [(1.7 × 10 J) + 10 J]. The minimum 2 S safety margin at this test energy would be 17 J.

Greater precision can be obtained with the 3 S protocol. Its distribution along the defibrillation success curve is similar to the decreasing-step DFT protocol. Thus, errors in overestimating the safety margin are comparable, $0.5 \times E_{50}$. For both tests, a DFT or 3 S at 10 J could be used to program the device to energies 25 J or greater. These protocols require a 15 J measured safety margin for the device. Further improvements in testing are obtained with the DFT+ protocol mentioned above. A DFT+ at 10 J would permit AICD programming to 20 J or more, corresponding to a safety margin of 10 J. Among these various protocols, those involving more detailed testing and greater number of defibrillation episodes will permit the use of smaller safety margins. These more involved protocols have the precision to allow greater latitude in programming the AICD defibrillation energies.

The continued efficacy of AICD therapy depends on proper defibrillation testing. The prime goal of this process is to verify that there is an adequate safety margin for the AICD system under test. Safety margins serve as an energy buffer between the defibrillation threshold (DFT) and the output of the device. Setting the AICD to the DFT energy for the purpose of defibrillation is not appropriate, since only a small shift in the defibrillation curve to higher energies could prevent the device from converting the patient on the first shock. An adequate safety margin (10 J) between the DFT and device output should be selected to provide a safety buffer in case defibrillation requirements are elevated (due to prolonged fibrillation [for the second or later rescue shocks], disease progression, changes in drug regimen, etc.). When the safety margin is large, a DFT protocol is adequate for proper assessment of patient safety and defibrillation requirements. If safety margins are near 10 J with high DFTs or with aggressive AICD programming to low energies, the variability of the DFT may result in overestimating the safety margin. Additional testing at the DFT energy (DFT+) will help clarify whether the measured safety margin is an accurate reflection of the actual margin. If this testing indicates that overestimation errors will compromise the safety margin (DFT−), then the lead system should be revised or the AICD energy programmed less aggressively. Testing protocols involving a limited number of test shocks at one energy (1 S or 2 S) necessitate larger safety margins due to their low precision.

References

1. McDaniel WC, Schuder JC (1987) The cardiac ventricular defibrillation threshold-inherent limitations in its application and interpretation. Med Instrum 21:170–176

2. Schuder JC, McDaniel WC (1985) Defibrillation threshold – normal distribution initial shock. Proceedings of the 38th Annual Conference on Engineering in Medicine and Biology 27:316
3. Lang DJ, Cato EL, Echt DS (1989) Protocol for evaluation of internal defibrillation safety margins. J Am Coll Cardiol 13(2):111A
4. Rattes MF, Jones DL, Sharma AD, Klein GJ (1987) Defibrillation threshold: a simple and quantitative estimate of the ability to defibrillate. PACE 10:70–77
5. Davy JM, Fain ES, Dorian P, Winkle RA (1987) The relationship between successful defibrillation and delivered energy in open-chest dogs: reappraisal of the "defibrillation threshold" concept. Am Heart J 113:77–84
6. Jones DL, Klein GJ, Guiraudon Gerard M, Sharma AD, Yee R, Kallok MJ (1988) Prediction of defibrillation success from a single defibrillation threshold measurement with sequential pulses and two current pathways in humans. Circulation 78:1144–1149

PART VI

Living with the Implantable Defibrillator

Management and Follow-up of the Implantable Defibrillator Patient

S. Nisam, R. N. Fogoros

Introduction

A great deal has been written, both in this book and elsewhere, about the patient indications, results, surgical aspects, and technical developments related to automatic implantable cardioverter defibrillator (AICD) therapy. But now that this modality has been extended to several hundred implanting centers around the world, the obligation for assuring proper post-implant management and follow-up to the many thousands of implantees has become a major and growing problem.

For most of the first decade following Mirowski and co-workers' initial implant in 1980 [1], follow-up was simplified by the fact that nearly all implantees had AICD devices from one manufacturer (CPI, St. Paul, MN, USA) [2, 3]. The rapid proliferation of the therapy has naturally been accompanied with the introduction of several manufacturers' pulse generators, leads, programmers, and equipment for system telemetry/analysis, making the problem of patient follow-up far more complex. The geographic mobility of the typical 55- to 60-year-old implantee, versus the need to follow him or her closely and the growing sophistication of the equipment all add still further dimensions to this challenge. In this chapter, we offer a brief overview of the issues and considerations involved in the management and follow-up of the patient with the AICD.

General Considerations: Requirements of the Typical AICD Patient

It is important to emphasize that there is considerable difference between patient follow-up in a "Pacemaker Clinic" and the follow-up procedures and care required for most AICD patients. The most important difference, of course, emanates from the *gravity* of the tachyarrhythmia for which the latter patients are being treated. In general, the AICD patient has highly deteriorated ventricular function, with a left ventricular ejection fraction between 20% – 40% for the great majority. Not surprisingly, many such patients are receiving vasodilators and diuretics for their heart failure. Management of ischemia as a ventricular tachycardia/ventriculator fibrillation (VT/VF) "trigger" is a concern for the roughly 75% of AICD recipients who have advanced coronary artery disease [3, 4]. Beyond these clinical considerations, there is frequently need for psychologic support for the implantable defibrillator patient [5, 6]. They are acutely aware of the lethal nature of their arrhythmias, many of them having actually been resuscitated *in extremis.* Thus, apart from technological aspects, the very nature of the arrhythmias being treated dictate a special approach in following these patients.

The Early Post-implant Period

In the first hours and days post implant, these patients are often prone to *transient* arrhythmias, which require special attention: atrial fibrillation/flutter, non-sustained VT, and sustained ventricular tachyarrhythmias. During this critical phase, appropriate programming of the AICD device will generally prevent its discharging into supraventricular and/or nonsustained arrhythmias, while we attempt to stabilize them.

There are a number of important pre-discharge instruction we must give our patients. They need to check the site of wound healing and inform us immediately in case of signs of infection. In their home and work environment, they need to avoid excessive, sudden upper abdominal exertion or pressure. Driving is a difficult issue, depending on the patient's hemodynamic tolerance of his arrhythmia(s), but also on his state or country laws. The patient's need for psychological support may be provided by staff clinical psychologists as well as patient support groups, which many implanting centers have set up [7]. We warn our patients to avoid strong magnetic fields, and to leave an area if they hear beeping sounds coming from the device. Patients should advise airport security of their implanted AICD device: ideally, the security guards should check without using their magnet-containing metal detectors wands, or at least limit to a few seconds the applications of these wands over the patient. Testing by nuclear magnetic resonance is absolutely contraindicated. Treatment with diathermy or electrocautery may permanently damage an *active* AICD, so should only be carried out after consultation with the implanting physician. The dentist should also be aware when he has a patient with an AICD. What the patient should do when he receives a shock and what he and his family should do in emergencies is covered later in this chapter. The patient manuals available from the manufacturers provide further details on such questions.

In one such manual [8], many of the points above are summarized in the post-implant instructions to the patient. The patient is instructed to call his or her doctor as follows.

Remember to call your doctor if:

- You receive an AICD shock at home or when you are not in the hospital.
- The area around your pulse generator becomes sore to the touch or has a bruise that will not go away.
- Any of your incisions from surgery become reddened, swollen, and/or begin to drain fluid.
- You have a fever that will not go away after a few days.
- At any time you have signs of your abnormal heart rhythm.
- You plan to take a trip or move to another place.
- Your hear beeping tones coming from the pulse generator in your abdomen.
- You have questions concerning your AICD or heart rhythm medications.
- You notice anything unusual or unexpected, especially things for which your doctor has told you to watch.
- You need to have any surgery during which equipment to be used may affect your device.

The first 8 weeks or so following the AICD patient's discharge from the hospital are often key to assuring satisfactory long-term results. Proper wound healing is a particular concern due, firstly, to the sheer volume of the hardware implanted and, secondly, because infection is potentially catastrophic, usually requiring repeat surgery for removal of the total system [9]. It is also in this early period that the incidence of shocks delivered to the patient is the highest [10, 11]. Receiving shocks from the AICD device is of no major concern *per se*, since that was why this form of therapy was prescribed, but it does require rapid evaluation (see "Evaluation of Shocks").

Routine Follow-up

Routine periodic follow-up visits are essential to the management of patients with implantable defibrillators. The purpose of such visits should be not only to ensure the optimal function of the AICD itself, but also to monitor and assess the patient's underlying cardiac disease, the frequency of recurrent arrhythmias, and the patient's physical and psychological functional status.

The steps to follow in carrying out these routine follow-ups are outlined in the following:

1. Evaluate general medical condition. Review all of the following:
   - Status of ischemic heart disease
   - Dyspnea
   - Exercise tolerance, functional and work status
   - Current drug therapy
   - Symptoms of recurrent arrhythmias
   - Frequency of shocks
2. Interrogate AICD
   - Shock counters
   - Charge time
   - Evaluate battery life
   - Reform capacitors
   - Lead impedance
3. Make decisions regarding change in therapy
   - Does AICD need to be reprogrammed or replaced?
   - Do medical conditions need to be reassessed?
   - Does antiarrhythmic therapy need to be changed?
   - Does patient require formal psychiatric/emotional support?
4. Final interrogation of AICD to assure device is active and programmed to appropriate parameters.

As many of the procedures in the above list are self-explanatory, we will only elaborate on elements of points 2 and 3, which are fairly unique to AICD therapy. The *shock counters* provide information not only on the absolute number of shocks, but also on their chronology, energy levels, and result. For example (see Fig. 1 A), for a patient with a relatively stable VT and whose AICD has been programmed to an initial low energy shock, in this case 5 joules, we can determine how many such episodes occurred since the preceding follow-up visit, how many of them successfully converted the VT, and how often additional, higher energy (30 joules) was needed. The actuarial incidence of shocks and whether they occurred alone or in clusters has also proven to help in determining their "appropriateness" [10]. A second example (see Fig. 1 B) shows the information available from the print-out of another device.

Charge time for AICDs indicates both the state of the battery and of the capacitors which enable the device to charge up to approximately 750 volts in a matter of seconds. Thus, verifying this parameter provides information on the relative *battery life* and, just as importantly, on the ability of those heavy-duty capacitors to charge up when needed. The *reform capacitors* procedure is related to the same requirement and

```
A
********************************
PATIENT
PHYSICIAN
DATE
********************************
        VENTAK P
       MODEL 1600
    PULSE GENERATOR
 PRESENT PARAMETERS
********************************
MODE          ACTIVE
RATE          155 BPM
PDF           ON
DELAY
  1ST         2.5 SEC
  2-5         2.5 SEC
SHOCK ENERGY
  1ST         5  JOULES
  2ND         30 JOULES
  3-5         30 JOULES
********************************
CHARGE TIME
              6.1 SEC
LEAD IMPEDANCE
              50 OHMS
PG BATTERY STATUS
   EVALUATE ERI
  CAPACITOR FORM
       SEC
COUNT
1ST SHOCK          10
2-5 SHOCK           3
TOTAL PATIENT      13
TEST SHOCKS         9
********************************
      NOTES
```

```
B
GUARDIAN 4202
  SN 0000000 / ON
DEFIBRILLATOR
  ON
DATE LAST PROG'D
  MAY 25, 1989
PATIENT SHOCK
  COUNT=1
TOTAL SHOCK
  COUNT=7
DEFIB ACTIVATION
  COUNT=6
PACER CELL TEST
  IMP<5 kohms
LEAD IMPEDANCE
  = 510 ohms
TACHY DETECTION
  ON
TACHY DETECT INT
  352 ms (170 BPM)
INITIAL ENERGY
  30J (650V, 12ms)
MAX NO. SHOCKS
  IN A SERIES 7
MIN SHOCK DELAY
  5 s
SENSITIVITY
  1.0 mV
STANDBY RATE
  50 PPM
REFRAC PERIOD
  250 ms
HYSTERESIS
  0 ms (50 BPM)
PULSE WIDTH
  0.50 ms
PULSE AMP
  5.0 V
```

Fig. 1A,B. AICD pulse generator data print-out. **A** CPI Ventak P Model 1600. **B** Telectronics Guardian Model 4202

reflects the fact that these components, when not "exercised", tend to lose their physical configuration, and therewith the ability to fully charge up.

Analysis of this information generally permits us to decide whether the device needs to be *reprogrammed*, and/or the patients *antiarrhythmic therapy* altered, etc. For instance, evidence of artrial fibrillation and associated shocks might lead us to give the patient beta-blockers, retest him in the electrophysiologic laboratory, and possibly program down the AICD's cut-off rate.

Evaluation of Shocks

Patients are instructed to contact their implanting cardiologist to report all shocks. For the first few such shocks, we always insist on seeing the patient in order to carry out a thorough evaluation. Thereafter, in many patients we verify, over the telephone, the circumstances and don't require their coming in until their next scheduled follow-up. The exception is when a patient has received a "barrage" of shocks and/or shows signs of worsening heart failure or other clinical problems. The most important questions we must try to answer are:

- Were the shocks appropriate?
- What symptoms, if any, did the patient experience prior and during the shocks?
- How was the patient's post shock recovery?
- Were there factors (e.g. drug compliance, electrolyte disturbances) which might explain the onset of the patient's arrhythmia?

Evaluation of shocks is unquestionably the most difficult aspect of AICD patient follow-up. Several newer devices currently undergoing clinical evaluation will have some kind of a built-in Holter monitoring function or retrievable electrogram storage, or both [12]. These enhancements will significantly facilitate the determination of whether shocks were delivered for ventricular tachyarrhythmias, for supraventricular arrhythmias rapidly conducted to the ventricles, or were precipitated by some type of lead fracture or connection problem, etc. But even these sophisticated advances will not always clarify the situation, since they will only be monitoring *ventricular* signals. For that reason, as well as the simple fact that, for several years to come, there will be many thousands of patients without these telemetry enhancements, we have summarized the following series of suggestions to help evaluate shocks for this great majority of presently implanted patients.

1. "Interrogate" the device to ascertain if shocks were delivered; for most currently available devices, additional information is provided on the number of shocks (since the last follow-up) and the detected ventricular rate triggering device discharges. Fig. 1 provides examples of such interrogations.
2. Determine the circumstances and symptoms surrounding the AICD discharges. Did the patient (or witness) note dizziness, syncope or pre-syncope, palpitations during or just preceding the shock(s)?
3. Evaluate the patient for sources of arrhythmia provocation: ischemia, exacerbated heart failure, electrolyte imbalance.
4. Perform 24-h Holter monitoring, including during exercise stress testing, and look for signs indicative of arrhythmia initiation [13]; if unrevealing, utilize one of the commercially available "event recorders" with a memory loop in an attempt to obtain electrocardiogram (ECG) tracings during shock(s) [14].

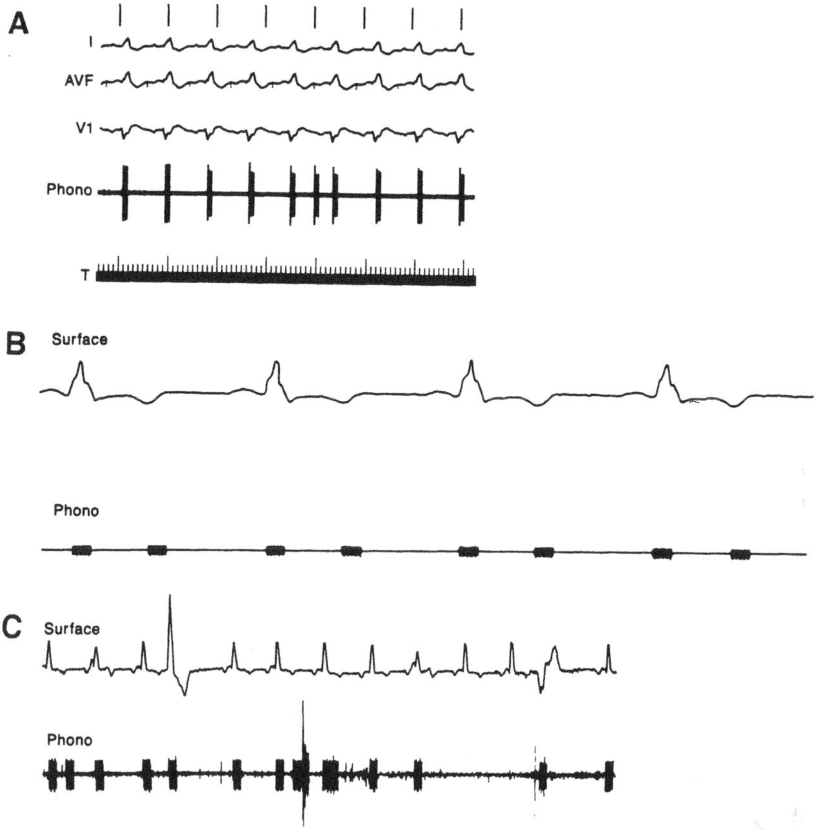

Fig. 2A–C. Examples of use of phonocardiogram to help in evaluating shocks (for CPI devices). **A** Intermittent sensing of atrial pacing spikes (Courtesy of Peter D. Chapman, MD). **B** T-wave sensing: beeping tone evaluation reveals T-wave sensing. Post-stellate block QT, 342 ms (Courtesy of Robert G. Hauser, MD). **C** Abnormal beeping tones during upper extremity exercise. Normal beeping tones are obtained while patient is at rest. Note AICD under- and over-sensing during upper extremity exercise (Courtesy of Jay W. Mason, MD)

5. Use the 'beep-o-gram' technique [15] to check on sources such as double-counting of P-waves or T-waves (see Fig. 2A, B) or artifacts arising from lead discontinuities (see Fig. 2C) [16].
6. Use chest X-rays to check for lead fracture or migration and to verify whether the lead is firmly within the pulse generator connector block.

Twenty-four-hour Holter monitoring [13], "event recorders" [14], and the use of a phonocardiogram probe to record "beeps" from the AICD [15, 16] are commonly used methods to determine the nature and appropriateness of shocks. Figure 2 illustrates several examples of how the "beep-o-gram" techniques helps in diagnosing the source of problematic shocks.

Generally, this evaluation simply reinforces the fact that the anticipated tachyarrhythmia did occur, the system detected it appropriately, and the programmed therapy was delivered to terminate the episode. On some occasions, the assessment points to the need for reprogramming the device's detection algorithm and/or output, or to modifying the patient's drug regimen.

Timing and Frequency of Patient Follow-up

The scheduling of procedures described heretofore depends both on the patient and or AICD device technology. Most implant centers carry out pre-discharge tests, typically 1 week post-implant, to verify that the system is operating correctly. Also at this occasion, the programmable parameters are finalized. In many centers, but not all, a pre-discharge electrophysiologic test, including repeat DFT testing, is performed during this pre-discharge test. Thereafter, patients are called in for follow-up every 2–3 months. As we indicated earlier, the generally serious nature of these patients' underlying disease requires us to see them on a fairly frequent basis. Furthermore, the current devices need to have their capacitors reformed approximately quarterly. As these devices approach their end-of-battery life, the interval between battery checks must be shortened to approximately monthly.

AICD Emergency Care Procedures

The handling of AICD implantees under emergency conditions warrants special mention, particularly since there is a higher than normal probability that such patients might need emergency care. Whether such a crisis is of cardiac or other origin, there are several guide-lines to follow in managing such situations.

Probably, most importantly, the procedures appropriate for the given emergency should be carried out as though the patient had no implanted device. Cardiopulmonary resuscitation (CPR), if needed, should begin immediately, without concerns about activating or deactivating the device or waiting for it to discharge. Most centers teach the patients and family in cough CPR, in case of light-headedness or palpitations. External defibrillation has been carried out in many AICD patients [17], e.g. in the early postoperative period when some institutions prefer to deactivate the device. Occasionally, it may be necessary to modify the position of the external paddles, e.g., anterior-lateral to anterior-posterior.

The use of the special AICD magnet provided by the manufacturer varies slightly for the various devices. It is important to be familiar with their use. For CPI devices, *activation* of an inactive pulse generator is achieved by placing the magnet over the upper-right corner of the device. Initially, and for 30 s, it will emit a continuous tone, thereafter followed by R-wave synchronous "beeps". The device is now in its active mode and the magnet may be removed. There are also situations requiring deactivation of the device (series of inappropriate shocks, series of true recurrences of VT which might be better treated with external cardioversion until the patient stabilizes, use of equipment which generates electrical interference (electrocautery). To *deactivate*, the magnet is positioned as above. The R-wave synchronous tones will be heard for 30 s, after which the device becomes inactive as indicated by a continuous tone, and the magnet can be removed.

With the arrival of newer devices, from multiple manufacturers, activation/deactivation can also be achieved via the respective programmers. Nevertheless, the magnets will continue to be available, as before, and to cover the very real possibility that the patient or attending physician may not be in the vicinity of the programmer.

Summary

Management of patients with the Automatic Implantable Cardioverter Defibrillator (AICD) has continued to expand rapidly, reaching tens of thousands of patients implanted in several hundred centers all over the globe. Consequently, the responsibility for following these patients now extends well beyond the staff at the implanting centers. It is precisely for physicians susceptible to come across such patients, in routine as well as in emergency situations, that we have outlined the major guide-lines for appropriate management and follow-up. In the early period up to and following the AICD implantee's discharge from the hospital, great care must be taken to assure the patient's physical and social rehabilitation. He, his family, and his primary physician must be made aware of what the patient can and cannot do. For instance, avoiding strong magnetic fields (which could turn the AICD off) is one of the most important "dont's". The routine follow-up of these patients must address not only the proper functioning of the AICD system, but also the patients' underlying malady. The shocks received by the patient from his AICD need thorough evaluation, to determine their origin and their significance. At such evaluations or following routine follow-up, decisions are taken concerning reprogramming the device (or exchanging it) and/or changing the patient's medications. The final section provides recommendations for handling emergencies, the most important of which is to react as though the patient had no AICD. Awareness of the few, substantial guide-lines in this chapter should facilitate the management and follow-up of the ever-growing number of AICD patients.

References

1. Mirowski M, Reid P, Mower M et al (1980) Termination of malignant ventricular arrhythmias with an implanted automatic defibrillator in human beings. N Engl J Med 303:322–324
2. Troup P (1989) Implantable cardioverters and defibrillators. Curr Prob Cardiol 14:675–843
3. Nisam S, Mower M, Moser S (1991) ICD clinical update: first decade, initial 10000 patients. PACE 14:255–262
4. Tchou P, Kadri N, Akhtar M et al (1988) Automatic implantable cardioverter defibrillators and survival of patients with left ventricular dysfunction and malignant ventricular arrhythmias. Ann Intern Med 109:529–534
5. Vlay S, Olson L, Fricchione G, Friedman R (1989) Anxiety and anger with ventricular tachyarrhythmias. Responses after automatic internal defibrillator implantation. PACE 12:366–373
6. Badger J, Morris P (1989) Observations of a support group for automatic implantable cardioverter defibrillator recipients and their spouses. Heart Lung 18:238–243
7. Winkle R, Stinson E, Echt D et al (1984) Practical aspects of automatic cardioverter defibrillator implantation. Am Heart J 108:1335–1346
8. CPI (1987) Patient manual for the automatic implantable cardioverter defibrillator system. Available from CPI, Saint Paul, MN, USA
9. Troup P, Chapman P, Wetherbee J et al (1988) Clinical features of AICD system infections. Circulation 78:155
10. Fogoros R, Elson J, Bonnet C (1989) Actuarial incidence and pattern of occurrence of shocks following implantation of the automatic implantable cardioverter defibrillator. PACE 12:1465–1473
11. Myerburg R, Luceri R, Thurer R et al (1989) Time to first shock and clinical outcome in patients receiving an automatic implantable defibrillator. J Am Coll Cardiol 14:508–514
12. Hook B, Marchlinski F (1991) Value of ventricular electrogram recordings in the diagnosis of arrhythmias precipitating electrical device shock therapy. J Am Coll Cardiol 17:985–990
13. Veltri E, Mower M, Mirowsky M (1988) Ambulatory monitoring of the automatic implantable cardioverter defibrillator: a practical guide. PACE 11:315–325
14. Luceri R, Habal S, Castellanos A et al (1988) Mechanism of death in patients with the AICD. PACE 11:2014–2022
15. Chapman T, Troup P (1986) The automatic implantable cardioverter defibrillator: evaluating suspected inappropriate shocks. J Am Coll Cardiol 7:1075–1078
16. CPI (1990) AICD system evaluation guide. Section 5:5–7. Available from CPI, Saint Paul, MN, USA
17. Pinski S, Arnold A, Maloney J et al (1991) Safety of external cardioversion/defibrillation in patients with internal defibrillation patches and no device. PACE 14:7–12

The Social and Economic Impact of the New Implantable Cardioverter Defibrillator Technology

S. Saksena

Rapid technologic advances are accelerating the widespread implementation of implantable cardioverter defibrillator (ICD) therapy for patients with life-threatening ventricular tachycardia or ventricular fibrillation. Multiprogrammable ICD pulse generator and nonthoracotomy lead systems can drive the process of catapulting this therapeutic modality from a last resort investigative option to a first-line choice option [1–3]. Clinical evidence continues to mount in favor of the superior therapeutic efficacy of ICD devices in prevention of sudden arrhythmic death as compared to empiric or directed antiarrhythmic drug therapy [4–6]. Controversy, however, exists on the overall impact of such therapy on total cardiac mortality in such patients.

Physician and patient acceptance of such therapy is expected to increase, however, at an exponential rate. This can be ascribed in part to the clinical efficacy and safety of ICD therapy but also in part to the perceived lack of a widely applicable competitive therapeutic alternative. Antiarrhythmic drugs, usually considered in the latter class, have been shown to have efficacy, albeit somewhat inferior, only in selected patients using provocative invasive electrophysiologic stimulation. Empiric therapy with several type I antiarrhythmic drugs has failed to show benefit in several patient populations identified to be at increased risk of sudden arrhythmic death [4, 5]. The overall social impact of such technology can be expected to be influenced by clinical issues, demographics, economics, psychologic factors, perception and philosophy. However, an overiding momentum may develop with respect to the use of ICD technology based upon the technical ease of its implementation widespread applicability in many patient populations and clinical acceptance of new technology. The long-term clinical efficacy and safety of new technology in this area remains under active evaluation. If current expectations with respect to its efficacy are met, the economic impact of widespread clinical application needs to be carefully considered.

Assessment of economic issues surrounding development of ICD therapy will have serious social and health care policy importance.

Table 1. Economic issues for ICDs

System cost	
Implant hospitalization	
	Duration
	Implant procedure
	Resources
	Total cost
Follow-up hospitalizations	
	Troubleshooting
	Pulse generator or lead system replacement

A variety of economic issues have been identified for ICDs. Concern regarding the overall economic impact of this new high-technology therapy has been expressed [7, 8]. Cost effectiveness is an important factor in the widespread adoption of any form of modern medical therapy. Analysis of the economic impact of ICD therapy is currently limited by the absence of a firm data base and the fluid nature of an evolving technology which has been continuously in various degrees of clinical investigation since its inception. Rapid transition from a nonprogrammable ICD with an epicardial lead system to a fully programmable hybrid ICD device with bradycardia and antitachycardia pacing, cardioversion and defibrillation capability with endocardial lead systems suitable for nonthoracotomy implant is now in progress. Nevertheless, Table 1 identifies three primary factors accounting for consumption of health care resources in this therapy:

(a) the ICD system,
(b) the implant hospitalization preceding and following device implant, and
(c) follow-up hospitalization related to the system's function.

System cost includes the ICD pulse generator and lead system. In 1990, cost estimates for a hybrid multiprogrammable ICD pulse generator range from $ 14500 to $ 17500 (manufacturer's quotations). Epicardial lead systems range from $ 2790 to $ 4350 and endocardial leads cost approximately $ 3600. This has led to total ICD system costs ranging from $ 16290 to $ 21850 (manufacturer's quotations).

Assessment of health care resources directly consumed by ICD implant hospitalization costs has been confounded by the current clinical practice of undertaking ICD implants at the tail end of a preexisting hospitalization. The hospitalization is usually prompted by a sudden arrhythmic event and subsequent noninvasive and/or invasive electrophysi-

Table 2. Implant hospitalization (1990 US $)

Duration
Hybrid programmable ICD with epicardial leads[a]; primary implant 26 ± 12 days; preoperative stay 11 ± 10 days
Nonprogrammable ICD: replacement 6 ± 2 days; endocardial leads[a] 16 ± 13 days
Implant hospitalization cost: $ 58400[b] – $ 53310[c]

[a] EHI-NBIMC data, Passaic and Newark NJ, 1988 – 1990.
[b] Krucoff et al. [7]
[c] Kuppermann et al. [13]

ologic evaluation of ventricular tachycardia or ventricular fibrillation [7, 9 – 11]. A previous NASPE position paper identified this issue and noted that actual hospital charges clearly exceed those related to device implant [7, 12]. The actual costs related to device implant are often not clearly identifiable. Health care charges in the index hospitalization are determined by the duration of this hospitalization, implant procedure costs, and resources related to needed support facilities, personnel and indirect costs. Current estimates at selected centers suggest that most hospital stays for hybrid multiprogrammable ICDs with epicardial leads average 3 – 4 weeks, with preoperative evaluation and electrophysiologic testing accounting for as much as one-half to two-thirds of this period (Table 2). Since current clinical practice is likely to maintain the need for such merged hospitalizations, reported charges have ranged from $ 53000 to $ 58000 in 1990 estimates corrected for inflation [7, 13]. Endocardial lead systems averaged 2 weeks for similar implant hospitalizations [14].

Follow-up health care costs for ICDs are related to system replacement and/or troubleshooting. Hospital stays for pulse generator or lead system replacement typically average 3 – 6 days and charges for such hospitalization have been estimated to average $ 16600 in one report (1990 US dollars) for the life expectancy of an individual ICD system [13]. The latter in current systems averages 2 – 3 years, suggesting an estimated annual cost of $ 6000 – $ 9000 per year for each surviving patient to the health care system [13].

Prospective comparison of the economic impact of ICD therapy with other approaches to antiarrhythmic therapy is presently unavailable largely due to the absence of prospective clinical trials examining this issue. Retrospective, uncontrolled data are available for a limited analysis. An early report, now adjusted for current costs, suggests that the average hospital charges associated with empiric antiarrhythmic drug therapy over 1 year can exceed $ 35 000 per patient [9]. The same analysis suggested that guided antiarrhythmic therapy using noninvasive or invasive selection techniques in the same period would have reduced annual health care charges to the $ 20000 range in 1990 [9, 10, 15]. Nonpharmacologic approaches such as guided surgical ablation and catheter ablation have comparable charges to ICDs for the index hospitalization [1, 10]. Cost effectiveness analyses of ICD therapy are also presently limited by absence of firm estimates of impact of all antiarrhythmic therapies on total mortality in this population. In the absence of prospective controlled clinical trials, projected estimates of average survival of ICD patients based on expert opinion have been quite variable. Estimates of improvements in total outcome of ICD patients as compared to guided drug therapy in current literature exist but remain tenuous [13]. Assumption of 2 and 1 year improvements would suggest an additional approximate economic cost of $ 20000 and $ 40000, respectively, per life-year prolongation in 1990. This would place current ICD therapy at 30% and 60%, respectively, of current economic estimates of other high-technology life-saving therapy such as renal dialysis or neonatal intensive care, or preventive medical therapy such as drug therapy for mild hypertension [17].

The clinical and economic impact of imminent new technology in ICD therapy is considerable. Hybrid ICD devices and endocardial lead systems can be expected to greatly enhance acceptance of this therapy for a variety of clinical reasons. A reduction in follow-up hospitalizations can be expected related to inappropriate device therapy, particularly for unknown clinical events, drug-device interactions, and demand pacemaker therapy. Ambulatory follow-up device assessment and outpatient device reprogramming can be expected. Pulse generator longevity is projected to nearly double. These trends will improve the economic profile during device follow-up. Endocardial leads are expected to increase implant safety. Earlier implementation of ICD therapy in the index hospitalization can be expected. Concomitantly, costs of ICD therapy can be realistically expected to substantially decline at implant and during follow-up. Suggested reductions in costs have ranged from 50% to 70% [14]. Thus, a number of clinical strategies could further reduce health care costs associated with ICDs (Table 3). These include identification de novo of appropriate candidates for ICD therapy, preferably based on clinical cardiologic characteristics. Limiting serial drug testing in such patients, would reduce preoperative evaluation costs. Implementation of imminent new technology and reduction in ICD system cost is also essential to this effort. The use of ambulatory facilities for device follow-up and system component(s) replacement should be encouraged. Solicitation of prospective information on each of these issues will per-

Table 3. Future strategies to reduce ICD costs

- Identify de novo candidates
- Limit serial drug testing
- Implement new technology
- Reduce system costs
- Ambulatory facility for follow-up EPS or device and endocardial lead replacement

mit objective analyses of clinical and economic impact. It is in the clinical and manufacturing communities' interest that information on these issues, for example through mechanisms such as a controlled clinical trial and/or device registry, is undertaken to permit a rational diffusion of this potentially important new antiarrhythmic therapy.

Wide application of such therapy can be expected with imminent technologic advances. Table 4 identifies clinical scenarios which may be influenced by such technologic advances. Such projections suggest that a wider patient population may be identified, particularly with safer and simpler device implant techniques. Hitherto untreated patient populations known to be at high risk for sudden arrhythmic death, such as patients with congestive heart failure or nonsustained ventricular tachycardia in the presence of advanced left ventricular dysfunction, may be con-

Table 4. Economic impact of new ICD technology

Programmability/device memory
- Decreased hospitalizations for inappropriate therapy, unknown clinical events, or drug-device interactions

Hybrid devices
- Avoid implant of two devices (10% of current population)
- Reduce hospitalizations for pacemaker therapy

Endocardial leads
- Increase implant safety
- Reduce implant procedure costs
- Reduce implant hospitalization costs
- Reduce costs associated with lead malfunction and replacement
- Wider application of therapy: (a) poor candidates to receive alternative therapy or epicardial lead system; (b) identification of hitherto untreated population, in whom risk/benefit of therapy with epicardial implant does not justify use, e.g., individuals with CHF, nonsustained VT with severe heart disease, high risk post-myocardial infarction, and/or syncope

sidered at ICD implant prior to the index event. Estimates of potential patient populations have been highly variable but, nevertheless, impressive. In North America, 300000 sudden cardiac deaths occur. While a significant proportion of these patients could be potential device recipients, limitations in emergency rescue efforts preclude the vast majority from initial resuscitation. Up to 100000 patients present with sustained ventricular tachycardia and an estimated 15% could receive such therapy in 1995. However, the largest potential group (1 million annually) comprises those patients who could receive prophylactic therapy, e.g., 400000 patients with congestive heart failure and 600000 survivors of acute myocardial infarction. While only a small proportion may be identified at the highest risk, usage in this group may equal or approach the previous two categories. Industry and analyst estimates suggest that 35000 ICD implants may be expected annually by 1995 in the USA. The estimated direct device system costs would approach $ 800000000 exclusive of hospital and professional charges. These can be expected to contribute to an aggregate cost to health care system up to and possibly in excess of $ 1.5 billion. While such estimates may seem extraordinary in 1990, achieving a significant fraction of such growth can be an economic embarassment for an unsuspecting health care system. Efforts to reduce costs at all critical links in the economic chain appear vital for the long-term growth of the therapy. New strategies to reduce device, implant and hospital costs acceptable to manufacturers and health care providers alike need to be devised. Such efforts remain in the long-term interest of all individuals and organizations involved in this arena.

References

1. Lehmann MH, Steinman RT, Schuger CD et al. (1988) The automatic implantable cardioverter-defibrillator as antiarrhythmic treatment modality of choice for survivors of cardiac arrest unrelated to acute myocardial infarction. Am J Cardiol 62:803
2. Saksena S (1989) The impact of implantable cardioverter-defibrillators on cardiovascular practice. Cardiovasc Med 8:131 (editorial)
3. Fogoros RN, Elson JJ, Bonnet CA et al. (1990) Efficacy of the automatic implantable cardioverter-defibrillator in prolonging survival in patients with severe underlying cardiac disease. J Am Coll Cardiol 16:381
4. The Cardiac Arrhythmia Suppression (CAST) Investigators (1989) Preliminary report: effect of encainide or flecainide on mortality in a randomized trial of arrhythmia suppression after myocardial infarction. N Engl J Med 321:406

5. Aronow WS, Mercando AD, Epstein S et al. (1990) Effect of quinidine or procainamide versus no antiarrhythmic drug on sudden cardiac death, total cardiac death, and total death in elderly patients with heart disease and complex ventricular arrhythmias. Am J Cardiol 66:423
6. Tordjman-Fuchs T, Cannom DS, Garan H et al. (1990) Out-of-hospital cardiac arrest: improved long-term outcome in patients with automatic implantable cardioverter-defibrillators (AICD). Rev Eur Tec Bio 12:395
7. Krucoff M, Chu F, McCallum D et al. (1987) New medical technologies in a cost containment environment: implantable antitachyarrhythmia devices. PACE 10:2
8. Furman S (1987) New medical technologies in a cost containment environment: implantable tachyarrhythmia devices. PACE 10:1
9. Ferguson D, Saksena S, Greenberg E et al. (1984) Management of recurrent ventricular tachycardia. Economic impact of therapeutic alternatives. Am J Cardiol 53:533
10. Ross DL, Farre J, Bar F et al. (1980) Comprehensive clinical electrophysiologic studies in the investigation of documented or suspect tachycardias. Circulation 6:1010
11. Saksena S, Greenberg E, Ferguson D (1985) Prospective reimbursement for state-of-the-art medical practice: the case for invasive electrophysiologic evaluation. Am J Cardiol 55:963
12. Saksena S, Camm AJ, Bilitch M et al. (1987) Clinical investigation of implantable antitachycardia devices: report of the Policy Conference of the North American Society of Pacing and Electrophysiology. J Am Coll Cardiol 10:225
13. Kuppermann M, Luce BR, McGovern B et al. (1990) An analysis of the cost effectiveness of the implantable defibrillator. Circulation 81:91
14. Saksena S, Tullo NG, Krol RB et al. (1989) Initial clinical experience with endocardial defibrillation using an implantable cardioverter/defibrillator with a triple electrode system. Arch Intern Med 149:2333
15. Graboys TA, Lown B, Podrid PJ et al. (1982) Long-term survival of patients with malignant ventricular arrhythmia treatment with antiarrhythmic drugs. Am J Cardiol 50:437
16. Morady F (1988) A perspective on the role of catheter ablation in the management of tachyarrhythmias. PACE 11:98
17. Drummond MF (1987) Economic evaluation and the rational diffusion and use of health technology. Health Policy 7:309

Outlook

E. Alt, H. Klein, J. C. Griffin

Ten years of defibrillator therapy have changed the cardiology scenario dramatically. Although the initial defibrillator device was not programmable, its longevity was rather limited, and its indication was restricted to patients who had survived more than one episode of aborted sudden death, experience has shown beyond any doubt that no other approach is as effective in preventing sudden arrhythmic death as defibrillator therapy. Although it had initially been considered an aggressive and intolerable mode of treatment by many cardiologists, defibrillator implantation gained widespread acceptance worldwide and became *the* armamentarium in many of the larger cardiology centers for patients at risk for sudden death.

In the meantime technological progress has improved defibrillator devices considerably, and second-generation systems with programmable features have been implanted in almost 20000 patients. For the first 7 years, there was only one manufacturer for approved devices; today six manufacturers offer highly complex devices that are able to defibrillate or cardiovert, provide antibradycardia pacing, deliver programmable modes of antitachycardia pacing, store electrograms of the tachycardia event, and recall the therapy history. There is one question which automatically arises: Will the physician be able to understand and put to proper use what the field of electronic engineering has availed him of? Does the increasing complexity of the defibrillator provide more safety and useful flexibility or does it produce a greater risk for failure and unforeseen harm?

There is no doubt that the programmability of various parameters was necessary and essential. Probably the most important features added to the mere cardioverting/defibrillating system were antibradycardia and, more recently, antitachycardia pacing facilities. Today already all six manufacturers (CPI – PRX; Medtronic – PCD; Intermedics – ResQ; Ventritex – Cadence; Telectronics – Guardian; and Siemens – Siecure) offer antitachycardia pacing modes with their devices. However, the question of how many patients will actually require antitachycardia pacing cannot be answered yet. Comparing the number of patients successfully treatable with reasonable pacing modes with those just requiring immediate cardioversion or defibrillation clearly favors the latter. Successful antitachycardia pacing requires a reliably terminable ventricular tachycardia with sufficient hemodynamic tolerance, permitting numerous pacing attempts without frequent acceleration or degeneration into ventricular fibrillation. To date the majority of patients who have survived a cardiac arrest, and especially those with poor ventricular function, just do not show such "electrically stable" ventricular tachycardia. Unless the indication for electrical devices is liberalized, the ratio of patients requiring antitachycardia pacing to those who do not will be two out of ten.

Prior to the initiation of antitachy pacing, thorough pre-implant electrophysiologic testing is necessary; intraoperative testing is extremely limited and unreliable; and pre-discharge testing of the optimum antitachycardia pacing mode quite often demonstrates noninducibility of the tachycardia or inappropriate pacing modes, thus necessitating antitachycardia features to be switched off. This problem has been clearly revealed by the clinical trials presently being performed with various antitachycardia devices. One of the reasons for this may be that no one antitachycardia pacing mode is generally recommendable.

It has become obvious already that patients with antitachycardia pacing and defibrillating devices in general require more sophisticated follow-up visits and more frequent hospital readmissions, with repeated testing and more often additional antiarrhythmic drug therapy, to keep the ventricular tachycardia pace-terminable. Why, then, should a patient receive a device with the highest number of flexible antitachycardia pacing features if it is easier, less troublesome, more cost-effective, and simpler with respect to follow-up, if the tachycardia can be safely terminated by "simple" low-energy cardioversion or even defibrillation? Even if antitachycardia pacing has improved defibrillator therapy significantly, caution should be excercised to ensure, however, that the same mistakes that have often been encountered with antibradycardia pacing are not made, i.e., the device contains highly complex features that will never be used or, quite the opposite, even be abused, thus harming the patient.

The future impulse form of the defibrillator shock will certainly be a biphasic one in all devices. Limited testing procedures will render extended programmability of the various biphasic impulse modalities unnecessary. Biphasic impulse shocks reduce the energy requirement. The significance of sequential shock delivery needs further evaluation.

The availability of endocardial pacing and shock leads with smaller diameters permitting easier insertion will be most important in the future. It may well be that bi- or multi-directional spread of shock energy can be achieved without placement of a subcutaneous patch electrode. Lead configuration and material will have to be improved, and the question of thrombogenesis of endocardial leads has not sufficiently been answered.

We shall need improved longevity of the pulse generators. Battery and capacitor technology is calling for further improvement and more reliability. Although component failures have been relatively rare, they will occur again in the future; it is our wish, however, that the problems that have occurred with pacemakers and have necessitated explantations on a larger scale will not be a complication in defibrillator patients.

Future devices will offer complete therapy-history storage with digital electrogram print-out facility. This feature will enable us to get more insight into the tachycardia mechanisms or events, and it is not unrealistic if we ask for devices offering complete Holter functions as they are available already in some specific pacemakers.

Currently every medical society sets up its own guidelines for defibrillator implantation. The usefulness or applicability of these guidelines is currently pending evaluation. They will continuously remain behind technical and medical progress in device therapy, and it may even happen that health care systems may arrive at wrong decisions from these guidelines, thus preventing improvement of therapeutic approaches.

Smaller device size, easier implantation and follow-up, reduced costs of the devices and of the medical procedure, and better selection of appropriate recipients, not to mention the increased actual implantations, will favor a more widespread use of defibrillators cardioverters in the future. This might help to reduce the currently existing gap between those who actually receive a defibrillator and those who really need it.

Implantable cardioverters/defibrillators are not just larger pacemakers. However, they have some similarities in that there will be enormous competition between various manufacturers in the future. Today the implantation of devices of more than two manufacturers would already seem to be impossible in one center, as handling and management of defibrillator devices often differ considerably. This may incur risks and pitfalls both for patients and physicians.

Would it be too ingenuous for physicians to ask for uniformly applicable programmers for all devices available, and for patients to receive software containing disks that can be read by and are applicable with all devices and programmers? This is a dream which to date has failed to come true with pacemaker therapy. Could it not be different with defibrillator therapy?

Subject Index

SPRINGER NATURE

GPSR Compliance

The European Union's (EU) General Product Safety Regulation (GPSR) is a set of rules that requires consumer products to be safe and our obligations to ensure this.

If you have any concerns about our products, you can contact us on ProductSafety@springernature.com

In case Publisher is established outside the EU, the EU authorized representative is:

Springer Nature Customer Service Center GmbH
Europaplatz 3
69115 Heidelberg, Germany

FSC
www.fsc.org
MIX
Papier | Fördert
gute Waldnutzung
FSC® C083411

Kolibri 360 GmbH
Ferdinand-Jühlke-Straße 7
99095 Erfurt, Deutschland
produktsicherheit@kolibri360.de